2006

Beyond Morning Sickness:
Battling Hyperemesis
Gravidarum

To order additional copies, please contact us.
BookSurge, LLC
www.booksurge.com
1-866-308-6235
orders@booksurge.com

ASHLI FOSHEE MCCALL

BEYOND MORNING SICKNESS: BATTLING HYPEREMESIS GRAVIDARUM

2006

Beyond Morning Sickness: Battling Hyperemesis Gravidarum

CONTENTS

Appendices

I WOULD LIKE TO THANK

- My children, all of them, for breathing joy into my life

- My husband for enduring

- My in-laws for babysitting

- James and Elise Foshee for being the grandest parents ever

- Uncle Garry for the laptop and endless geek support

- Madeline Pecora Nugent (aka Super Mentor) for total encouragement, faith, countless edits, kicks-in-the-fanny and general invaluable help

- Dr. Jeffrey Wall for editing the medical content in memory of his precious son Conner

- The Motherisk Program and Dr. Koren, Director, for permission to reprint the awesome algorithm

- Miriam Erick for the motivational chats

- Karen Heying, for thorough information regarding the services provided by Child Care Aware

- Pharmacist Michael Moore for enthusiasm and lots of drug information

- Attorney Darren A. Schwartz for providing free legal research

- LB for the thrill of being in the "G family loan loop" and so much more

- Steve Lewis for domain assistance

- Christel Michaud for the kickin' Web site

- Daniels Harper and Krancer for graphics support

- Dr. David Dixon for providing truly excellent medical care that saved my daughter and enabled me to write crucial parts of this book

- Melissa, Ben & Kelsey, Diana & John, Maribel & Aja, A&C and many others for the unbelievable privilege to serve and the priceless gift of friendship

- All the HG moms who have submitted their stories and shared their joy and sorrow to help others

- And God, most of all, from Whom the children come and to Whom the children go.

In Memory Of
Tennessee Elija McCall

You Did More In Fifteen Weeks Than Many People Do In
A Lifetime.

FOREWORD
Dr. Jeffrey Wall

I received an odd and presumptuous email one day. It was unsolicited, there was no "hello," no introduction, not even an explanation, just a frantic demand for information. It seems the woman who sent it had suffered from severe hyperemesis gravidarum in her first pregnancy. Frankly, I was a little put out by it. There was however, something in the tone of the message, an urgency, a sense of desperation that moved me to answer her. That woman was the author of this book and so began a long correspondence that has ultimately resulted in me writing this foreword.

Ashli McCall has a terrible story to tell. It is a story of suffering, hopelessness and anguish, a story that brings us to the edge of human endurance and to the decision that no new mother-to-be expects to face. Unfortunately, it is not her story alone but the story of countless women worldwide. Hyperemesis gravidarum takes its terrible toll every day. As a disease it is under-studied, poorly understood, and fraught with the myths of years of misinformation and misunderstanding from the medical profession. We as doctors teach it to our students poorly and have handed down years of tradition founded on suspect science and bad medicine. We tell our patients to just "get over it;" we tell them it's all in their head. We are trained to make our patients better but in reality are poorly armed to do so. In our frustration it becomes easy to blame the patient. I know. I've done it.

This book is a step in the direction of understanding a horrible condition. The first time I read it I was astonished at the depth of information it contained. It is extremely well researched, and the clear, concise writing provides a firm basis of understanding for those wanting, *needing* to learn more about this condition. But this book is more than just a collection of medical facts. Those who read it will gain real insights into the human suffering that women with hyperemesis endure. Readers will also find hope and wisdom for those experiencing the condition and understanding for those who live with and love them.

As a medical educator, I am humbled and grateful for the knowledge and wisdom that Ashli McCall and the women who helped her write this book have given me. It is a great gift and now it is my assignment to make sure that this gift is passed on to those doctors whom I teach. It is my task to help unravel the years of misinformation and to ensure that those who train under me know the facts about hyperemesis gravidarum, and most importantly, that they understand the human toll of the disease. This book makes my task much easier.

Ashli McCall was faced with a terrible decision. She has lived every single day since then with the pain of that decision. Yet from her pain have come works of great love, the greatest of which are her beautiful children and this book. I think she has done the memory of little Tennessee McCall great honor. I hope she thinks so too.

Jeffrey Wall MD, FACOG
Kansas City, February 2005

PREFACE

This book is for informational purposes only and is not intended as a substitute for consulting qualified health care professionals. Medical information is in a constant state of flux; by the time you read this book some information may already be outdated. Circumstances will vary with each sufferer. Consult your doctor before taking medications or implementing any treatment options or methods mentioned in these pages. Only a physician can confirm and prescribe pharmaceutical doses and schedules recommended by manufacturers. *The contents of this book should be regarded solely as food for thought.*

You will notice that feminine pronouns are used throughout these pages. This is only to avoid the confusion associated with continuously alternating "he" and "she" when describing unknown or hypothetical persons.

If you are too sick to deal with terms and books, then <u>Beyond Morning Sickness</u> can help your caregiver, family member, friend or any other person advocating for you.

This publication offers an overload of information on hyperemesis gravidarum (HG), and some of the technical terms expose you to "official terminology" that medical professionals use. I don't include these terms to be vague. Grasping certain medical concepts can help you to better understand and communicate with your doctor, and correctly using a few terms may impress upon your physician that you have cared to acquaint yourself with your illness and treatment options. This may give you an edge that actually improves your health care.

Although the names have been changed for the purpose of anonymity, <u>Beyond Morning Sickness</u> includes the stories of real women who suffered through HG. I am one of them. When I went through HG initially, people did not know how to comfort me. Most of them didn't know anything about the disease and couldn't give me anything real to cling to. In fact, some of their attempts to help hurt very much. In my first pregnancy, I searched but never found anyone else with HG. I didn't know the first thing about it and felt like the only one in the world with such an illness. When it was over and I was able, I went looking for some serious answers.

Initially, I spent days following every HG link that popped up on the Internet. There were scads of sites, but none of them were completely accurate or gave a satisfactory snapshot of what it is like to live with HG. I couldn't find one personal Web site devoted to HG, so I designed one myself, sharing the information I found. To my surprise, I began hearing from people on a daily basis. Eventually, I decided to write a book because I was meeting more and more people who needed a convenient source of information. Sufferers felt they didn't know enough about HG and found it difficult to convey the experience during a time when others most needed to understand it. No one can adequately explain HG in a mere moment of conversation. It would take days. It would take a book.

For nearly ten years I have made annual trips to the medical library of a teaching hospital roughly four hours away. I have buried myself in hundreds of articles and abstracts dating as far back as 1994. I have accumulated a photocopied mountain of information, which includes historical references to HG and represents over a decade of the latest research on the illness. However, I find more comfort and healing in the personal stories of other women who don't use complicated terms and whose official definition of HG is: feeling like crap that got crapped on for a long, long time. I believe the personal stories are the most valuable part of my research, and I hope you find something meaningful in them too.

When I talk with other sufferers I feel "normal." I don't feel defensive having to watch everything I say lest it be misconstrued. When no one understands, they do. We have laughed together, cried together, battled HG together, and we have even been in the delivery room together. Connecting with other sufferers has been an amazing experience that none should go without. In the beginning, when I didn't really know where the content of this book was headed, I was certain that it had to consist heavily of personal stories, because they meant so much to me. In addition to validation, I felt encouraged by the fact that women had been through HG and survived. Their stories were part of the reason I tried again and again to have a living child. These women had been there. When they said I could do it, I believed them.

I am convinced that the women in this book must be allowed to share their experiences in their own words, and I strived for minimal editing. For this reason some stories may seem elaborate in length while others may appear remarkably short. Some may be graphic or emotional, while others may come across as lacking in detail or may appear stoical. Women are different. An array of perceptions and philosophies is represented while the experience of living with HG remains the awful, common thread.

Publishing what was quite possibly the first detailed online personal account of HG-related termination frequently attracted people who had tragic stories of their own. For this reason, the majority of the stories you are about to read involve some type of devastation or another, although most have at least subsequent outcomes that are successful and encouraging.

The last thing I want is for a mom to notice the high frequency of complication and loss stories, compare that to the general population of women with HG, and think that something similar is going to happen to her. *Tragic accounts are overrepresented in this book.* It makes sense. Most people who have had only positive pregnancy outcomes are not lurking around the Internet trying to find information on HG. Their children survived; their focus is on being good parents and trying to forget HG as much as humanly possible. *Please keep this in mind and do not allow yourself to think that major complications or loss are a frequent part of the HG experience, because they aren't.*

Take heart in the overwhelming message that you and your baby can survive HG and that you are not alone.

HYPEREMESIS GRAVIDARUM
An Introduction

MY STORY

In 1996 I married my steady of six years. Three months after the wedding, we lucked out. I always wanted children, and we succeeded in pregnancy without even trying. We had a lovely home, good careers, a strong relationship and a beautiful new life! We were very blessed.

At first I didn't know I was pregnant. I had no symptoms until Thanksgiving Day when I was six weeks along. I was busying myself with the annual preparation of ambrosia when the thought occurred to me that if I smelled one more orange I would vomit. I supposed I had the flu, but my husband's grandmother joked that I was pregnant. We all had a good laugh.

The flu was getting worse, and the pink stuff wasn't working on the day that my best friend called. I told her about the flu and she ended up on my doorstep with a pregnancy test. She had desperately been trying to have a baby with her new husband and related all things to the making of babies, so I humored her knowing that I was not pregnant. The positive result came up immediately. I was surprised and elated! The elementary school teacher was finally going to have a child of her own!

My friend went home and the silence was divinity. I didn't want to tell anyone for a few hours. I wanted to be selfish with my precious secret. I knew this would be the only time that my baby belonged solely to me. I got down on my knees, thanked the Lord, and felt an overwhelming sense of excitement and peace. I felt simple and somehow holy.

When my husband got home I told him. He was wide-eyed and smiling like a kid at Christmas. He kissed my tummy and we spent a content sleep curled around each other. It was one of the last times.

The next day I was bursting with the news. I told everyone at work, and they were all excited for me. It's a small town, and the news spread like wildfire. Parents (of my second-grade students) sent me gifts for the baby, and we held a celebratory dinner with my husband's family.

My grandparents raised me for the better part of my life because my birth parents were ill equipped for the job. My grandparents had both just died; how I wanted to tell them the good news! In lieu of that, I took a risk and called my birth dad. Foolishly I imagined the baby would somehow touch his heart. When I got him on the phone I told him, "I'm going to have a baby, Daddy." He replied, "Well… are you going to keep it?" I was crushed. It strengthened my resolve to be a better parent than he was.

Everyone kept teasing me about morning sickness; had it come on yet? I felt queasy 24-hours a day but had not thrown up and was disappointed. I wasn't doing it right. I worried that I would miss out on the "pregnancy initiation" that is morning sickness. We went to the doctor and got our first ultrasound. On the screen was a kidney bean with a flashing heart. It was incredible! We nicknamed the baby "Pinto."

I got up for work the next day and opened the fridge for a little breakfast. The light flooded over me, and I fell into the sink retching. I died laughing after it was over and went to work bragging to all my co-workers that I'd had my first glorious bout with "morning sickness."

A few days later the joke was on me. I was vomiting six times a day. These weren't just any episodes. Each one lasted around fifteen minutes, and involved projectile vomiting and dry retching. I couldn't eat or keep anything down when I tried. Everything made me vomit. I couldn't watch TV because the moving pictures made me vomit. I couldn't walk for more than a few minutes or I would throw up. I was so constantly nauseated that it physically hurt. I couldn't sit up for long periods of time. I couldn't read for more than a moment because the presentation of so many letters and words visually over-stimulated my brain and made me throw up. I could smell the ink and paper. I could smell the water in the tap. I could smell the coils heating up in the oven two rooms away. All of it made me hurl. Even thermal fluctuations would cause an emetic episode. This was beyond morning sickness.

I begged the doctor to admit me to the hospital. I knew something was wrong. I couldn't work or brush my teeth or even bathe. I hadn't eaten anything in days and was vomiting up all fluids and bile. My doctor phoned in Phenergan and Reglan. My husband picked these up from the pharmacist who said I should try my best not to take the medication because "drugs aren't really safe in pregnancy." It scared me, but I took them. They didn't work and made me feel worse. Still the doctor wouldn't admit me. I thought she must know best and that I was probably just overreacting. I kept vomiting and calling every day. Finally, when all the doctors in the practice were unavailable, a nurse took my call at the hospital and said I needed to be admitted right away.

My urine was flooded with ketones, I had an electrolyte imbalance, and I was severely dehydrated and thoroughly frightened. Needless to say, I was a little depressed from all of this. The nurses were appalled that I had not been admitted sooner and told me I had some kind of illness with a long name and two words: hyper-something. They assured me that I would never be delayed or denied admittance again as I had been diagnosed and looked severe enough.

I still vomited in the hospital on IVs. However, I felt less anxious in the care of medical professionals. If something bad happened, I was sure they would save me. I was also very excited about getting another sonogram when they checked for twins or a molar pregnancy. There she was at ten weeks moving all around with a strong, beautiful heart beating the soundless music of two loves made one. The delicate hand was waving. The nurse captioned the image "Hi, Mom!" My cheeks were warm with the ecstasy of motherhood. How could I have imagined that the life would not be? And how in the world could I have imagined that it would end at my hand?

The doctors in my practice were insensitive. One had eight children and never felt better than when pregnant. In the hospital they had me in the room next to the coffee pot at the nurses' station, and Dr. Mom refused to relocate her coffee upon entering my room. She was amused and laughed that it made me vomit.

My main doctor was having a nervous breakdown at the time of my treatment, however she only confessed it after my pregnancy was over. I should have recognized the signs when I asked her about antiemetics and teratogenic effects and she went ballistic, actually yelling at me. She sharply reminded me that she was the doctor and I was the patient and asked me if I'd chosen an OB by randomly sticking my finger on any old name in the Yellow Pages. She had been my gynecologist for seven years.

I made excuses for the female doctors in this nefarious practice because, in the initial patient info packet, they actually warned us that they would be tired, hungry and sometimes cranky. I tried to be compassionate and understanding. And I really wanted to trust these people, because I needed their help so badly. Who better to put my faith in than my doctor?

I barely ever saw her (no more than three times during countless visits) and was shuffled between nurses, midwives, someone different every time. All of them told me glaringly different things. The contradictions confused and frightened me. Their only consensus was that I might be this way for six more months. Six more months with that level of illness and medical response? I couldn't bear the thought.

I begged to go home from the hospital. First they wouldn't let me in, and now they wouldn't let me out. It was ridiculous. It was Christmas Eve though, and they took pity on me and issued my release. I went home to start the downward spiral of vomiting, starvation and dehydration all over again.

My boss called and implied that I was going to lose my job soon, and my birth dad came over twice and told me my baby was going to die or be born severely retarded. "This is not good," he repeated like a mantra. He worked in developmental health; he was very convincing as an authority on mental retardation. He was scaring me with all his talk. He suggested termination because he said I was going to lose everything: my job, my baby and possibly my life. I told him over and over that two of our loved-ones recently died and hadn't we had enough of death for a while? I told him I loved my baby as she was. He argued, "It's not a baby." "It" felt like a baby to me.

My doctor's solution was to offer two-hour IVs and send me home to repeat the cycle. It became obvious that the medical staff were getting fed up with my inability to get well. The first trimester was over, and I was still puking my guts up and starving. I could get the occasional Ensure pudding down and on very good days, a piece of cheese toast (three pieces in eight weeks). I'm 5'7" and started the pregnancy at one hundred twenty-six pounds, but by the end of the fourteenth week I had lost eighteen pounds. My skin was flaky and yellow, I had scleral discoloration, and the house reeked of vomit and bile.

My husband worked all day, and I couldn't take care of myself at all. I could barely get out of bed. I literally survived on the small amounts of Ensure that I could keep down. To be out of the situation I went to bed at seven PM but woke up at four AM every morning. I opened my eyes in the darkness of my strange new life, and fear engulfed me. I prayed and took my anxiety-inducing Reglan. I threw up and fell back into bed where I would lay for the next fifteen hours with nothing to do but try and remain as still as possible in the space between various vomiting spells. At seven PM the sweet, numbing "Prozac" of sleep would carry me off beyond the world of tremendous discomfort. Four AM would come too soon, and I would mourn my diseased consciousness.

No one would help me. I began to lose a pound a day. My birth dad's foreboding voice echoed in my head. Images of my dying grandparents floated in and out of my mind's eye. Their suffering, the loss of appetite, the pain, the lethargy, the anxiety and depression... it mimicked my own symptoms, and lest we forget: *they died*! I was terrified. I came to believe that debilitating illness was an unbeatable foe; I knew that I was as mortal as my folks and that life was a temporary affair. Clear-thinking was difficult.

My lovely child... the one that I sang to, the one that I'd been hoping for all my life, the one that I loved and wanted and named... she was transformed into little more than an illness that was torturing me. Eventually my silent tears turned into wailing upon waking. My husband felt inadequate and helpless. He didn't know what to do. He thought I was either going to die or lose my mind, and everyone was telling us how abnormal it was except the doctors who took the blasé attitude that I was pregnant not sick.

Outside of my husband I had no support whatsoever. His parents stayed out of it. Later they said they had been afraid of what might happen if they led us in any particular direction. Besides, it was "our business" and they regarded me as strikingly independent.

My best friend hated me from the moment the pregnancy test was positive. I chalked it up to her secondary infertility issues. She called me once to tell me how rude I had been when it took me five minutes to get out of bed and answer the door. I tried to explain, but she just hung up and I never heard from her again during the pregnancy. I prayed endlessly, but my idea of God was corrupt. I had no one.

I began to get the feeling that something pretty bad was going to happen, because my doctors weren't doing much of anything and no one seemed concerned that I was turning yellow and beginning to have mild hallucinations. I began to see faces coming out of the stucco walls and plush carpet. I had never experienced anything like that, and it was disturbing. I worried about my job and how we would pay massive hospital bills if something drastic occurred.

One morning I woke up and snapped. I felt I just couldn't go on. I was completely debased and functioning on a primitive level. I adopted an attitude that one of us had to go and it wouldn't be me. My heart was gone; I wanted to get well by any means. No more hospitals, no more throwing up, no more worrying, no more drugs, no more panicky side effects, no more judgements, contradictory opinions or pain or anything... no more. "Uncle."

My doctor told me I was obsessed with my pregnancy and needed to seek mental help, so I mustered the strength to visit a counselor. If I was crazy and they could make the HG stop by fixing my mind, then I was all for it. I wanted them to fix me, because I wanted my baby to live. Perhaps this was my child's reprieve. The counselor had my OB prescribe Zoloft, an anti-depressant. I kept the first pill down for a little while but then woke up with projectile vomiting. I vomited throughout the night. I called the counselor. After piecing everything together it became clear that there had been a mix-up, stemming from the HMO, resulting in an overdose. I had taken four times the prescribed amount through no fault of my own. My counselor was horrified. I wasn't physically able to pursue more counseling, and I lost my faith in the process after the overdose.

In a last-ditch effort I called my doctor one more time but got one of her partners as usual. I laid it on the line for her and demanded care. I told her that if she wouldn't do something to help me I was going to terminate the pregnancy, because I was reaching a physical threshold. I tried one last time to get admitted to the hospital because I was afraid that I was in such bad shape that even if I did go for an abortion I might die in the middle of it. This particular doctor told me that there were women in the hospital with worse problems than mine, and that I would only disturb patients with "real" illnesses, because they actually wanted their babies.

Bewildered, I angrily demanded again to be admitted. She laughed at me. She informed me that the hospital was not a hotel and that I couldn't just book a reservation when I felt like it. I argued with her some more, and she finally told me to go into the ER where she would have a nurse meet me for an evaluation. My husband packed a bag because we knew anyone who looked at me would admit me.

When we arrived at the ER we noticed the nurse didn't take my vitals as expected. Instead she asked questions about the baby and if this was a planned pregnancy. We were shocked to discover she was a psychiatric nurse. I was so disappointed and humiliated that I started crying. I tried to defend my unplanned pregnancy. Ever since I had been diagnosed with HG the doctors had made the "unplanned factor" a major issue. I told the nurse that my husband and I never wanted to plan a pregnancy; we just wanted it to happen spontaneously. In my medical record she basically wrote: "Patient says she never wanted children." A male doctor walked by the exam room and heard me crying. He poked his head in and said, "Wow, you're dehydrated. You need an IV."

I looked at the nurse and said, "Listen, I love and want this baby, but no one will help me so I've got to get it out of me!" The nurse ended the consultation by telling me that if I didn't immediately go and voluntarily admit myself to a local psychiatric unit she would have me forcibly admitted. It scared me to death, but part of me thought it might still be some sort of chance for the baby, so I went.

When I got to the mental facility it kind of freaked me out, because it was a lock-in situation. There was a big gate-like door and you could see people pacing the floor in their pajamas. Some of them were very obviously disturbed, and I worried about being so sick with all that going on around me. The intake administrator took one look at me, interviewed my husband and me very briefly and just shook his head in disbelief. He said, "You're not crazy, you're sick! You don't need to be here; we can't give you the medical care you need." Then he said, "You need to go to the hospital." My husband threw his hands up in despair and said, "We just CAME from the hospital!" The man was flabbergasted that medical professionals at the hospital had told me to go to the mental facility. I lamented that no one would help us, that they had overdosed me on medication and tried to send me to a lock-in mental facility. I felt that we were getting shafted and lost in the cracks. The guy actually made some remark about it all being our baby's way of saying she didn't want to be born, and I remember wondering if he was really just a patient at the mental facility. We went home and made the appointment.

I was in the second trimester by that time and had to go five hours away to abort our baby. Protestors stood outside imploring, "Please don't kill your precious little child!" Inside, the clinic workers were transparent, manipulative salespeople. They were weird and fake in the worst, most obvious way. The room was packed with women and teens aborting their second trimester babies. If you stood up, you lost your seat. The "counselor" was eighteen-years-old and only wanted to know if she could sell us some birth control pills after the abortion. The staff all called me "sweetie" too much and lied to me about the development of my baby when I asked. They told me not to worry and that I could always have another baby. I told them I wanted this one. They just shrugged their shoulders and moved me down the line.

The abortionist did a sonogram and jerked the screen away when I tried to look. He told me "the fetus" was bigger than he thought and said he would need my credit card again. I was on auto-pilot, not there, a stunned zombie, helplessly obeying orders so that I could somehow find my way back to "life before HG." He removed the small bell jar from the room and came back with a bigger one. I eyed it with horror and revulsion yet did not move. I told him I was sick and that I didn't want to kill my baby. I used those words. He said I could leave if I wanted to. I sat there. He asked me if I was ready; I handed him my arm. The needle pricked, the lights went out, and "life before HG" became an impossible dream.

The abortion was complicated. I woke up in the middle of it and now deal with flashbacks of the abortionist tugging out parts of my child. It was not a delicate procedure; my whole body rocked back and forth as he untenanted me. I lost consciousness. When I woke up again it was over. The "nurse" stood me up, and what was left deluged out of me forming a bloody puddle on the floor. I looked down and passed out in it. I awoke on the table with a shot in my rear and a fist in and out of my stomach to stanch the flow. Too much bleeding. They told us not to leave town and sent us a hotel where we waited to see if I would live through the night or bleed to death in the tub. My record from the clinic says I experienced "scant" bleeding five minutes after the procedure and then "none" seven minutes after that. I bled for months and sustained a permanent incompetent cervix. I contacted the proper authorities, but no one would touch it.

I went back to my OB/GYN for my two-week post abortion check up. She told me she would have aborted the baby herself if I had simply asked her to. She also told me how "substantial" my empty uterus still was, that the baby must have been a good size, and that I hadn't wanted her as much as other women want their babies. She made her point by citing moms with cancer who insisted on having their babies even when she told them not to. I went into hysterics. She told me

I needed to do as she did and see a therapist for counsel and anti-depressants. She confided that she had been under a lot of stress, was taking Prozac for it, and locked herself in her private office to cry on a daily basis. All at once I realized I had put all my faith into the hands of someone who couldn't manage her own life much less the life of a sick patient. I could have killed myself on the spot.

The following year my second pregnancy ended in a missed miscarriage right around Christmas. The year after that, after twenty-eight weeks on strict bed rest (due to the combination of HG and the incompetent cervix) I had a living child who means the world to me. When he was five, a daughter joined our family after my most severe HG experience ever. I couldn't eat or drink for 77 days and was on TPN for over a month. I was in the hospital for five weeks, had three PICC lines in ten days, and added a fourth after staph infected the third. I kept a diary of the entire ordeal, and you can read it at: http://www.hyperemesisgravidarum.blogspot.com

We would like more children, but HG compels us otherwise. My battle with this illness has come to an end, yet it has cost me a child and much of myself and will continue to cast long shadows over the remainder of my life.

ONE
What Is Hyperemesis Gravidarum?

Hyperemesis Gravidarum is a pregnancy-related disease that approximately five women out of a thousand will experience.[1-2] While no standard definition exists, HG usually starts by six weeks of pregnancy and results in extreme nausea, vomiting, malnutrition, weight loss and dehydration. It is debilitating, can be very difficult to manage, and *significantly* interferes with daily life. In the past, before the advent of IVs, it was not terribly uncommon to die from HG. Today medicine is advanced, and HG is generally referred to as a "sheep in wolf's clothing." That is, HG is so bad that many people wonder if they and/or their baby will survive, but medically speaking, it isn't generally considered a killer anymore. Maternal death due to HG is nearly unheard of, and the risk of anomaly and death to the HG baby is small and relative to the risk in any pregnancy. Do not lose hope!

When Will It END?
Though many (including some physicians) will tell you that all this "morning sickness" will end by the twelfth week, there is evidence that HG generally resolves by the twentieth week.[3-4] It is rare for it to continue throughout the entire pregnancy, but research suggests that between ten and twenty percent of women with HG still have some nausea and vomiting up until the end of the pregnancy.[5] The good news is that by the end of

the pregnancy, Mom may only vomit once or twice a day and may be able to eat relatively normally.

Varying Degrees

Each HG experience is unique. Some women diagnosed with HG work fifty hours a week, vomit less than a handful of times (but can't eat), resolve in six weeks, or are "cured" by taking vitamin B6 or homeopathic remedies. Other women are so sick that they cannot read, watch TV, or tolerate odors, bright lights, noise, movement or pretty much *anything* without throwing up so much that they eventually need a feeding tube to deliver "formula" directly into their blood stream to keep them alive. Whatever the form of HG, it is distressing.

Moderate

Moderate HG may be described as a mild version of the illness, but still involves significant nausea and vomiting and will beat the socks off the worst food poisoning or stomach virus. It can cause a mom to become dehydrated and lose at least 5% of her total body weight.[6] It is troublesome but does not thoroughly prevent food consumption. If mismanaged or left untreated, moderate HG can quickly evolve into severe HG.

Severe

Severe HG not only causes dehydration but has been defined as losing 5% or more of the total body weight[7] and consists of numerous vomiting episodes throughout the day without any symptom-free periods. Severe HG usually requires hospitalization for metabolic disturbances and involves supplemental feedings and other more aggressive interventions.

It is important for physicians to differentiate between moderate and severe HG, because severe HG requires more aggressive care. If treated improperly (or not treated at all) severe HG can eventually lead to death, but this is almost unheard of today. Severe HG is a test of endurance because it lasts day in and day out for *months* with little to no respite. This severe illness causes such a remarkable amount of suffering that it has literally driven women to abort children they want. HG-related therapeutic abortion rates are unknown but have ranged from 1.5-3.4% in individual study populations.[8-11] That a woman would abort the child she wants speaks volumes of the debilitation of HG.

Effects of HG

A hyperemetic mother can vomit between four and twenty (or more) times a day for months. If, starting at six weeks, a particular woman vomits an average of fifteen times a day she will have endured several hundred emetic episodes by twenty weeks. Imagine the discomfort of vomiting that much in such a short span of time! The vomiting can be so frequent that the stomach acid erodes tooth enamel. The emesis itself is often bile-filled and blood tinged (the blood usually comes from small tears in the esophagus, stomach or duodenum), and the cycle is self-perpetuating and relentless. In addition to the excessive vomiting, a severely hyperemetic mother suffers from weight loss, dehydration and metabolic disturbances.

Weight Loss

The nausea and vomiting of HG make it nearly impossible for the mother to eat or drink much, if anything. Obviously, if you don't eat you lose weight. Again, losing greater than 5% of your total body weight is one clinical indication supporting a diagnosis of severe HG.

Dehydration

Fluid, which makes up around two-thirds of a person's body weight, is vital, because every single process in our bodies occurs in a fluid medium. Surprisingly, dehydration can cause nausea and vomiting, and that's the last thing a hyperemetic wants more of. Some symptoms of dehydration are lowered blood pressure, headache, blurred vision and fever.

Electrolyte Imbalance

Electrolytes are chemical compounds that break down into such elements as potassium and salt in the body fluid, and they play a vital role in stabilizing body systems. Electrolyte imbalance may manifest as a tingling sensation in the hands and feet, general weakness, decreased reflexes or reaction times and other symptoms.

Carbohydrate Depletion and Ketonuria

Carbohydrates include sugars, starches, and fibers. They are the body's main source of energy, and if carbohydrate levels are inadequate, a person's body begins to break down fat for energy and may take energy from muscle and even organs. This can disrupt the nervous system.

The central nervous system refers to the brain and spinal cord and conscious motor activities like walking and talking, while the peripheral nervous system involves automated functioning such as the heartbeat and digestion. Your body needs energy to function. Carbohydrate depletion causes weariness with a capital "W", and it can make a three-step trip to the toilet feel like world travel.

Additionally, when the body must break down fat for energy, this creates substances called ketones, which can make the blood too acidic. If your urine is flooded with ketones it is a sign that you are in a period of starvation.

If you are living with the suffering of HG, don't let your physicians tell you that you're not sick but only having a baby. You *are* sick. HG is not a normal pregnancy experience. However, be encouraged; there is good news!

HG and Pregnancy Outcomes

With so much nausea and vomiting, adequate nutrition is obviously an issue. A good diet and vitamins during pregnancy have been so fanatically drilled into society that many of us *incorrectly* assume that a woman who eats negligible amounts and hyper vomits for months is going to have a malformed, severely retarded baby if the little one even survives. Fortunately, nothing could be further from the truth. The body has a miraculous compensatory ability, and a severely hyperemetic woman with sufficient medical care has as much chance at a successful pregnancy outcome as anyone. In fact, some studies have shown that hyperemetic mothers have a reduced risk of miscarriage[12] and no increased rate of birth defects.[13-14] However, alternative nutrition is often considered in cases involving a total body weight loss of 10% or more, in order to prevent low birth weight and prematurity.[15]

The Influence of Nausea and Vomiting

People (who are not sick) underestimate the biological power of nausea and vomiting. Cicero said, "I would rather be killed than again suffer the tortures of seasickness."[16] It wasn't hyperbole. In my own family, a cousin had a motorcycle accident and was lying in the street with a compound leg fracture. A bone was literally sticking out of his leg. Did this deter the man from ever riding on a motorcycle again? No. Yet the same fifty-year-old man hasn't touched a plate of spaghetti since he threw it up when he was four. In light of the important biological purpose nausea and vomiting serve, it comes as no surprise that they are extremely potent.

The human body has a built-in safety mechanism by which toxins, if consumed, can be expelled. Nausea and vomiting have prevented countless deaths and are generally very beneficial for survival. The purpose of nausea and vomiting is to rid the body of ingested toxins and deter you from consuming items that may be risky to your health.

The protective mechanism of nausea and vomiting can backfire. When one is ill, one can develop an aversive, conditioned response to stimuli that are not toxic (such as spaghetti). When something goes haywire, and one experiences this stimulus in unavoidable overabundance, the result can be devastating.

Vomiting Triggers
When you have HG, keeping the vomiting at bay is a 24-hour job. Anything and everything can trigger a vomiting episode. Some of the most notorious triggers (in no particular order) are:
- Scents
- Heat
- Humidity
- Mold/fungus in a building's air ducts
- Noise*

- Motion
- Vitamins
- Intense visual stimuli
- Intense physical/emotional stimuli
- Dehydration

Why Me?

HG is nasty stuff. If you're reading this book, chances are you've won one crummy lottery. You may be angry and confused. Why did this have to happen to you when others get to have normal, happy pregnancies? There is no answer to this question, but you must understand that it is not your fault, and you are not alone.

*Noise has been studied in the military for its ability to induce nausea.

Vivan's Story

I was on a ski trip in Utah when it began. I was nauseous, and I thought it was altitude sickness. I threw up once and waited for my period, which was one day late. Depo Provera (the birth control shot) and a scare with cervical cancer had kept my periods very limited and irregular in the previous three years, so I still didn't suspect anything.

When I returned home I vomited for nine days. After that I was fairly certain what was going on. I had a history of false positive home pregnancy tests, so I went to my doctor for an actual blood test.

My OB confirmed that I was pregnant, prescribed prenatals, and sent me off with a big bag of stuff. I threw up over and over again and thought it was the vitamins, but discontinuing them didn't help. I tried homeopathic formulas, teas, nutritional supplements but nothing worked. I tried staying home on the couch, but I felt worse there, and the dog always wanted my attention.

I couldn't read, because it made my head ache. I couldn't watch TV, because the food on the commercials made me ultra-nauseous. Radio commercials did the same thing. My eyes were dry, my lips were cracked and bleeding, and I was losing weight quickly.

I have heart problems and had to discontinue taking my heart medication for the baby. A book I was reading had lots of information on women, heart problems and being very sick. I wondered if it was a good decision to continue with my pregnancy.

I started my pregnancy at one hundred sixty-eight pounds and lost 18 pounds by the time I was nine weeks pregnant. Eventually I lost 29 pounds. The day I was hospitalized I showed up in my doctor's office unannounced. The vessels in my eyes had burst and bright red blood pooled in them. My hair was dry and limp, my skin was scaly, and my fingers were pruny and wrinkled.

They asked for a urine sample. I was lucky to be able to provide it, as I wasn't really urinating much anymore. The sample was like orange syrup. I watched the nurse test it. "Oh my God," she said. "I've never seen such high ketones in a living person." I asked her what that meant and she pointed to the doctor's office. "Go in there," she replied, pointing to the doctor's personal office as she knocked on one of the exam doors. Without waiting for an answer she handed the doctor the little color stick. He walked out of the exam room saying, "Excuse me," to the patient.

"Why don't you lay down right there on my couch, my dear," he said as he called Cedar-Sinai and asked them to prepare a room. He had the director of OB admit me in advance because I'd be coming alone.

He tossed me two pillows and asked me how I felt. I told him I felt like barfing. He laughed and pointed to a picture of his three daughters and told me I'd have one of those soon enough. I asked if I was being hospitalized and he said yes. Then he let me use his phone to call my husband or whomever

I needed and offered to have the nurse call my sister who worked nearby.

When I got to the hospital I went to the director's office and told her that my doctor told me to come directly to her and she fumbled around for a minute and then remembered that she'd just spoken to him. She walked me to the nurses' station and sat me down until my room was ready. The nurse who got me into my room said they weren't supposed to start my IV yet because I wasn't officially admitted but that she was the best at putting them in and was leaving soon, so she'd hook me up while they were sorting through the paperwork.

She laid big white towels over my chest, belly and legs and then got out the needles and stand. She said that sometimes she makes a mess when she's putting an IV into someone who had collapsed veins and mine all looked collapsed. I was so perplexed by the towels and her behavior that I didn't even notice that she had put the needle in the back of my forearm. She laughed, pulled the towels off and said that she was just kidding. They put me on antiemetics and fluids for two days. I ate and didn't vomit, so they released me with some prescription antiemetics.

I felt stronger, like I could get through it, but my husband maintained that it was more important to him to keep his wife than it was to have a child. He wanted a child, but not if it meant losing me. By all appearances, he wasn't sure I would live.

The prescription from the hospital did not work so I was given another one in suppository form. After a couple of days on that, I was doing fairly well until I had a particularly gassy morning. I went to the restroom and found a bloody mess in the toilet. Evidently, I had burst an internal hemorrhoid and had to discontinue the suppositories.

My doctor gave me Compazine next. It stopped the nausea but had me climbing the walls. I could not sit still or get comfortable. It was as if my skin was an outfit purchased two sizes too small and there was no way of removing it. I stopped taking it for one day and realized that it had been the medication and not the pregnancy that was making me feel insane. My doctor (who I was still seeing twice a week) said he had an identical response to it when he was doing his residency.

At just over five months pregnant I could pull my jeans off without unbuttoning or unzipping them. I couldn't wear a belt because the pressure was uncomfortable, so I got teased about needing suspenders a lot. Finally at six months pregnant, my clothes began to fit again. I could still wear my normal clothes but they were starting to get tight. At seven months I went shopping for maternity clothes.

At eight months pregnant I had my first desire for food. I ate a double-decker supreme taco without lettuce, and it was the first thing that didn't gag me and tasted good. Out of sheer gratefulness I sat there and cried in the fast food booth while I crunched away. I WAS EATING!

I continued to vomit off and on but by maintaining a steady supply of revolting sour gummy fruit candy and Dr. Pepper I managed to make it through my pregnancy. My doctor told me not to be too concerned about the caffeine, that it was more important that I retain fluids.

My labor was long, but not hard, and after thirty-five hours when I was finally ready, I pushed twice and my baby was born at nine pounds and one ounce.

"No two pregnancies are ever alike," every doctor told me. "You may not be sick at all the second time around." Everyone seemed to have a theory about why I had had HG, and all offered that theory as evidence that I could get pregnant again and not get sick.

Again, I was traveling when the nausea set in. I was in New York for a wedding on the hottest week of 1998. It was humid and hot and I was pushing my eighteen-month-old son around the city in a stroller and loading him into town cars for various wedding duties. My husband ended up having to stay home so I was going solo. I tried to convince myself that feeling ill and tired was a result of the weather, but after I flew home, the vomiting began. At work we had a unisex bathroom that everyone had to pass by, and the walls were thin. After a couple of days of vomiting I was pretty sure I was pregnant and knew I needed to try to prevent dehydration. I bought the home test knowing already that I had to be pregnant. I called my OB in the morning and told him that the vomiting had begun.

I had just seen him the month before to tell him we were considering having another. He had prescribed vitamins, which I had not yet picked up. He told me to come in. After nine days of throwing up I had already lost weight. He told me to be careful, to do what I could, and to come in every week.

As my weight dropped, the visits became every other day. He was reluctant to prescribe anything so early. My sister, also his patient, had had four miscarriages, so he was extra careful with me.

One night I was upstairs throwing up when I started to feel dizzy. Our tiny bathroom was at the top of the stairs and, expecting to pass out, I thought I had better fall to the side of the toilet closest to the wall and not closest to the open door at the top of the stairs. I slumped over and passed out. When I came to, I felt like I was stuck in that position. I was shaking, freezing cold, but I didn't feel like I could move. I felt like I'd had a seizure. I couldn't get up but I was shaking and aware that I was on the floor. Eventually I got up and went downstairs where my husband was holding our sleeping son and watching hockey with a neighbor. I told him that something needed to be done and went back upstairs to bed.

At five weeks pregnant my skin was pruny, my lips were cracked and my eyes looked bloody again. I told him it was time. I had barfed fifty times at work the day before. By three PM I stopped counting. My doctor asked if I wanted him to book a room at Cedars and I told him to go ahead. I called my sister to come take care of my son and pets. My husband drove me in and called my boss on the way to the hospital. My boss hadn't known I was pregnant. He never noticed how many trips I made to the bathroom.

After fishing around in my veins for a little while the hospital nurse managed to get my IV in. They gave me Droperidol, saline and other stuff. All I could do was sleep.

After a night I began to keep fluids down and eventually some food. When they decided to take me off the IV and send me home, the attending gave me a prescription for another drug. I had it with my previous pregnancy in suppository form but now they had a pill. They thought that if I got on the pill before the IV drugs wore off I would likely be able to keep the pills down and maintain the cycle.

My husband had been caring for our eighteen-month-old and working, so my father-in-law (FIL) brought me home. My FIL picked up my prescription and some mashed potatoes (painless to regurgitate) while I got myself in order at home. My mother-in-law (MIL) wanted to wait until I took my medicine. I said she was being silly. She tends to be nervous, which in this case was a good thing. My son was in bed, and my in-laws were about to leave when my tongue felt funny. Then my jaw felt tight. When I found I couldn't move my jaw I paged my doctor. As I began to feel like I was having trouble breathing, my FIL loaded me in the car while my MIL stayed with my son and waited for the doctor to return my page.

As I got into the hospital the triage nurse seemed unconcerned and told me to sit down. I wondered if he could understand me, so I wrote down the name of the IV drug I had taken and put it with the bottle of pills I had also taken. Just as I sat down I had to run to the bathroom with diarrhea. As I walked out the nurse called me in. I was feeling somewhat panicky. I was no longer able to talk. She said, "Don't worry, this is a common response with both these drugs. We are going to put another IV in, give you medicine, and you will feel better very quickly."

She didn't even take my personal information. She led me into a room right across the hall and a longhaired guy walked in with the IV setup and got the needle in. A woman walked in at the same time to tell me that she'd be getting my info. I nodded to my purse, and my FIL pulled out my license and insurance cards. After a few seconds of mumbling I realized I could talk again. The hippy-haired nurse told me he liked me better with the locked jaw and made me laugh.

Whatever I was reacting to stayed in my system for a few days. I had to take Benadryl regularly. The day after my hospital visit, I was watching my son and husband having breakfast, trying to eat biscuits and gravy (another easy-to-barf food), and making trips to the bathroom to vomit. Some of the Benadryl came up, and my jaw began to tighten again. I took the Benadryl and left the room because I didn't want my son to see me so anxious. After two days of vomiting again, I knew I was getting dehydrated. There was nothing I could do.

I called my OB and said I was going to the hospital where my primary worked. In the morning, my husband went for his daily jog with our son in the jog stroller and the dog trailing behind. I sat in the shower and cried until the water turned cold. I thought about driving myself to the hospital. I could just pull over and vomit on the side of the road like I'd often done before. Sometimes I threw up in large plastic "zipper" bags, because it was too exhausting to get out of the car to barf. I threw up in grocery bags at the store, trashcans at the park, and even the planters at work. Vomiting in public was no longer humiliating to me. Still, it wasn't safe to drive because of my HG history of passing out.

My sister came to take me to the hospital because my husband had to go to work. My son came along and slept in the stroller while I sat with the little pink emesis basin in the waiting room. My sister and I thought the little kidney-shaped bowl was laughable. If I threw up in that basin, bile would have gotten everywhere.

Once I got admitted to the E.R., a man in the bed next to me was very stinky. When he coughed it was worse. I didn't think I could get any sicker until I smelled him. After the nurse got my IV in, she started to hep-lock it and asked me to hold the end. Her eyes were watering; she coughed and turned to spit in the trash behind her. When she returned, she apologized for throwing up in front of me. She said she wasn't sure what it was. I kind of chuckled and raised my eyebrows. I told her maybe it was the smell next door. She nodded.

My sister sat outside the ER with my son until he woke up. By then, I had gotten half way through my drip, so they let them come in to say hello. My son climbed up and snuggled with me on the bed and shifted when the nurse took my blood pressure. I couldn't relax because I was sure they'd ask him to leave, but the nurse said he was fine. After about twenty minutes my sister decided to take him home for a while. The nurse told her that I'd be able to go home as soon as I'd gotten two bags of fluid and that they would call her. It was pretty uncomfortable. Someone came to take my blood twice, which I thought was odd, but I wasn't really ready for a debate. The third time someone came I told them that I'd already had two people take my blood and she look at my chart with a puzzled look. "Sorry, we only needed to do that once. Good thing you said something."

The next day I got a call from my HMO. It was the case-nurse assigned to me because my pregnancy had been designated an at-risk pregnancy. She was calling to talk about my first hospitalization and to give me a number where I could call to speak with a nurse at any time and numbers where I could reach her in the daytime. I told her that I had been to the hospital two more times. She told me that she was calling to tell me that the HMO would authorize me to have a home nurse. I was surprised.

She said that it would be cheaper for them and easier for me, especially since I had another child to care for. I didn't have a problem with that and figured it wouldn't be long before I needed it because I wasn't on any medication and continued to vomit. She asked me how my food intake was and I told her that I wasn't able to eat or drink anything.

I told my doctor that I had been authorized for this service but he told me that it could be a bad thing and that he wanted to check out the company they used before he recommended it. I was driving an hour and a half each way every other day to weigh in and have my urine tested with him. I was almost out of sick days and we were in escrow for a new house. I had signed the loan papers the first day that I had been hospitalized. Our lender, who I spoke with on my cell phone from the hospital, told me that we would not be able to complete the loan if I went on disability.

After a few days my doctor decided that since I couldn't keep any fluids down, I needed an IV again. The supplies came in two boxes by UPS. A nurse called to confirm that I had all my supplies. It was very odd to have so many medical supplies on my kitchen table. At about 11:15 that night my IV stand arrived.

The next morning the nurse came while my husband was having breakfast with our neighbor and son. I was feeling very hopeful. She brought me a scale, weighed me and showed me how to test my urine. She gave me a toilet collection thing I had to use to measure all output. Then she gave me a log in which to note everything I ate or drank and when I threw up. She told me all the things I should do to avoid throwing up, all of which I had read online except that I could not brush my teeth for thirty minutes after I threw up. That one killed me but I knew my teeth were decalcified. My dentist had prescribed a special tooth treatment to help keep my teeth in good shape.

The nurse looked at my arms. I told her that the veins in my left arm were supposedly harder to get into but all the recent IVs had been in my right arm. She sent me into the bathroom to heat up my left arm in the sink hoping the heat would bring the veins closer to the surface. Then she poked in and hit a knot. She decided to try the vein higher up. I told her it wasn't hurting, that she could take her time. She proceeded to fish around in my arm. I started to watch the clock. She paused and said, "Are you sure this is okay? We can take a break." I asked her to just go ahead and so she did. After twenty minutes she pulled the needle out and told me she'd just have to put it in the crook of my elbow.

She asked me to put a towel on my abdomen, which I did. Then she put one of those blue, ultra-absorbent pads under my arm and popped the needle in. She thought she had it, but then no blood came out. She said she was going to have to try again and stepped back to the kitchen to get something. As she did, the blood flowed out and down my arm. The blue pad filled with a pool of blood more than a foot long. "Uh," was all I could say. "I'm in!" she exclaimed. I wasn't feeling really great about her performance, but I paid close attention when she showed me how to flush the vein before I disconnected.

Later that day, I was rushing to get to the phone after a trip to the bathroom. Just as I answered the phone I stepped on my line. I clamped it off as I saw blood running up the tube. The needle had been partly pulled out and by that evening it was so uncomfortable I had to remove it. Nothing felt as good as pulling that needle out of my arm.

The next day, the same nurse came. She got an IV in quickly, revved it up, and went into the kitchen to clean up. The IV started to burn, and I thought that maybe I was just being sensitive. Then I noticed that there was a bulge forming. "Is this supposed to be happening?" I asked, unable to think of a better way to get her attention. "Oh no, I blew a vein," she said as she stood there. I reached up to shut off the IV before she thought of it. The bulge was slightly larger than a half of a golf ball. She never even addressed it. Before she left, she told me she'd be requesting another nurse because she was pretty sure she had blown my confidence in her. I didn't argue. It hadn't helped that her coffee breath was nauseating and my dog didn't like her.

The next day my right arm was swollen all over. The golf ball bulge spread across my arm. It was purple, yellow and red. The nurse I called every morning (to report my vitals) told me to put moist heat on it. By nighttime my whole arm was fat and by morning I had fever. That lasted for another couple of days until I got a better nurse.

When the good nurse called to schedule her arrival I asked that she not wear her nurse's coat or uniform. My son had started to cry when he saw the nurses arrive. He said that he thought they were hurting me. He was a trooper. He learned to be very careful about my arms, and while there were tubes and blood everywhere for weeks, it never really seemed to bother him.

She came and was great. She only used pediatric needles for dehydrated patients and had me lay down for an audio. She identified the baby's heartbeat; it was comforting to hear before I got poked again. After spending some time looking and feeling my veins she said she wasn't going to touch my "golf ball" arm, which was still bruised and swollen, but asked to insert the new IV without gloves. I told her I didn't mind.

She was into a vein very quickly, and that line lasted the longest. I didn't throw up when I was on IV fluids but I still felt sick and couldn't eat much. At night I ran an IV, hep-locked it in the morning, went to work, and then hooked up again when I got home. It was a pain in the neck. My husband was working nights, so I had to have help at around four AM to change my bag. It was the only thing I couldn't do one-handed. We had a friend staying with us for a couple of weeks, and he got up early every morning to change my bag and get me rolling.

When I finally did pull out that line, I was disappointed because it meant someone would likely have to struggle with a new location. The most annoying thing about the actual IV at home was my son's cat. She was evil. If I got up to get a drink or something to eat I would have to do it in stages. There was a step into my kitchen and I once knocked over my IV pole trying to tackle it, so I had to reach over the stair to put my drink or food onto the fish tank and then reach back for the IV pole. The cat would always appear from nowhere and begin sampling whatever I had put down. She did the same thing when I went to the bathroom. I ended up having to use sippy cups or bottles with tops so that she wouldn't get into whatever I was trying to consume. Pets can make HG harder to deal with.

The good nurse went on vacation. Home health care was having some difficulty finding a replacement. Finally they got one to agree to come to my work. I found an empty office and laid out my needles, lines, heparin, saline and sharps container. I only brought the pediatric needles. The nurse arrived and I took her into the office where we found a friend of mine on the phone.

I had a short window of time with the nurse, and my friend didn't mind the procedure so we got started. The nurse said that it was going to be difficult so I offered to heat up my arm. She said she didn't think it would help much, but it did. I hadn't even offered my right arm, as it was still painful. After a few minutes she got into a vein on the back of my hand and I put my bag on a hanger and went back to my office.

She seemed pleasant enough, but she called her office and refused to see me again. She said that I was going to need a PICC line. They called my doctor and my doctor called a line technician. By the time I got home I had an appointment to have a PICC. I thought it was excessive until my discovery.

I hep-locked my line early that night because I had been able to get enough fluid during the day. I read a little and then turned off my nightstand light. When I was setting my alarm I knocked something off my nightstand. I turned the light back and leaned over to pick it up. As I did I saw the blood. Blood was flowing through the hep-locked valve on the back of my hand. The nurse had covered the back of my hand with tape and gauze so that the IV wouldn't rub. With all the tape, I didn't even feel the blood.

It turned out to have been a faulty valve. Had I not knocked something off my nightstand I would have likely bled to death during the night. It was then that I grabbed my son and snuggled up closely with him. I had to remind myself that it was all going to be worth it. It scared me to think that I might not have been there for my little boy. I was already feeling like I wasn't doing enough for him.

One of my health care professionals took it upon herself to try to prevent the PICC line. She noticed in my record that I had never tried Zofran. It wasn't related to the drugs that I was allergic to. She called my HMO case nurse, my OB and my perinatologist and convinced them to let me try it. My doctor phoned in the prescription and I started taking it that night. I was scared I might have a bad reaction, so I called my son's babysitter to babysit *me*. I was hopeful and determined. My doctor wanted me to keep the appointment for the PICC line but I had already decided against it.

Saturday I ate. Not only that but I drank. I ate normally and didn't vomit. I was elated. We were even able to go on a family vacation to Costa Rica when I was six months pregnant. I regained my appetite and was able to do some mild activities like kayaking and hiking with my husband and son.

At about thirty weeks I went into mild labor. I continued having contractions until I was around thirty-two weeks pregnant. At that point my doctor said I could deliver, and of course my labor stopped.

At my next perinatologist appointment I was huge and fed up. The husband-and-wife team argued about how far along I was but agreed that I could be induced because of the baby's size. My doctor agreed because the baby might weigh more than ten pounds if I went full term. The labor went quickly and my second son was born weighing eight pounds and seven ounces. He was healthy and happy. I made it through two pregnancies with HG and have two wonderful boys.

Update: Vivian recently had a third HG pregnancy that came dangerously close to ending in termination. However with the love and support of family, friends and different doctors she was able to get through the worst of it and deliver a beautiful, healthy baby girl.

TWO
What Causes HG?

Roughly 80% of women experience nausea during pregnancy while 50% experience actual vomiting.[17] No one knows why. Some have proposed that women suffer from nausea and vomiting during early pregnancy in order to limit fetal exposure to dietary toxins during the teratogenic stage. There is also some evidence that supports the theory that undernourishment in early pregnancy stimulates placental growth, which is beneficial to the baby.[18] One interesting theory wonders if morning sickness is a primitive positive pregnancy test that tells a woman's family that she will need more food and heightened protection. It may also be a way to reduce sexual intercourse during pregnancy.[19]

As with normal morning sickness, there is no lack of theory regarding the cause of HG. In fact, HG has been called the disease of theories, and there is no real consensus. Different studies suggest that women at risk of developing HG are: nutritionally deficient,[20] underweight,[21] or even heavy.[22] Some studies conclude that miscarriage rates are lower for women with hyperemesis[23] while others say the rate of miscarriage is slightly higher.[24] Varying literature shows a slightly increased risk of central nervous system malformations,[25] testis cancer,[26] prematurity[27] and lower birth weight[28-29] in the offspring of hyperemetic women, while other studies show no increased risk of any type of defect whatsoever.[30-31] At least one study actually shows a *decrease* in certain birth defects.[32]

Treatment is based on experience and conjecture, but it is clear that we really don't know too much about what causes or cures HG. All the theories can be filed under one of five subheadings: endocrine, allergy (immunity), metabolic, neurologic and psychogenic.

Endocrine Theories (Most Studied)

The absence of nausea and vomiting during pregnancy has been associated with an increased rate of miscarriage.[33] The hypothesis is that low hormonal levels may contribute to the loss of the baby and account for the lack of nausea and vomiting. There are at least thirty hormones needed to maintain pregnancy.[34] Who knows which one might cause a specific individual sensitivity? Maybe it's not *one* hormone but a combination of different hormones. The possibilities are endless.

hCG

Many people believe HG is caused by a reaction to high levels of human chorionic gonadotropin (hCG). HG has also been linked to higher hCG level pregnancies such as multiple gestations (twins and so forth) and molar pregnancies (where the developing cells have turned into cancer).[35] Direct injection of hCG, however, does not reproduce nausea as one might have expected (though one woman contacted me and said the injections did make her vomit). Different studies have found differing levels of hCG in hyperemetic patients compared to controls and have implicated and not implicated it.[36] So much conflicting evidence is frustrating.

Progesterone

The hormone progesterone is another suspect in the HG mystery. It has an inhibitory effect on the gut which delays gastric emptying, reduces esophageal sphincter pressure, decreases gallbladder motility, and slows gastrointestinal transit time. These are all things that are believed to contribute to HG. Still, they don't necessarily cause HG, for as nausea and vomiting subside (sometime after the first trimester) progesterone levels are actually *increasing*.

Another progesterone factor may be the position and size of the corpus luteum. Once a month a little ovum-containing blister forms on an ovary. When the blister bursts, the ovum or egg is released. What is left of the blister is a yellow glandular mass that serves as a temporary endocrine organ which secrets progesterone (a steroid hormone that prepares the uterus to receive and develop a fertilized egg). This vessel is the corpus luteum.

One study found an association between nausea and location of the corpus luteum.[37] If the egg popped out of the ovary on the right side, women tended to have more nausea and vomiting. The proposed reason was attributed to differing hormonal drainage between the right and left ovary. If the corpus luteum were on the right side, a higher concentration of steroid hormones would supposedly reach the liver increasing nausea/vomiting. If this theory is fact, it might explain why some women have nausea in one pregnancy but not the other and how one HG pregnancy can be more severe than another. However, I have heard from women who experienced HG in pregnancies initiated by invitro fertilization (IVF), which involves no corpus luteum at all. One might then argue that the

IVF drugs cause the HG, yet if that were so, the illness should always end after cessation of pharmaceutical administration (at around twelve weeks), but it doesn't. That leads us back to other theories and other hormones.

Estrogen

Estrogens have been noted as mildly toxic and have been shown to cause vomiting in test subjects.[38] Some suspect a physical, maladaptive reaction in women with HG. It is theorized that a pregnant woman may produce more estrogen in nine months than in three non-pregnant years.[39] Perhaps some women's bodies have a difficult time dealing with such high levels. In fact, women who are very sensitive to the estrogen in the contraceptive pill do seem to be prone to developing HG in pregnancy.[40]

Another estrogen theory holds that some women make too much estrogen or related substances. Some reports claim a significantly greater level of total serum estradiol and non-protein-bound estradiol in their study group of hyperemetic women.[41] Other articles look to examine the sex of the offspring in an effort to test the double estrogen theory.[42]

If estrogen is the catalyst as some believe, it is theorized that a woman carrying a female child would experience not only her own estrogen but that of her growing daughter and thus be bombarded with a double dose of estrogen. This has been studied and, although some literature demonstrates that HG moms do have a slightly higher tendency to carry girls, many HG moms carry boys. Therefore carrying a girl cannot be said to be *the* cause of HG. The increased ratio of girls to boys is interesting, though no one really knows what the relationship means. There are many facets yet to explore.

Statistically, there do seem to be contributing components that predispose a woman such as weighing more than 170 pounds, nulliparity (never having completed a pregnancy beyond miscarriage or abortion), age and even non-smoking status.[43] These may be estrogen-related components.

Hyperthyroidism

Some women with HG present with hyperthyroidism, a condition that involves an overabundance of thyroid stimulating hormone. This hyperthyroidism is usually transient (short-lived), first appearing with the onset of HG and disappearing with the resolution of HG. Because HG can cause transient hyperthyroidism, some professionals prematurely diagnose HG as Graves' disease. Distinguishing between Graves' and the transient hyperthyroidism caused by HG can be problematic.[44] However, Graves' has certain clinical and immunological features that HG does not.

In Graves' the vast majority of sufferers has experienced symptoms for at least a few months before diagnosis. Some of these symptoms are heat intolerance, weight loss (in spite of increased appetite) and warm, moist skin.[45] Although Graves' induced hyperthyroidism *can* technically appear for the first time in pregnancy, it's unusual.[46] The transient hyperthyroidism resulting from HG is usually not treated because treatment is ineffective in suppressing symptoms.[47] It would be like taking an aspirin to alleviate a headache caused by a woodpecker actively boring a hole in your skull. You have to get rid of the woodpecker to get rid of the headache!

Allergy Theory (Least Studied)

In this theory, an individual sensitivity to a particular endocrinologic agent (or combination of agents) of pregnancy could cause HG. Histamine poisoning, an allergy to the semen of a particular partner, or even an allergy to the baby herself has been hypothesized.[48]

One study suggested that the cause of HG might be related to a mechanism that increases fetal DNA in maternal plasma. Perhaps the mom's immune response fails to tolerate the biological interface between herself and the baby.[49]

Another intriguing study examined the fact that cell-mediated immunity is elevated in cases of HG.[50] In normal pregnancies the mother's immunity is depressed so the baby won't be rejected as she grows in her mother's body, but in moms with HG this immunity is actually enhanced possibly making it harder for the maternal body to accommodate the baby without an allergic response. Could HG be that response?

Yet another interesting study found more cow milk allergies in the offspring of mothers who had more severe nausea and vomiting.[51] This prompted scientists to wonder if the nausea and vomiting were actually linked to *fetal* sensitivity.

Metabolic Theory

Some suggest a vitamin B6 deficiency, as vitamin B6 has treated cases of hyperemesis with some success.[52] However, evidence to support this theory is conflicting. Other scientists have found low plasma levels of zinc and magnesium in women with HG. [53] Are low levels the cause or consequence of this illness?

Another theory is that women with HG may possess lower functioning livers that have difficulty metabolizing even a fairly low amount of circulating sex steroids while women with higher-functioning livers may have no nausea at all even with a fairly high amount of sex steroids.[54] However, how does one explain the fact that HG usually diminishes by twenty weeks when some sex steroid levels are on the rise?

Neurologic Theory

Some hypothesize that HG is caused by a hypersensitive "vomiting center" in the brain or by defective vestibular function. In one study, more pregnancy-related vomiting was reported in subjects who suffered from a history of motion sickness.[55] Generally, the neurologic theories are vague and have little or no specific research to support them. Much research needs to be done.

Psychogenic Theory

This is the dangerous theory that HG is a neurosis, and a whole chapter of this book is devoted to it.

Who Gets HG?

All types of women of childbearing age suffer from the condition in every area of the world, whether the pregnancy was planned or not, be the women rich, poor, married, unmarried, religious, non-religious, professional, non-professional, black, white or different in any other way. HG does not discriminate.

HG often recurs with similar symptoms in subsequent pregnancies.[56-57] Each pregnancy is different however, and the levels of severity can differ as well. Although not the rule, familial trends can be seen as in Dora's family:

> "I had it for five months with my first baby. One of my sisters had it for three months with her first and seven months with her second. The other sister had it for seven months with her first and didn't have HG at all with her second."

Interestingly, the overall rate of HG has decreased over the years, but the severity seems to have increased.[58] Related disability is substantial.

A Brief History[59]

Those of us who suffer from HG today may not realize how fortunate we are compared to women of yesteryear. In eras of limited medical technology, many of those who suffered from HG literally vomited themselves to death.

Vomiting in pregnancy was first recorded on an Egyptian papyrus dating 2000 B.C. Later, both Hippocrates and Soranus wrote about and attempted to treat pregnancy-related nausea and vomiting. In 1706 Kerkring gave the first *report* of an HG-related death, and in 1863 Muenoit reported forty-six deaths out of one hundred eighteen patients with HG.

It is not surprising to learn that in 1813 physicians began prescribing therapeutic termination as treatment for HG.[60] Not everyone opted for this "therapy" however, and in 1855,

Charlotte Bronte, author of Jane Eyre, died in her fourth month of pregnancy along with many other mothers of the day.[61] So the next time you feel unlucky about getting HG, remember these poor gals, and thank your lucky IV!

Ginger's Story

Though I am a scientist it is not the sum of who I am. I am also a person, a woman, a wife, a mother… and my experience with reproduction has had perhaps the biggest impact on my life. My husband and I planned our first pregnancy, succeeded on the initial try, and felt very lucky. About five weeks into it I woke up one morning and threw up. My husband and I laughed and thought, "So this is morning sickness!" I hadn't vomited since I was a little girl. How soon I found out that this was no laughing matter.

Within the week I was vomiting or on the verge of vomiting for most of the day and night and was admitted to the hospital for IV hydration. I was so dehydrated that my veins kept collapsing, and between two nurses and seven attempts, they could not get the IV into me. Finally, I told them to just give me a cup of water. I drank it down and they sent me home without the IV.

I took a leave from my work and wasn't able to leave my house for the next eight weeks because of extreme nausea and fainting spells. I moved into the guestroom because I could no longer stand the smell of my husband. I spent my mornings in bed reading <u>Clan of the Cave Bear</u> where, coincidentally, the main character actually gets severe morning sickness. Around noon I was able to get out of bed and eat some fruit on my porch. Then I would walk to my living room (usually vomiting along the way) and spend the afternoon watching TV or videos. Videos were better because they didn't contain food commercials, which would set me off vomiting again. Most of the time my brother, who was a graduate student, would come in the afternoon with videos and would give me something to try to eat and take it away quickly so I wouldn't have to see it when I felt the urge to throw it up. I existed on Tums, fruit, lemonade, corn pops, and things like goldfish-shaped crackers, and I usually had to change foods every three days. Forget about prenatal vitamins. Vitamin B and acupressure wristbands didn't help. My doctor had nothing else to offer. I lost fifteen pounds (going from one hundred five to ninety pounds) and was miserable the entire time. I would vomit all times of the day, couldn't eat any of my favorite foods, and couldn't even choke down a plain toasted bagel.

Luckily, I was able to return to work at fourteen weeks, and the nausea was gone by the end of my fourth month. The only good thing I can say about it was that I was not the least bit scared about the delivery like most first time moms are. People say that having a baby is the most painful thing a human can experience. My labor and delivery was nothing compared to my severe and prolonged morning sickness.

People who haven't gone through it don't have the slightest understanding of how horrible it is to wake up in the morning and just suffer non-stop, waiting for the day to end. One woman told me I was "so lucky" and that she wished she had severe morning sickness so that she wouldn't have to worry about getting fat during pregnancy! Unbelievable. But I have to say that even though I thought I would never let myself go through such suffering again, after having my baby, I understood it had all been so worth it. I read a study about people with severe morning sickness having a higher risk of post-partum depression, but I was never happier in my life than those few months after the birth of my son.

Two years and five months after he was born, I thought it was time for my little prince to be dethroned. Again I got pregnant on the first try. This time I held onto the words of others "Every pregnancy is different. Maybe you won't even have morning sickness this time." I never for a moment thought it could be worse. I had never heard the words that describe hell: "hyperemesis gravidarum." But at five weeks it started again. Two days into it I told my boss I was pregnant and needed a leave of absence. A week later I was too dizzy and dehydrated to walk unassisted and wanted to see my OB/GYN a week before my first appointment was scheduled.

My insurance forced me to see my general practitioner before I could see my OB. My husband and I begged her to let him go in and get the referral papers because I felt too sick, but she said she had to see me first. I moved to Los Angeles a year before and had never seen either doctor, having been perfectly healthy before this point, so why should I expect any compassion, trust or favors from a doctor who didn't even know me? I leaned on my mother as she brought me into the office and they did a pregnancy test to confirm what I already knew. When they did a lying down, sitting, and standing blood pressure I passed out, and the doctor sent me to the hospital for IV hydration. I also got my OB referral.

After a full bag of fluids, I felt stronger, but was still extremely nauseated. They had me in a shared room where others were eating, and every smell hit me like a poison dart. The nurse called my OB, and he put me on IV Zofran followed by another bag of hydration. I was sent home with a prescription for Zofran pills every six hours, and went to see my OB for the first time the next day.

My new OB gave me a picture of my baby and told me that I didn't look so bad. He also said that he and a friend did a study that showed that women make their morning sickness more severe to prove to their doubting husbands that they really are feeling bad. It really offended me. I knew that this was not the case but had no energy to argue. I was worried about taking Zofran, having not taken any medication in my previous pregnancy, but my OB said it was harmless and showed me a picture of his "Zofran baby."

I spent the next week too nauseated to get out of bed except to use the bathroom. My retired parents and my son's nanny took care of my little boy and me, because I quickly lost the ability to eat and drink without throwing up. In an entire week I ate two slices of toasted white bread (sometimes with peanut butter) and a half a glass of water a day. By the end of the week, of course, I was severely dehydrated again.

Feeling too weak to go to the hospital, I asked for a home IV. Matria, a home nursing company that specializes in the care of pregnant women, came to teach my husband and me how to change the IV bag. My Zofran pills were getting harder and harder to take and didn't stay down, so Matria got me started on a Zofran pump. They put this subcutaneously in my thigh. Day after day the Zofran dose was increased, but I still couldn't eat or drink. My blood pressure was down to seventy over thirty-eight. I could no longer get up, not even to pee, and had to use a bedpan (luckily for everyone nothing solid made it to the other end). The nurses came once a day to take my vitals and finally decided to put the Zofran directly into my IV. They thought that maybe it wasn't working because I didn't have enough fat on my thigh to absorb it.

I was on the highest dose of IV Zofran possible for my weight and started to get very painful sores in my throat and mouth from the acid, vomiting and dry heaving. HG is very different from prolonged stomach flu; I felt *worse* after vomiting instead of better. I couldn't clean up or put a toothbrush in my mouth or even rinse with water without vomiting again. I gave up trying to eat or drink anything. I spent my days and nights fighting extreme nausea and trying as hard as I could not to throw up. Sometimes in the middle of the night I would wake up and already be in the middle of vomiting before I had any chance to try and somehow stop it. I had nothing in my stomach to vomit, so my body just tried harder to get rid of whatever agent was making me so sick. I vomited often, all the way down to my intestines, and I couldn't breathe. It was horrible.

My sense of smell became so sensitive that my husband joked that he could rent me to the police as a sniffer dog. I could tell, by scent, which of seven nurses was coming to visit me before they even entered my room. I could smell what shampoo people used and what they ate for their last meal. And when friends sent flowers, my husband would show them to me from outside of my room and whisk them away before the smell hit me too hard. Every smell made me sick. I also got all these extra side effects like ptyalism, which is awful. I couldn't swallow my saliva without vomiting, and when I spit it out it was so acidic that it burned my lips and face. I got a suction machine like they have at the dentist's office, and that helped a lot. However, when I was sleeping I would swallow and then wake up vomiting saliva and stomach acid. In addition to ptyalism, I got severe acne all over my face, and my skin became flaky and yellow.

I could no longer see my little boy without getting sick, because his movements were too quick and his voice too loud. My husband would carry him in once a day to say goodnight to me. My parents took him to their house to sleep so that I would have peace during unbearable nights and mornings of fighting the relentless nausea. My poor little two-year-old had suddenly lost his mother; he told my husband, "Daddy, you are my mamma now." My sickness was taking its toll on my family.

My husband was getting worn out from having to wake up three times a night to change my IV bags, my Zofran syringe, pump batteries, etc. I had no energy to worry about anyone but myself. At this point I was too weak to see my doctor and too weak to speak to him on the phone, so my very worried parents would report to him daily. He got fed up with that, demanded to speak to me, and then told me his latest theory: I was getting worse because my parents were giving me too much attention! As if I enjoyed asking my father to change my bedpan! I told my doctor that he was wrong and that without my parents I wouldn't be able to make it through this. Dear doctor hadn't even *seen* me, so he didn't have the slightest idea about how ill I had become. He didn't know that I could no longer even lift my head or hold up a book. I could not even turn to my side without vomiting. I just lay there day after day on my back unable to move. I kept thinking each day and night that I had been through the worst, but every day was worse than the last.

After not keeping any food down for several weeks, I was not only getting too weak to fight the constant suffering, but my veins could no longer retain the IV. After two home nurses failed to reinsert the IV, my doctor said I would have to go to the hospital to get a PICC line put in. My father took me to the hospital where I was wheeled to the labor and delivery ward to get my PICC line. Unfortunately, it was the day off for the woman who puts it in. They called her at home, and I waited in the hospital all day with no hydration and no Zofran. She arrived around four PM and put in the PICC. I had to have an X-ray to be sure it was in correctly. The radiologists started to take the X-ray without covering my baby, and I had to ask them as they were running out of the room, "Shouldn't I have a shield on me, I'm pregnant?" The shocked technician ran out to get a shield. You can't count on anyone to do her job correctly. You have to constantly look out for yourself. This type of thing really shakes your faith in the people you are trusting with your life. I had to wait several hours for the radiologist to read the results of the PICC line placement from my arm to just above my heart. My doctor didn't come see me while I was in the hospital and gave no orders to have me hydrated.

When I got home, my parents had to arrange with the nursing company to come at nine PM to start up my IV fluids through my PICC line. I was severely dehydrated at this point and dizzy, but I didn't feel more nauseated than usual even though I hadn't been taking the Zofran. Because of this I asked not to be restarted on the Zofran. I think this was a big mistake. That night was totally unbearable. I dry-heaved non-stop for seven hours straight until the nurse arrived and put me back on Zofran. That is how I knew the Zofran was actually helping. With Zofran I still couldn't eat or drink, but at least if I lay still, I wouldn't constantly throw up and could relax a little. Even so, after that night of constant torture, I had had enough. I was literally starving to death and was getting delirious. I decided I couldn't take it any longer and over the next few days, when the nurses came or my parents or husband came into my room, I told them I wanted to terminate the pregnancy. I didn't want to abort my little baby, but I wanted to end the suffering. I couldn't take it anymore. The interesting thing is that I was too weak and nobody could hear me. I remember the nurse saying, "What, Sweetie?" and then coming right up to my mouth so she could hear me, which of course, made me sick. I could never request termination loud enough to be heard without getting sick.

Even though I was on the PICC line, my doctor still didn't start me on the thousand-dollar-a-day IV nutrition (TPN) but instead just kept increasing the Zofran and giving me fluids through the PICC line. Because I was too weak to project my voice, I had to have a buzzer to signal when I needed my bedpan, a Zofran change (approximately every three hours), or a new IV bag. I don't remember the last few days very well, but at some point my parents called my doctor and I motioned that I wanted to talk.

I got on the phone and told my doctor that I had to end this and that I was dying. He said I wasn't dying, that abortion is a permanent decision, and that he wanted me to talk to a friend of his first. After several hours his friend called who was a female gastroenterologist. She told me she couldn't help me with my decision, but she could prescribe other drugs to try. That afternoon my nurse reluctantly put me on at least six different drugs per my doctor's orders. I was on IV Zofran, Zantac, Benadryl, Prevacid, Reglan, and something rectally which burned and didn't help at all. I had a bad reaction to something (probably the Reglan) and was twitching and panicking and was put on extra Benadryl. Eventually, all medications were stopped except IV Zofran, Zantac and Benadryl, and I was started on TPN through the PICC at long last.

This was very difficult in the beginning because my blood had to be drawn every other day, and my veins would collapse. The nurses would have to poke around under my skin to search for a vein with a pediatric needle, which made the blood draw so slow that it seemed endless. As I felt myself turning green, the nurses would say, "It's OK if you faint, you aren't going anywhere," and continue the needle writhing under my skin to catch a rolling vein.

I couldn't tolerate the full dose of IV vitamins. When I was on them I would wake up every two hours at night dry heaving. My gastroenterologist didn't believe this and would actually *yell* at me on the phone. He didn't understand why I couldn't come in to see him or why I couldn't tolerate swallowing pills either. The IV nutrition started giving me the strength again to deal with this. I began to be able to hold up a book and to use the computer in my bed while lying down. I could tolerate a much-needed sponge bath and, a little later, a shampoo. Not every day but every week I was improving, though still not eating or drinking. The suffering was tolerable, and now I knew I was going to make it. By my thirteenth week I could sit up a little, and by the fourteenth week I was able to walk, once every other day, to the bathroom.

My family and I monitored my urine output daily. One day we noticed that the urine had turned a very strange fluorescent orange color. The nurse and doctors said this artificial color must be from the IV vitamins. Then in my fifteenth week, after peeing in my bedpan, I noticed what looked like blood on the toilet paper. I called the on-call doctor and she said this was normal. The next morning I was spotting a little and I called and left a message for my doctor. The day dragged on without hearing from him. It was nearly lunchtime on the day before Thanksgiving, and the office was going to be closed for a four-day weekend, so my energetic and aggressive mother called again and demanded that he speak to me. He suggested that I come in for reassurance that everything was fine.

Before I could leave, my home health care nurse arrived. She didn't hear the baby's heartbeat, which she claimed was normal at fifteen weeks, but she also no longer heard my heartbeat in the placenta. That was when I knew something was very wrong and started to panic. The nurse told me to get to the doctor right away.

My mother and sister got me a wheelchair and drove me to the office with my PICC line and my Zofran pump hanging out of me. On the drive there I didn't feel that nauseated, and I was begging myself to feel worse so that I would know the baby was still alive. I was still so weak that I couldn't sit upright in the wheelchair. After waiting in the waiting room for twenty minutes my mother started to yell at the nurses, "Can't you see how sick she is? She is bleeding and needs to lie down!" I didn't want to rush. I wanted my husband to be there. And most of all, I didn't want to know the truth.

My doctor saw me for only the second time and said I looked like I had been through a war. He had no idea. My husband arrived and the doctor did the ultrasound and told me the baby was dead. The whole world must have heard me howling. My suffering was intense and came from a deep place inside that I didn't even know existed. The doctor told me I needed to have a D&C and gave me the choice of doing it in his office or at the hospital across the street. It depended on my threshold for pain. I didn't deserve any more pain with this pregnancy, so I went to the hospital where my physical pain was *not* over. The nurses couldn't get the IV in. After seven digging sticks the anesthesiologist made four more attempts in my arm, the back of my hand and my fingers, and finally got it in. I was put to sleep.

I went home that night, and the next day, which was Thanksgiving, I ate for the first time in almost two months. It tasted *so good*. How did something as easy as eating become so difficult? My urine was back to a normal color even though I was still on the IV vitamins and the PICC line nutrition for several more days, so nobody knows what was really wrong or what caused the fluorescent orange colored urine.

The next month I was doing pretty well; it was so nice to be able to play with my little boy again, to sleep in the same room with my husband, to eat, to go outside for a walk. But once the novelty of being normal wore off the reality of what happened hit me. I am now at a point of being very sad, very angry, and very frustrated about what happened.

I went to my OB for a follow-up appointment and he recommended surrogacy. He said that I should not get pregnant again unless I am willing to abort. Ridiculously, he suggested that Prozac might help. He claimed that a dozen of his patients with "bad morning sickness" got on Prozac and had no morning sickness in subsequent pregnancies. Highly doubtful. It was obvious that he thought of HG in terms of a psychological problem. He's not the only one. My female boss, an MD Ph.D department chair at a prestigious medical school, was annoyed that I never signed sick-leave papers and said to my face, "Everyone has morning sickness; it is all psychological."

The results of genetic testing revealed that my baby was a karyotypically normal little girl. I will never know why she died. It is strange how quickly the suffering from HG becomes a blur in my head, but the pain from my loss just does not go away. People say when you miscarry you only feel better when you have the next baby in your arms. I think forgetting the suffering in pregnancy must be instinctual so that you have the urge to try again. But I know I should not get pregnant again and have resolved to try gestational surrogacy. HG has robbed me of the usual experience of having a child. I will not let it rob me of additional children.

Update: Less than two years after the loss of her baby Ginger was blessed with twin girls via gestational surrogacy. Surrogacy wasn't easy, and the price tag was around sixty-five thousand dollars, but in a picture she sent she is holding a gorgeous little boy and two adorable baby girls and wearing a smile on her face that says it was worth it all.

THREE
Diagnosing HG

To treat HG a physician has to rule out any other condition that might emulate HG. These types of conditions can be referred to as mimics. Some of the mimics are:

gastrointestinal conditions:
hepatitis, appendicitis, peptic ulcers, gallbladder disease, etc.

genitourinary tract conditions:
pyelonephritis, kidney stones, uremia, etc.

metabolic conditions:
hyperthyroidism, Addison's disease, diabetic ketoacidosis, etc.

neurologic disorders:
vestibular lesions, migraine headaches, brain tumors, etc.

pregnancy-related conditions:
multiple gestations, molar pregnancy, preeclampsia

fetal anomalies:
carrying a child with Down syndrome

Once the mimics are ruled out, a general diagnosis of HG can be made. Run-of-the-mill HG is currently associated only with pregnancy itself. It is an anomaly, and the cause and cure are unknown. Interestingly, if the vomiting begins after nine weeks, it is usually not HG.[62] Also, HG is often accompanied by aggravating symptoms like the sensation of ptyalism (excess saliva production) and hyperolfaction (grossly heightened, nauseating perception of odor). Neither one of these is treatable, but there are suggestions for reducing discomfort in chapter fourteen of this book.

No Universal Diagnosis

There is really no standard definition of HG.[63] Typically, HG involves excessive nausea and vomiting, total body weight loss $\geq$ 5%, ketones in the urine, dehydration, electrolyte imbalance and carbohydrate depletion. Some authorities say the $\geq$ 5% weight loss alone is enough to justify a diagnosis of HG. Some doctors simply refuse to hospitalize for HG, so of course, hospitalization is not necessary to establish a diagnosis. Since there is no set standard for diagnosis, women need to advocate for themselves if they have the typical cluster of symptoms.

No Universal Protocol

Just as there is no standard diagnosis for HG, there is no standard treatment. As the authors of one study write, "The question as to how and when to treat [HG] is still open."[64] This should not be. Some doctors consider HG to be a mental disorder while others know it is a physical disease. Some physicians will administer an alternative method of nutrition when a woman loses 5% of her body weight; others will allow a patient to lose over 14% of her total mass without administering anything more than a two-hour IV with a Phenergan suppository. As one doctor put it, "I have never ordered a PICC for HG, and I'm not about to start now." Some moms get hospitalized for medical treatment while others get hospitalized for psychiatric treatment. Some hyperemetics get life-saving corticosteroids and some get the pepsin-flavored pink stuff. Until standardized diagnosis and treatment become convention, women with HG must advocate for themselves or appoint others to advocate for them.

Benefits of Standardizing Care

A standard treatment protocol is sorely needed to increase medical accountability. HG treatment is typically expensive.[65] With a standard, it may be easier to get insurance companies to pay for necessary treatments, and the patient may get better treatment faster.[66] Unfortunately, if a physician has learned that an insurance carrier routinely declines payment for certain pricey treatments, there is at least a chance that she will not offer her patient viable treatment options. Additionally, there is the sinister possibility that an unethical physician might deny expensive treatments in order to benefit financially from an insurance company that offers certain perks for keeping medical costs down. Capitation can involve this type of scenario.

In capitation the insurance company gives the doctor a fixed amount of money to care for the patient. If the cost of treatment goes over that amount then the physician makes up the difference. If the cost stays under that amount then the physician pockets the extra. Check to see if your care has been capitated. Widely recognized standards would make it easier to hold unethical physicians accountable.

Well-defined standards would also enable patients to have a better understanding of their illness and necessary treatment options. Confident self-advocacy has the potential to increase the odds of a successful pregnancy outcome.

For now, all that sufferers have is what little information we can glean from our experiences with physicians, medical studies, family, friends, the Internet, our own individual pregnancies and books like this one. From these varied sources we can gain insight into the availability and appropriateness of treatment options such as prevention (the best medicine), natural remedies, antiemetics, IVs, nasogastric enteral feeding, percutaneous endoscopic gastrostomy and percutaneous endoscopic jejunostomy, total parenteral nutrition and termination. Bear in mind that anything and everything you learn, particularly from non-medical sources like me, *must be thoroughly discussed with your physician prior to implementation.*

Dr. Brenda's Story

During my medical career I have delivered hundreds of babies in four different countries on two continents. As a result, I have counseled hundreds of mothers through their pregnancies. Through all of this I always considered myself an understanding physician. I was patient with nervous parents and compassionate with women whose pregnancies were difficult. And then I became pregnant.

I now realize that although I treated patients with respect, it was nearly impossible for me to understand what they experienced. I could sympathize, and I could support, but I could never really understand the roller coaster of a difficult pregnancy. During my training I encountered several women with HG. I remember discussing these cases during early morning hospital rounds. The protocol was nearly always the same. These women were presented as "overly emotional" often with "clear psychological components" to their illness. I was able to treat these women with compassion, but I also felt frustrated. I believed what I was taught: on some level they had brought their illness on themselves.

I was halfway through a month-long stretch of working nights and was feeling tired and worn out. I assumed it was simply because of the hours, but a nurse suggested a pregnancy test "just in case." In my mind there was no way that I could be pregnant. My husband and I had been talking about starting a family, but we had not decided when we would actively begin pursuing this goal. When the results came back positive, I was shocked but also thrilled.

When I returned home the next morning, I vomited twice. I joked with my husband about how exciting it was that I had morning sickness and that we were now officially pregnant. The next morning, however, the nausea got worse and the joking stopped. The next day, I was worse still. I continued working long hours at night, and I eagerly anticipated the weekend so I could get some much-needed rest. But when Saturday arrived, everything I ate came right back up. Even small sips of water would send me frantically running to the bathroom.

Soon this doctor became a patient, and I thought I knew what to do. I self-prescribed two popular anti-nausea medications and sent my husband to the pharmacy that same afternoon. They didn't help. After a long weekend of vomiting, I called in sick on Monday morning and made an emergency appointment with my OB/GYN. "Relax," I was told, "Women get sick in the first trimester." He was following the same protocol I had followed so many times before. He gave me a liter of IV fluids, prescribed a third anti-nausea medication, and sent me home. The fluids did improve my condition but only temporarily. The new medication didn't help either.

Now I was beginning to worry. They say that doctors make poor patients, but I knew that things were getting serious. I continued to eat, forcing myself to hold down foods as long as I could so that the baby would get the needed nutrition, but the vomiting worsened. Desperate, I tried everything I could, including alternative therapies. I went to an acupuncturist, but found the treatments painful and more importantly, unhelpful. I scheduled a visit with an herbalist to experiment with different natural remedies and this too failed. I was less than six weeks into my pregnancy and I had already lost ten pounds.

At this point I called my doctor and explained that I was sure I had HG. He asked me to come in again and try IV fluids one more time. Upon arrival I gave the nurses a urine sample that was dark and cloudy, a sure sign of dehydration. A nurse attempted to attach an IV, and my veins were so lacking in fluid that it took her several tries to get the needle in. Remarkably, the results of my urine test proclaimed that my fluids were fine. I was sure that somehow there was a mix-up of samples, but my doctor determined that I must have not been vomiting as much as I claimed and again sent me home asserting, "Lots of women have morning sickness. It's just a part of pregnancy. You'll be fine." I *wasn't* fine. By this point, my weight loss had reached fifteen pounds. I promptly made an appointment for the next day with a different OB.

The next day I was feeling a little bit better. I was still nauseous, but I was able to keep down fruit juices and a bit of yogurt. I went to my appointment with the new doctor hopeful that the toughest times were behind me. To her credit, my new doctor listened to my story carefully and was concerned about my condition. She did an ultrasound to make sure the baby was fine, offered a new treatment regimen, and instructed me to come back weekly for regular visits. I left her office feeling pretty good. I had a doctor I liked, I was feeling less nauseous, and I had my first picture of our baby. But in a pattern that would repeat far too often, I was vomiting again by morning. I spent the entire weekend on the couch barely able to move. My husband went to the store multiple times to buy a variety of things I thought I could eat. Nothing stayed down. On Monday morning I went back to my OB. My weight loss was now twenty pounds. I was immediately admitted to the hospital.

I was very familiar with the workings of a hospital, but not as a patient. I felt powerless. They tried multiple medications and still nothing helped. I was re-hydrated and given vitamins through a line. My blood was drawn twice a day and my blood sugar levels checked around the clock. I was beginning to feel like the proverbial pincushion, but I was relieved that our baby was finally receiving the nutrition she needed. By the fifth day in the hospital, a new drug regimen finally started to take effect, and I was no longer vomiting several times a day, although my nausea remained intense. Unable to eat, my doctors decided to place a PICC line in my arm to provide around the clock nutrition and hydration. By now, my weight loss had climbed to thirty-four pounds. I wanted to go home.

I lasted a week before things got worse. I was unable to keep anything down so I just stopped trying to eat. I continued vomiting even when I avoided food. I had difficulty getting out of bed because any movement made me sick. My sense of smell became so acute that ordinary household odors made me vomit. I couldn't even stand the smell of my husband and I forced him to sleep in the other room. Beyond this, the side effects of the anti-nausea medication made it difficult for me to concentrate even for short periods of time and my arms and legs became jittery. My entire day consisted of lying in bed depressed and staring at the ceiling. I could feel myself slipping away. We exhausted option after option and I began to pray for a miscarriage. I was getting to the point that I was ready to give up my baby to be free of the HG. Every day I thought about terminating the pregnancy, but I just couldn't seem to find the energy to arrange it.

I called the director of my department at work and asked him if he knew of any other treatments that I hadn't tried. He suggested a psychiatrist and an anti-depressant since HG was considered a psychological problem. He reported facts I already knew: women with HG often had negative feelings about their pregnancy and were more likely to suffer from depression. He was not entirely wrong. I certainly had negative feelings about my physically intolerable pregnancy, and I was indeed becoming more and more depressed. But these feelings were the *result* of my illness, not the cause. Even so I began to wonder if, on some level, my emotional perceptions had preceded my physical symptoms. Maybe I *had* brought this on myself after all. In addition to constant vomiting and nausea, this rationale made me feel guilty and confused. Finally, one morning before my husband left for work, I told him that I couldn't take it anymore. I wanted to terminate. I *needed* to terminate. I knew this was my only chance to have *this* baby, but I just couldn't continue. My husband called my doctor and made an appointment for that day. I was 10 weeks pregnant and in a downward cycle that I could not break.

I arrived at the doctor's office in tears. Normally a strong-willed and independent person, I had lost my ability to cope. My doctor tried everything to encourage me. "You're at ten weeks," she reminded me. "Most women feel better at the end of the first trimester. You are almost there." Over and over she insisted that women felt better by twelve weeks. She also did another ultrasound so that I could see my baby. This became a pivotal moment in my pregnancy. On the ultrasound screen there was this little person with a beautiful head and distinct arms and legs. She was no longer a peanut; she was our baby. This gave me the needed strength to continue with my pregnancy. I vowed to try harder to make it through. My spirits were higher but my physical condition continued to decline. Instead of sending me home, my doctor sent me back to the hospital. This time I went with my prized ultrasound picture clutched tightly in my hand.

The second hospitalization was even more awful than the first. I laid in the fetal position and barely moved. Again, the doctors were able to control my vomiting with IV medications but the nausea continued. I begged to go home. If I were going to be miserable, I would rather be in my own bed than in the hospital. I went home on high doses of IV medication because I could no longer take my medicines by mouth.

My husband continued researching possible treatments. He read several references to the effectiveness of hypnosis and we decided to try it. We found a hypnotist with experience treating HG and he agreed to see us. We drove an hour to his office; I vomited all the way. The hypnotist assured us he could help. He had treated many women with my condition and had been successful *every* time. He spent three hours with us, and we left feeling very hopeful. In an all too familiar scenario, this treatment was also ineffective. I saw him three more times, but nothing changed. He told me that my subconscious was rejecting the baby, and through hypnosis we could discover why and resolve the conflict. Again I was told that it was all in my mind and somehow under my control. In the end, when there was no improvement he said to me, "You know, maybe there *is* a physiologic component."

Throughout this entire time well-meaning friends and family would call to offer support and advice. They told me about other women that they knew who had "bad morning sickness" and what medications or herbs they had taken. My mother insisted I would feel better if I just got out of bed and got some fresh air. I couldn't make them understand what I was experiencing so I isolated myself, no longer answering the phone or returning phone calls.

I was almost twelve weeks pregnant-the magic number. I was counting the days hoping that suddenly I would feel better overnight. I didn't. In fact, my twelfth week was one of my worst. I lost all hope. At thirteen weeks, I wished I had gone through with the termination. I felt that beyond twelve weeks it was too late. It was now Christmas, by far the worst holiday season we'd ever had. I cried most of the day. My husband didn't know how to help me. How was I going to survive this way for six more months?

Long days stretched into long weeks and the hoped-for improvement still seemed remote. My doctor continued to push back the time at which everything would improve. We went from twelve to fourteen to sixteen and finally, to eighteen weeks. Each day was an enormous struggle as the emotional pressure combined with my physical decline to nearly make my life impossible. But my story does have a happy ending.

At the end of my eighteenth week, the vomiting trailed off and I began eating for the first time in nearly three months. The nausea would never completely disappear, but it did lessen. Gradually I was able to eat enough small amounts that my doctor removed the PICC line in my arm. I hoped that every day for the rest of my pregnancy I would continue to improve until I felt like myself again. Unfortunately, that didn't happen. I did get a bit better though, and by my twenty-fourth week, I had reached a kind of stable level of sickness that was at least manageable. I remained on medication and continued to be nauseous every day until the day I gave birth.

My pregnancy was extraordinarily difficult, but as I write this, I am looking at our beautiful three-month-old baby girl. We are both healthy and happy, and now I can block out the most painful memories and conclude that it was all worth it. I still have difficulty looking back on my pregnancy. I get annoyed when I tell people I had a trying pregnancy and they say, "Oh yes, I had a lot of morning sickness too." And a medical community that continues to insist that HG was all in my head *really* bothers me. For me, one of the most difficult things I faced was the feeling that I was alone. No one could help, no one could understand, and I felt more and more isolated in the midst of my suffering.

My hope for those who struggle with this condition is that they will know there is help. Hopefully this book will convince people to support women with HG, but more importantly, I hope that sufferers will be able to read these pages, find some comfort in them, and know that they are not alone.

TREATING HYPEREMESIS GRAVIDARUM

FOUR
Prevention

Outside of pregnancy prevention, we really don't know enough about HG to be able to prevent it. Some things that may help include:

Vitamins

Taking multivitamins prior to conception reduces neural tube defects in a subsequent pregnancy (if the vitamin contains folic acid). Similarly, multivitamins taken before conception (periconception) may reduce the risk of getting HG.[67-69] I had severe HG in my first pregnancy. Six months prior to my second and third pregnancies I took prenatal vitamins (with folic acid), and my HG never attained the level of severity that it did in my initial pregnancy. I took vitamins again before my fourth pregnancy, and it was my most severe HG ever. I suspect that the differences between my first, second and third pregnancies had more to do with the level of medical care than any nutrient deficiency prior to pregnancy, and while it couldn't have hurt, I don't feel that prenatal vitamins had much to do with the level of suffering in my experience with HG.

Low Fat Diet

Saturated fat intake may be a strong risk factor for HG because saturated fats may influence estrogen production during pregnancy.[70] If this theory is correct, a diet low in saturated fats could prevent the onset or lessen the severity of HG. Personally, I was a low fat freak prior to my first severe bout with HG and a high fat junkie prior to my second and third "mild" pregnancies. I didn't change a thing with my fourth pregnancy, and it was the worst.

Antibiotics

The bacterium helicobacter pylori are the culprit behind stomach ulcers, and a few women with HG were given antibiotics to treat such ulcers. Surprisingly, in some women, the HG disappeared with the antibiotic treatment.[71]

In later studies doctors found that roughly twice as many HG patients test positive for the bacterium compared to the normal pregnant population,[72] and the levels of H. pylori may be directly related to the degree of gastric complaints.[73]

Most people with an H. pylori infection don't have any symptoms. Before you get pregnant, go out and get a blood or breath test (breath is more effective) for H. pylori. If you test positive for the bacterium, take the full course of antibiotics your doctor prescribes. Get pregnant with a clean slate! If you're already suffering from HG you can still test for and treat the infection. Erythromycin is one of the popular antibiotics used to treat the H. pylori infection. It is drug category B for use in pregnancy, which means it is not likely to harm the growing baby. Treating the H. pylori infection may result in a full resolution of the HG.[74]

Unilateral Ovary Incapacitation

One theory holds that the right side position of the corpus luteum may cause HG.[75] If this theory were correct, then it might make sense to incapacitate the right ovary in order to prevent or lesson the symptoms of HG. Supposedly, if there's nothing wrong with the left ovary, this would not affect fertility or hormone excretion. Evidently, the ovary that remains compensates for the one that is missing. It pumps out twice as many hormones, and instead of spitting out one egg every other month it doubles the workload and releases one egg per month. This way the fertility and cycle would remain intact.

This theory is so radical and unproven that such a personal alteration should probably never be considered. Besides, I know a woman who has had severe HG in every pregnancy and she never even had a corpus luteum since she conceived via invitro fertilization.

A Final Word on Prevention

Although we can't be sure to prevent HG, we are able to prevent some of the stresses that can arise when embarking upon such a pregnancy unprepared. If you know you have a propensity towards hyperemetic pregnancies, then detailed plans for medical and social support should absolutely be outlined prior to pregnancy. Knowing when treatments are necessary and, more importantly, that your doctor is willing to offer such treatments, is important.

Having social support in place for children is monumental. If HG spirals out of control, it could be very helpful to have somewhere for them to go and stay for a while. Grandma and Grandpa can come to the rescue here. Many women have found that their parents were able to offer a child-friendly environment where nutritious meals were always at hand.

Daycare, pet care, finances and the like can all become issues in the hyperemetic pregnancy. If at all possible, plan for these things ahead of time. We have little control over HG, but we should wield all the power we can over the manageable aspects of life, aspects that, while perhaps not making HG better, may help to avoid making it worse.

Arin's Story

I gave birth to my daughter eleven months ago after enduring a horrible pregnancy. At one point in the pregnancy, I remember stating to my whole family, "It's either me or the baby that is going to live; I want it to be me." I even asked my doctor when the last legal date in our state was to have an abortion. I was so sick that I was ready to terminate. The only way my daughter was brought into this world was through my unbelievably supportive family that researched for me and stayed by my bedside.

After reading a story about a hyperemetic woman who lacked support and terminated, I realized for the first time that the people who supported me were my daughter's angels; there is no way I could have done it on my own. I am so sorry for women that do not have the type of support I had. HG is HORRIBLE and, unless they've been there, NO ONE understands what it is like to feel physically forced to consider terminating a child they want because of an illness. Thank God I was one of the lucky ones and got the support I needed. I can't even imagine the grief moms feel at terminating children they love and want.

My HG was so awful that it was shocking. I became severely depressed by the physical suffering and cried all the time. Because of this, they prescribed Prozac. I wondered where God was. Luckily, my husband is a physician and has medical knowledge and access to research. What he discovered allowed us all to at least not be scared that I was going to die, because that's what HG feels like. My husband actually diagnosed me before the doctors. There were so many times when he came to the rescue. For instance, my HG caused hyperthyroidism, but my endocrinologist told me I had Graves' disease. He wanted to put me on medication that causes "cosmetic disorders" in the baby (but told me not to worry about it)! Thankfully, my husband handed him some studies that related HG with hyperthyroidism and told the doctor we wanted to wait and see before I took any medications for Graves'.

I wish I had had more information when I was going through everything. It seems like such a mysterious disease; a lot of the doctors treated it that way. They didn't know what caused it, cured it or how long it would last. Everyone was just guessing. Information is so important for those enduring the nightmare. If someone at my doctor's office had been able to hand me even a pamphlet...you can't imagine how helpful it would have been.

Eleven months after my daughter's birth, I am still in shock. I can't really believe that the whole experience is over and my body is back to normal just like nothing ever happened. The illness was so life-altering that I still think about it every day. We want another child so badly, but I am absolutely scared to death of going through HG again. I can't stress enough that it was so bad that I considered destroying my child. If caring people had not fought for my daughter and me, I guarantee she would not be here today.

FIVE
Alternative Treatments

While women desire "natural" pregnancies, it may not always be possible. In fact, refusing intervention when it is clearly indicated can actually be detrimental to the pregnancy. Depending on the severity of the HG, moms may be able to delay or prevent more aggressive types of treatments by taking advantage of alternative therapies. Such therapies may alleviate some of the symptoms of HG without compromising the goal of a "natural" pregnancy. There are several options to choose from. Among these are herbal teas, natural medicines, ginger, enemas, acupressure/puncture, aromatherapy and other treatments.

Natural remedies don't always equate safe remedies, so be sure and check with your doctor regarding the safety of *any* intervention. You might also check with a certified, licensed homeopathic practitioner. You can find more information on where to find such a homeopath in Appendix B of this book.

Natural Medicines

Of the natural medicines available, some are homeopathic in nature while others are herbal. Homeopathy treats an illness by administering small doses of an agent that, in a healthy person, would actually cause symptoms similar to the disease. And the best part? No one knows how it works (or even *if* it works). I purchased a homeopathic medicine myself. Before full-blown HG developed in my first pregnancy, I went to the local health food store in order to find a natural aid. The "naturopath" on duty handed me a small bottle of little white pellets labeled "Sepia" (Cuttlefish ink). I bought the bottle (under three dollars) and took it to my doctor who refused to approve the use of the drug, because she had never studied it and had no knowledge of its interaction with other drugs or effect on the baby. It scared me at the time, so I never took any of the pellets. Several doctors may have the same lack of knowledge, and that may hinder your decision-making process.

Herbal Teas

Herbal teas can be helpful; however, some caution is necessary. The following herbal teas are **not** known to cause birth defects: ginger, peppermint, red/black raspberry, spearmint, slippery elm and dandelion. Chamomile must be taken with caution because of possible rare yet serious allergic reactions. Fennel contains a good amount of vitamin A, and vitamin A supplements have been linked to fetal anomalies. However, fennel tea is a natural source and is not as likely to cause problems as synthetic forms of vitamin A.

If you are interested in herbs for use in pregnancy, get your hands on a copy of Penelopy Ody's book, <u>Herbs for a Healthy Pregnancy: From Conception to Childbirth</u>. It contains charts that clearly state which herbs are safe and which herbs to avoid.

Ginger

Ginger is prescribed so often for nausea and vomiting that it deserves special mention. This natural antiemetic has been used in the Orient for centuries. It improves production and secretion of bile from the liver and gallbladder, improves gastrointestinal motility, and stimulates digestion. Lots of folks immediately think of ginger ale but, even when hyperemetics can drink without vomiting, many cannot tolerate soda. The carbonation can cause nauseating pressure in the stomach. Fresh ginger tea is a non-carbonated alternative that can be easily prepared at home. Your advocate can find fresh ginger root in the produce section of most grocery stores, and following this recipe makes tea:

Fresh Ginger Tea
4 C boiling water
2 T fresh, grated ginger root
honey & lemon to taste

Boil water in a pot. Grate the fresh root, skin and all, until you have two tablespoons of mushy, fibrous, lemony smelling stuff. Steep this amount in the boiling water for ten or more minutes. Pour the solution through a strainer. Once the tea is clean, pour it in a mug and add lemon and honey to taste. Conversely, the ginger can be cut into thin "coin" slices instead of grated, but some say this makes a less potent tea.

Ginger is spicy, and it burns all the way down. Still, sometimes the burn is enough to replace the nausea for a moment or two, and that is a welcome effect. Be liberal with the lemon and honey because, unless you're used to it, ginger tea can be NASTY tasting stuff. You might wonder if you could bypass the foul brew by taking powdered ginger capsules. Doctors themselves have studied the use of powdered ginger capsules in cases of hyperemesis gravidarum, and approximately

70% of women preferred it to a placebo (fake sugar pill). This preference seems to indicate the effectiveness of ginger. Still, some sources advise women to avoid medicinal doses due to a component in the powdered form (thromboxane synthesase inhibitor) that may or may not affect the baby.[76] Ingesting any substance during pregnancy may carry an associated risk and should be a decision that is ultimately made by you with help from your doctor.

Herbal teas, homeopathic medicine and ginger are fine assuming you are at the point where you can still keep a swig of something down. If you are beyond this point, there are other natural alternatives.

Enemas

Theoretically a warm water enema *can* add fluids, and I've heard midwives discuss enemas with such things in them as molasses or Pedialyte. However, some doctors question absorption rates and are anxious about the risk of diarrhea. If you think you would like to try enemas as a method of rehydration, consult your physician.

Acupuncture

Acupuncture uses needles to puncture the skin at certain points on the body according to the standard healing categories of traditional Chinese medicine. Formal validity has never been established. One study concluded that acupuncture wasn't any more effective than placebo (fake) acupuncture[77] while another study found that it was effective in alleviating some of the symptoms of hyperemesis when used to compliment conventional treatment. [78]

Acupressure

Acupressure is a therapy in which pressure is applied to those areas of the body used in acupuncture. For the treatment of nausea/vomiting, pressure is applied at the P6 (Nei Kuan) point, which is basically located on the inner wrist, three fingerbreadths up from the wrist joint. The theory is that stimulation increases the release of endorphins. One product available over the counter at drugstores and travel agencies is Sea-Bands. They were created for motion sickness and are basically sweatbands with a plastic button on the underside. The bands are tight and keep the button pressed firmly on the inside of your wrist. Possible side effects of this product are the sensation of finger numbness, caused by constant pressure, and redness under the button. Also, the bands can be so uncomfortable that the stimulation can aggravate nausea in the HG sufferer.

On a personal note, when I'm traveling, Sea-Bands seem to be effective for reducing my motion sickness. When I'm suffering from HG they only serve to exacerbate my discomfort.

Aromatherapy

Aromatherapy is based on the theory that certain aromas can affect the emotional/physical state of the sniffer. The two scents recommended for HG are fresh lemon and peppermint oil. Some women have claimed great relief from smelling these. There have been women who have carried around a cut lemon in a plastic baggie or even on a rope around their neck, and when they got nauseated, they sniffed the lemon for comfort. Perhaps the lemon acts as a sort of "white" scent that blocks out all other annoying smells that might provoke a vomiting spell.

Peppermint oil may work on the same principle as fresh lemon. However, peppermint oil taken internally may cause liver problems and supposedly nullifies the effects of any other homeopathic you might be taking, so use it for smelling only. Personally, smelling *anything* made me puke, but everyone is different.

Electrical Stimulation

In one study moms with HG were willingly experimented on with electricity.[79] Doctors created a headset and neckband that had electrodes in them and involved stimulating the area behind the ear (electric stimulation of the vestibular system). The study was not controlled. Physicians merely applied the unit, delivered the "electrical stimulation," and then asked the women if they felt at all better. Some women reported some relief during this therapy. Another study concluded that a product called the ReliefBand, an electrical stimulation wristband device that resembles a watch, might be helpful to reduce some symptoms of HG.[80] I tried it for motion sickness, and for me it was as effective as Sea-Bands. Although the electric current can cause your fingers to twitch during use, it is not uncomfortable. The sensation is tingly as if your hand has "fallen asleep," and it cycles every four seconds. The coin cell battery only lasts about one hundred fifty hours though, so stock up. The "morning sickness" version of the band used to require a prescription but doesn't appear to now. You can find ordering information in Appendix B of this book.

Natural remedies are not harmless placebos. They can be quite potent. When considering any remedy, find out the associated risks, be particularly cautious about anything you read on the Internet, and always seek the advice of your physician.

Courtney's Story

I'm no wimp. I've always been extremely active and adventurous. I've been skydiving, ultralighting, and hot air ballooning. I started my own business at twenty-one and completed both my undergrad degree and master's degree while working full time. I am, by all accounts, a type "A" personality with tremendous energy and a "can-do" approach to life. Give me an obstacle and I'll solve the problem. This strategy has served me well in life and in business, but it couldn't touch HG.

Nausea and vomiting in pregnancy run in my family. I saw my older sister become sick during her pregnancies, but I never knew how bad it could be until I became pregnant myself. With my first child, I managed to go to work and school, taking breaks to vomit and regain my composure, but functioning more or less. My OB was compassionate but offered little support, medication or otherwise. I was miserable but not totally incapacitated. I delivered a little girl, full term, and the HG finally ended. My husband brought me my first real meal in eight months that evening and I enjoyed every bite! I remember hoping that this was a one-time ordeal, and that my next pregnancy would be normal.

My second pregnancy was much worse. I didn't need a pregnancy test because by the fifth week I once again had a terrible taste in my mouth and nearly constant nausea. I prayed it wouldn't get worse, but by the next week I was vomiting constantly and losing weight. I took a leave of absence from work and spent most of my days in bed. I wondered what "morning sickness" meant, because my nausea worsened as the day went on. At four PM the worst of the nausea and vomiting would begin. By seven weeks pregnant I had lost twelve pounds.

The days went by so slowly that I thought I wouldn't get through it. Although I had changed OBs to get better medical support, none of the conventional drugs they prescribed (Compazine, Phenergan, Vistaril, Unisom) worked. I was losing weight and hope daily. As I lay there feeling just awful, sometimes I didn't care if I lived and sadly, I admit I prayed to God for a miscarriage.

By eight weeks I'd lost over seventeen pounds and was so dehydrated that my OB had me hospitalized. She consulted a GI specialist who put me on the latest remedy at the time: Reglan. I felt better for about a day but uncomfortable side effects began. I wasn't able to sleep, I felt like pacing around, my mood was really poor, and still the nausea and vomiting persisted. At that point, I had no hope for a cure. Time was the only thing that would stop it, and it was standing still.

I was released from the hospital after a few days of IVs, and I gradually worsened. At ten weeks I knew I really needed help. On top of the almost constant nausea and frequent vomiting, my thinking became very uncharacteristic for my normally optimistic spirit. I got really depressed and even suicidal. I was so sick I wanted to die. I just wanted the misery to end.

Eventually, I phoned my OB who referred me to a psychiatrist in charge of mood disorders at our local university. This doctor saw me a few days later and quickly diagnosed me with severe clinical depression, a condition that occurs in approximately one in ten women during pregnancy. I had heard of postpartum depression, but never depression during pregnancy. I was truly shocked at the diagnosis. I had never been clinically depressed before in my entire life. I was already miserable with the nausea and vomiting of HG but depression brought a new dimension to my suffering.

I hesitated to take medication I knew nothing about, but the doctor said that without it the baby and I might die. The HG finally improved at around eighteen weeks. Like the first pregnancy, I remained mildly nauseated and still vomited from time to time, but I could function both at home and at work to some degree. My daughter was born at thirty-seven weeks and was healthy. The HG left me immediately, and I was put on Zoloft for the depression, which disappeared after the pregnancy was over and I was well again. I was back to myself! I loved being a mom, and life was good.

When the baby was about nine months old I came down with the flu. Or so I thought. When the funny taste in my mouth appeared I took a pregnancy test and was shocked to find that, even though I was on birth control, I was pregnant again.

I can't describe my overwhelming fear. I simply didn't think I could make it through another pregnancy. Within several days, the HG was raging along with the newly emerging depression. At five weeks I was a basket case. I became desperate and felt I couldn't endure more suffering. I was terrified of leaving the care of my two small children to someone else for months at a time. I felt I was missing out on so much of their lives. I had absolutely no positive or hopeful thoughts, not even about the beautiful baby I might hold someday. I was FIVE weeks; it was just too far away. My anxiety and fear were high and the nausea was unbearable.

I phoned my OB and cried to him that I didn't know how I was going to survive this. Knowing the severity of my HG he said, "Well, have you thought about terminating the pregnancy?" I didn't know what to say. I don't think I even answered him. Abortion was not an option, but then again, I wasn't sure if I could endure HG even for another day. The doctor gave me a Zofran prescription and said that it was the latest arsenal for HG. I took it the first day and felt unbelievably good. Finally something worked! Unfortunately, by the third day, the Zofran seemed to wear off and I was back to vomiting countless times a day.

I began to weigh options and found myself ruminating over the doctor's question about termination. The only other time I'd ever heard of a woman terminating her pregnancy due to severe nausea and vomiting was in Miriam Erick's book No More Morning Sickness. I had read that book during my first pregnancy hoping for relief, but I found none. I remember being amazed that a woman would abort her child due to nausea and vomiting knowing they would eventually get better. At the time though, I had no clue how bad HG can get.

By week six, the HG was worsening along with the depression. I looked at my two little children and convinced myself that I just couldn't do this again, not after what I'd been through with the last pregnancy and not for the length of time I knew was to come. I felt trapped, desperate and hopeless. I decided that was either the baby or me, and in my weakened physical and emotional state, I convinced myself that I had no alternative but to terminate.

I made an appointment at the abortion clinic (a number I never in my life imagined I'd call) and was told that, due to a state law, I'd have to listen to a five-minute tape about the ramifications of abortion. I put the phone down while the tape played. I didn't want to have to think about what I was doing, because if I thought about it, I wouldn't be able to do it, and I desperately wanted to be well.

The next morning I arrived on time for my appointment. I was terrified and confused, but the nausea was already growing as the minutes ticked by. I was required to attend a "counseling" session where they gave me a lecture on birth control, and they gave me a ten-second ultrasound to "size up" the baby. I was morose, unlike most of the mothers there who chatted and talked openly about their reasons for aborting their children. Most of them didn't want their babies. One lady felt she was just "too old" to have another child. I sat there knowing that no one would begin to understand my reason for aborting a child I wanted. I can't even count the many times I've been told to have soda crackers and eat small meals. No one understood.

Staff called me in to undress and that's when the reality hit me. I knew I wanted my baby, but the fear of the HG and related depression overwhelmed me. I prayed that something would happen, that maybe the doctor would be sick that day. I wanted something to save us, because I knew I wasn't strong enough to do so at that point. But nothing saved us.

The nurse knocked on the bathroom door and said I was ready to go. I had already opted not to receive anesthesia so I could leave the clinic as soon as possible. The doctor came in the room and greeted me with a smile. I can still hear his voice in my mind today, and I cringe at the cheerful attitude he had just before killing my child. I will always be puzzled about that.

I was compliant; I did what I was told. The whirring of the machine they used to suck out my baby runs through my mind even as I write this. It is so barbaric. I have no idea how I did it, how any woman could do it, but it was over. In just a few minutes I became a grieving mother.

I was escorted to a recovery area where a group of us sat in recliners to make sure we weren't bleeding excessively. Once seated, I immediately started to cry, knowing the HG hell was over but feeling horrible, agonizing regret rather than relief. Physically I was healed, but emotionally, the pain was just beginning. As I cried, the woman overseeing us came over and asked me to please stop so I wouldn't upset the others. I muffled my sobs the best I could. The young woman next to me extended her arm and patted my hand. I was absolutely the only woman in mourning in that room at the time, but I wonder how many women suffered, after leaving that place, upon finding the mother in them.

I went home and immediately threw away the clothes and shoes I had worn so as to have no visible reminders of the abortion. Of course this did nothing. Each day the bleeding, cramping, and taking of prescribed, abortion-related medicine (antibiotics) were physical reminders of what I'd done. Aborting my child put me in a place mentally that I had never been, not even in the absolute worst moment of HG. The anguish and despair were something I could never have imagined. I didn't think it was survivable.

Within a couple of days, I went to talk to a priest/friend who always seemed to have the right words of comfort during difficult times. I explained HG to him as best I could and sobbed through my story of my prior pregnancies. Thankfully, my friend was very comforting. It took years, but I believe I have finally forgiven myself. However, this does not heal the grief I feel for having lost my child. Not a day goes by that I don't wish I had made a different choice. I miss my child and want that little one by my side.

Five years after the termination I gradually came to the conclusion that I *had* to have another baby. I adored my husband and children and didn't want to end my childbearing years in such a negative way. We created a "survival plan" for HG, something no HG mom should be without. This plan consisted of care for our children, meal support for my family, a leave of absence from work, and most importantly, an urgent discussion with my doctor and psychologist prior to becoming pregnant. In the presence of my husband, I told my pregnancy team that, under no circumstances, did I want to repeat a decision to abort. I might kick, scream and plead, but somehow, some way, they needed to protect my baby and me from myself. I entered this pregnancy with fierce determination; this time was going to be different.

Through exercise and nutrition, I had gotten myself into the best shape of my life. I had done research about the

Canadian drug Diclectin (another name for Bendectin), and its 95% efficacy for HG impressed me. I had even gone so far as to travel to Toronto, Canada where I could be seen and obtain four months worth of medication. I was prepared for HG this time and began taking Diclectin the moment I found out I was pregnant, as instructed by Canadian Motherisk specialists. In spite of every preparation I descended into the hell of HG by seven weeks, and this was the worst pregnancy of them all. Over the course of four months, I was admitted to the hospital four times for a total of twenty-one days. The medication arsenal included all of the regulars: Compazine, Tigan, Phenergan, Zofran, etc. By the third hospitalization I had lost twenty-one pounds and could keep nothing down.

The latest HG news involved corticosteroids. I discussed it with my doctor and during my last hospitalization I began receiving Solu-Medrol via IV. I was taught how to inject myself twice a day into different muscle groups so I could continue treatment at home. Like most of the other drugs, I felt some initial relief, but the HG came back within a matter of days in full force. Unfortunately, steroids need to be tapered down, so the injections needed to continue for almost two weeks beyond the point they were deemed ineffective. As I injected myself each morning and night with a medication that wasn't working, I knew I had reached a low point in the course of HG. It just couldn't get any worse than this.

By eleven weeks I had gone even further downhill in terms of weight loss and dehydration, so my OB decided I should have a PICC for TPN. This involved another hospitalization and a minor surgical procedure where a catheter was inserted through my right upper arm and threaded up to the superior vena cava, stopping just above my heart. The procedure was neither painful nor frightening, but the idea of something being placed so near my heart was kind of disturbing to me. At that point however, I think I could have had anything done and not protested. I was a literal zombie.

After an overnight stay in the hospital, a home health care agency was dispatched to teach me how to mix up my bags of nutrition and insert them in the line. This was another low in my pregnancy; I was spending an hour or more each day mixing up my food and then getting the pump ready to dispense it. Between pump alarms going off, wrapping my arm with plastic wrap to shower and trying to navigate around the house with an IV pole and bag, it was a hellish experience. However, the PICC did afford me two major positives: relief at knowing my baby was finally getting some nutrition, and comfort at knowing I wouldn't have to go back to the hospital again (unless a major problem with the central line arose). No medication was administered through the PICC as nothing had been effective in the past. It was now just a matter of waiting until the HG subsided.

At around seventeen weeks the PICC line was removed in the hospital. My OB patted my arm and said, "You're through the worst. At this point, the chances of anything going wrong are miniscule." We heard the baby's heartbeat and it was loud and strong. I went home relieved and grateful that I had made it through and that the baby was doing well. I had felt the baby's flutters at about fourteen weeks, but had noted in a journal I was keeping that I hadn't noticed much afterwards. The baby's heartbeat had been a relief. Even after the appointment I felt a little fluttering but noted again in my journal that at about eighteen weeks I didn't feel anything. Also around eighteen weeks I started to feel better as expected. I even remarked to someone at work that I felt unbelievable as though I wasn't even pregnant.

At my twenty-week appointment I lay on the examining table as the doctor checked the baby's size manually and said, "It's feeling a little smaller than usual." He took out a Doppler to check the heartbeat. The moment dragged on ominously as the doctor moved the handset around my swollen belly. I looked over at my husband and said, "This isn't good," as the realization that our baby may not be alive set in. The doctor fumbled around and grew more frantic as he searched for the heartbeat. He then did an ultrasound. No heartbeat was present. I wanted to die. I didn't understand how this could happen after everything we had been through.

My doctor recommended a D&E and said there was only one doctor in our area that he trusted to do this procedure. The only problem was that this doctor didn't do the D&Es at the hospital but in his own "surgical facility." My husband made the appointment for the following day and we arrived there in the morning. The façade of the building was indeterminate but I found myself getting increasingly uncomfortable as we turned in the driveway. When I saw protestors and signs I realized where I was. My doctor had sent us to an abortion clinic.

I was overcome with sadness and grief already, and the realization that we were at an abortion clinic hit me like a brick wall. What was my doctor thinking? What in the hell was he *thinking*?! As my husband ushered me into the back

door a protestor called to me, "Have you done everything you
can to save your baby?" I just cried.

In the procedure room I immediately called my OB. "I
need to speak with him," I cried into the phone. She told me
he wasn't in. I told her I couldn't do the D&E, not there, and
I asked her why he didn't tell me where he was sending me.
"Obviously he thinks that is the best place for you," she said
before adding, "If I were you I would trust his judgment." I was
shocked. I begged my husband to do something, but he didn't
know what to do. As I struggled with everything, I heard a
child being aborted in the next room. I heard the doctor's low
voice, the whirring of the machine and the doctor's voice again.
I was completely dumbfounded. The experience was surreal.

The abortionist came into the room and I was shaking and
crying. I said to him, "I think I got sent to the wrong place."
He told me that my doctor refers all late-term cases to him
because he has more experience removing late term babies than
anyone in town. I cringed and told him I decided to deliver my
baby instead. He told me this would be safer and was what he
would advise his own family member to do instead of delivery.
I was confused and in shock. He told me what it entailed and
that it might be a two-day procedure. He would start by filling
my cervix with seaweed sticks (laminaria) to dilate it overnight.
The next day he would "evacuate" the baby. I got sick to my
stomach. Where was the "faster, easier" procedure my OB had
promised? I was appalled at the thought of having to come
back to this hellhole. I phoned my regular MD who reiterated
that my doctor was very competent and that if this is what he
recommended she agreed with it. At that point, I felt helpless
and hopeless and resigned myself to the "abortion" of my dead

child. The abortionist inserted the laminaria, and I wanted to die.

The next morning I returned to the abortion clinic with more protestors and an escort there. I barely heard the verbal assault but didn't have the energy to let them know my baby had already died in a faultless miscarriage. As I waited for the doctor I was forced to sign abortion consent papers. I complained to the nurse, "My baby is already dead, so why do I have to sign these papers as though I'm having a voluntary abortion?" She replied, "State law." I shook my head and signed the damnable papers.

It took about half an hour for the doctor to see me. We'd already agreed on anesthesia and the anesthesiologist was beginning his work. It occurred to me suddenly that I wanted my child's remains for burial. "Uh, y-yes," she stammered in shock. Later I found out that I was only the second person to ask for her child's remains in the history of the abortion clinic. When it was over I left immediately. The emptiness was overwhelming. Neither my OB nor any of his staff called to see how I was during the two weeks after the D&E. At my two-week follow up I confronted him about sending me to an abortion clinic without telling me. He sheepishly replied, "I knew you wouldn't have gone if I had told you." He had intentionally tricked me. I felt betrayed and disgusted. A week after my D&E we buried our baby at our local cemetery. It still comforts me today to know that our child's body wasn't put in the garbage like the other babies who died at the clinic that day. If anyone reading this is ever in the same situation, I would recommend that you deliver your baby in a hospital where you can find out the sex of your baby, hold your baby, and where there is dignity. There is none of that at an abortion clinic.

After the experience, I initially wanted to get a tubal ligation so that I never had to endure HG or child loss again. As the months went on however, I didn't want to end my childbearing with death. Even enduring HG seemed more bearable than that. I talked with my husband who agreed to go through everything again, but he said it must happen within six months or that was it. We couldn't keep lingering, living our lives in pain and uncertainty. We had other children to think of. I agreed, and in three months I was pregnant.

HG returned and I was on home health care with TPN by eight weeks. It was a miserable, nightmarish experience and once again, I wanted to abort my baby, have a miscarriage, or be exposed to the blast of a nuclear bomb-anything that would get me out of the torture. I had gotten a new OB who oversaw me with great care and who provided support, talking me through my roughest days, days when I shrieked, "I just can't do this!" over and over again. She and my husband watched me retch, lose weight, and vomit blood from my burning esophagus, and yet reminded me that it would all be worth it. They helped me make it through each day. At one point, my doctor hospitalized me for several days knowing that I needed more medical support than just home care and knowing that at that particular time I would have somehow found my way to an abortion clinic to end my intense suffering. Can you even imagine? Knowing the mental anguish I had been through because of abortion, I was ready to do it again to get out of the HG. It is that torturous.

At around seventeen weeks the HG resolved and I rejoined the living. My beautiful baby was born at full term and she is an absolute joy to our entire family. Thank God for the support that allowed me to have her. In fact, out of gratitude, I named my daughter after my new doctor!

I was not in my right mind when I aborted my third child. If I could, I would gladly go back to that pregnancy and suffer through it to change the outcome. At the time a friend had warned me: "You can suffer for a little while with HG or suffer for a lifetime with abortion. Which will you choose?" But every day seemed like an eternity, and it was impossible for me to see light at the end of the tunnel or understand that abortion would be worse. Now I know what she was talking about, and I make the same appeal to anyone considering abortion for HG. When I reached the crossroads in this last pregnancy, the choice was ultimately mine, and I chose to fight. I chose the rest of my life with my daughter, and I'm so glad I did!

SIX
Antiemetic Drugs

U sing antiemetics was a source of anxiety for me in my first pregnancy, and I'll admit I was a tiny bit anxious the first time I took corticosteroids in my fourth. Many women experience reservations when prescribed medications during pregnancy. Sometimes these reservations can actually do more harm than good. I wanted to learn more about womens' perspectives in this area, so I was very interested to read a study on the perceived risk of teratogenicity (ability to cause congenital anomalies) of drugs used for nausea and vomiting during pregnancy.[81]

In this study, women who were exposed to non-teratogenic drugs generally believed they had a one in four chance of having a child with major congenital anomalies. They were very wrong; that's the actual risk of taking thalidomide, a highly teratogenic antiemetic that caused major birth defects in thousands of children in the fifties and sixties! Women also believed the risk of congenital anomalies for the general pregnant population was around 4%, which is just about right. This shows that the women were educated and realistic regarding the normal pregnancy risks. However, their perception of risk related to nonteratogenic drug exposure was six times higher than the real risk (of 4%)! Misinformation and misperception accounted for these unrealistic fears. This study is important because it illustrates that women may be worrying too much about taking medications and therefore foregoing necessary treatment. Why were women in the study so afraid?

We are inundated with misinformation, and it comes from surprising places such as pregnancy books, the Physicians' Desk Reference and even pharmacists and physicians themselves. There are cases where physicians have advised termination due to drug exposure that is clearly safe.[82] Either those doctors were misinformed or termination was the easiest way to prevent a lawsuit.

Even after the women in the perceived risk study were assured that the drug exposure was nonteratogenic, they continued to cling to the misperception that their risk was still higher than the normal population. A significant number of women are terrified of taking medications such as Phenergan. In many instances, they stop taking medication as soon as they feel the least bit better, which can lead to a relapse. Women need information and reassurance from their physicians that the medications are safe.

Your physician may opt to prescribe antiemetics. Basically, the goal is for the antiemetic to inhibit the reflex activity of the vomiting center in the central nervous system. This can help prevent maternal malnutrition, which can affect the size of a baby. Some research suggests that smaller babies are at a greater risk of developing abnormal glucose tolerance, premature coronary heart disease and hypertension later in life.[83] When considering antiemetic use, calculate the risks vs. the benefits. The benefit of taking a relatively benign drug that might reduce some of the severe nausea and vomiting of HG normally outweighs the risk of taking no drug at all and continuing to vomit uncontrollably, which can cause malnutrition and dehydration.

I have talked to countless women who took one or multiple combinations of antiemetics for extended periods of time beginning at the time the baby was most vulnerable to teratogens (substances that cause congenital anomalies) until the baby was born. Only one had a child born with a problem that probably would have been present whether antiemetics were administered or not. The baby had Gastroesophogeal Reflux Disease, and most children grow out of the condition. I had been on over twelve different medications of varying potency by the end of my fourth pregnancy, and my daughter is perfect in every way. By ten weeks of age she was already saying "Mama."

Some HG sufferers do miscarry or deliver stillborn, but these rates are comparable to the normal pregnant population and have not been shown to be the result of any antiemetic on the market today.

Drug Forms
Some drugs are only available in pill and/or syrup form. If you can't keep anything down, do not give up; other medicines can be injected. If these create knots, bruises, sore spots, a burning sensation or blown veins, antiemetic suppositories can help, though they may have a tendency to burn or sting. Describe any discomfort to your doctor and ask her if she knows of any way to relieve the pain.

Types of Antiemetics

Antihistamines, phenothiazines, benzamides, serotonin receptor antagonists, and other classes of drugs have antiemetic properties, and a *few* commonly prescribed for HG are (or have been) Bendectin, Phenergan, Reglan, and Zofran. A newer drug therapy for HG involves the use of corticosteroids, and results have been very promising. Additional information on antiemetics is listed in Appendix A.

Antihistamines

Antihistamines block the effects of histamine, a chemical in the body that can manifest as allergic reaction when released. Simply put, antihistamines relieve the symptoms of allergies. If HG involves allergy, antihistamines can be an effective treatment.

All antihistamines have a sedative effect. This may help relieve nausea and vomiting by sedating the vomiting center of the brain and making it less sensitive to the nausea and vomiting messages it receives. Hyperemetic moms can safely use antihistamines in pregnancy.[84]

Bendectin

Bendectin is a combination of vitamin B6 and doxylamine succinate (antihistamine). In 1979 the National Enquirer published an untrue story of a "drug company cover up" of scads of deformed babies. Lawyers began advertising in women's magazines encouraging women who had deformed children to sue Merrell Dow if they had taken Bendectin at any point in their pregnancies. Thousands of women contacted the March of Dimes saying they'd been advised to abort their babies if they had taken Bendectin (and at least seven actually did abort).[85] In 1983 Merrell Dow withdrew Bendectin from the market because legal fees were costing more than the drug was even making.[86] There were two interesting results:

1. The rate of hospitalization for severe nausea and vomiting doubled in the U.S.

2. The legal wrangling involved so much pharmacological scrutiny that Bendectin remains the most studied of antiemetics for use in pregnancy. Subsequently, these studies showed that it was safe and effective.

While Canada still distributes the drug under the name of Diclectin, it is not yet available in America. However, at the writing of this book, the Canadian drug manufacturer is seeking FDA approval in preparation of selling it in the U.S. In the Briggs' reference guide on drugs for use in pregnancy, Diclectin received an "A", the highest safety rating there is. No other antiemetic has demonstrated the low risk record of Bendectin.

For now, Bendectin (10 mg of vitamin B6 and 10 mg of doxylamine succinate) can be approximately reproduced over the counter (OTC) although the OTC version will not be a time-release formula like Bendectin. *Do not reproduce or ingest Bendectin, without consulting your doctor.* In some cases a pharmacist will be happy to formulate a batch of generic Bendectin for you, and it never hurts to ask your doctor.

Bendectin Recipe[87]
Under a physician's advice only:

In the morning and afternoon one would take:

- *ONE-HALF of a 25 mg tablet of Unisom Sleep Tabs (12.5 mg),* NOT Maximum Strength Unisom Sleepgels *and*
- *ONE-HALF of a 25 mg tablet of vitamin B6 (12.5 mg)*

At bedtime, one would take one WHOLE tablet of each (25 mg of Unisom Sleep Tabs and 25 mg of B6) as needed.

How does Bendectin work?

Some theorize that HG may be related to a deficiency of vitamin B6,[88] and B6 may be added to Bendectin as a supplement. The doxylamine component (Unisom Sleep Tabs) is an antihistamine so it may act to sedate the vomiting center of the brain. Phenergan is another antihistamine, but it is also a phenothiazine.

Phenothiazines

Phenothiazines block dopamine, a neurotransmitter responsible for sending messages in the brain. By blocking this "messenger" from delivering vomit-inducing information to the chemoreceptor area, nausea and vomiting can sometimes be relieved.

Phenergan

Also an antihistamine, Phenergan is often used to treat allergies and to cause sedation. The majority of doctors use Phenergan to treat HG.[89] Studies of Phenergan in human pregnancy are lacking so the Food and Drug Administration has given it a rating of C for use in pregnancy. (See Appendix A for a full explanation of FDA drug ratings for use in pregnancy.) This means they won't say it is safe and they won't say it is harmful. Adequate, well-controlled human studies are needed to determine this.

Phenergan comes in syrup, pill, injectable and suppository forms. If you can keep the syrup/pills down then super! If your veins don't completely blow during the intravenous administration then great! If you need a Phenergan suppository just make sure you insert it correctly. If the insertion is too shallow, you may wonder if you accidentally grabbed a habanero pepper instead of a suppository. Ouch!

Some common side effects of Phenergan are dizziness, drowsiness, dry mouth, increased sensitivity to light and surprisingly, nausea and vomiting. Interestingly, a few antiemetics list nausea and vomiting as a side effect.

Substituted Benzamide
A substituted benzamide is like a phenothiazine because it possesses an antidopaminergic quality. In other words, it works to block dopamine. (More about this in Appendix A.)

Reglan
Pregnancy causes a natural slowing down of gastrointestinal function. The stomach and intestines move more slowly during digestion, the stomach holds in its contents for a longer period of time, and the esophageal sphincter (the one between your stomach and esophagus) relaxes. All of these things can contribute to nausea and vomiting. Reglan works to bring ev-

erything back up to speed. In addition to blocking dopamine, Reglan also stimulates the rate of force of contractions in the stomach and upper intestine. It is supposed to get *everything* out of the digestive system so there will be nothing left to trigger the vomiting reflex.

Reglan is a category B drug. Theoretically, it's as safe as taking minimal doses of vitamin B6. Reglan comes in liquid, pill and injectable form, and common side effects are nausea, diarrhea, dizziness, drowsiness, headache, depression, fluid retention (swelling of hands or legs or bloating) and increased urination.

I hated Reglan more than any other drug I tried, because it made my stomach cramp up and gave me horrible, foul-smelling diarrhea, which dehydrated me further. However, my medical care was insufficient, and I was not given an antihistamine concomitantly. An antihistamine like Benadryl should always be given with Reglan to reduce side effects.[90] If Reglan doesn't work for you there are other drug options.

Serotonin Receptor Antagonists

Some types of chemotherapy cause the body to release extra serotonin into the blood stream. This can also happen after surgery. If a person's body detects an overabundance of serotonin it will attempt to rid itself of the excess substance. This is why a patient can vomit if not given a serotonin receptor antagonist such as Zofran.

Zofran

In simple terms, Zofran blocks serotonin detection. This is the *very* basic concept: if your body doesn't know extra serotonin is there, it doesn't try to get rid of it. In other words, you don't vomit. Since Zofran stops the vomiting of one type of patient, it is logical to attempt to use it to stop the vomiting of other types of patients.

In one study, Zofran proved only to be as effective as Phenergan,[91] which might suggest that HG doesn't actually involve an increase in serotonin levels. Despite this, some (not all) women say Zofran helped them significantly. Interestingly, many said that the Zofran provided relief initially but that its efficacy waned after a few days. Some found relief when doses were increased.

In my experience Zofran took me from vomiting forty times a day to no more than eight times a day. I tried once to discontinue the Zofran and I literally vomited about every eight minutes from the moment I woke up in the morning until bedtime that night.

Zofran is rated category B for use in pregnancy and comes in injectable and oral forms including a nasty tasting pill that dissolves on the tongue. In my opinion, the best way of receiving Zofran is via a pump. Matria, a home health care group that specializes in treating cases of HG, managed my Zofran pump at home.

This method of Zofran delivery is better than the pill, because there are no real fluctuations of the drug level. When you take a pill it takes a while to start working and not all of it is absorbed. Eventually its effectiveness peaks and then begins to wane. With the pill you may notice that symptoms worsen an hour or so before your next dose is due, in which case you just have to suffer until you can pop the next pill. The Zofran pump maintains peak effectiveness levels 24-hours a day, administering a small amount of the drug at set intervals such as every three minutes.

The pump is the size of an eyeglass case, and the patient loads a syringe of Zofran into a chamber once every twenty or so hours depending upon the individual dose. The attached catheter is as small as a strand of angel hair pasta and is placed subcutaneously. The bad news is that inserting the catheter requires poking yourself in the thigh (or tummy) fat with a needle. The good news is that you'll probably be way too sick to care!

Typically, a small knot will form where the catheter is. This area is often red, warm and sore but fully heals within a couple of weeks, at which point it can be used again. To reduce the risk of infection, the site must be changed every other day. The inconvenience is much less troubling than vomiting forty times a day. Once you get over the creepiness of having to jab yourself every other day, you will probably agree that the pump is terrific! For those of you who can stand Reglan, you can also get that in a pump. (See "Line Types" in Chapter 7 for an alternative to jabbing yourself.)

Anxiety, drowsiness, dizziness and headache are all common side effects of Zofran. This drug is also extremely expensive, making it difficult, if not impossible, for some women to get. I know that my pills cost over three hundred dollars for a three-day supply, and my Zofran pump cost four hundred dollars a day. Yikes!

Corticosteroids

Steroids are naturally occurring substances that include sex hormones, bile acids and more. Corticosteroids, steroids that have an anti-inflammatory effect, are used to treat HG. No one knows exactly how corticosteroids work to counteract the symptoms of HG. Maybe there is a steroid hormone deficiency in a body that can't keep up with the increased adrenal demands of early pregnancy. Maybe corticosteroids have an anti-nausea effect on the chemoreceptor area of the brain stem.

In one study, corticosteroids were used to completely stop the vomiting in seventeen out of eighteen severely hyperemetic women.[92] For those who couldn't tolerate the medication orally, injectable corticosteroids were available. In another study, corticosteroids stopped the vomiting for 94% of women.[93] Like others in similar studies, these patients were eating *meals* within three days of treatment. That's a miracle for women with HG.

There are several autoimmune disorders requiring corticosteroid use in pregnancy. Corticosteroids are commonly prescribed in cases involving severe asthma or Addison's disease,[94] and no adverse fetal effects related to the therapy have been reported. Bear in mind that such conditions differ from HG and so administration varies, but long-term steroid use has not been shown to pose significant risk to the baby.[95] The women in one HG study were on low doses of prednisolone for up to thirteen weeks without any negative effects to the babies.[96]

I don't know why some doctors are reluctant to administer steroids, but they are. Perhaps it's because steroids are rather systemic and generally considered more potent than other antiemetics. Mothers who are suffering so terribly that they are on the verge of unwanted termination might discuss this with their doctor. Do the benefits of steroids outweigh the perceived risks? Physicians must consider how seriously the abortion of the anticipated child could affect the mother, not only physically but also emotionally.

A woman needs to be given *all* of her options. She cannot make the best decision for herself and her child if only *some* of the options are presented. A good doctor is willing to consult other professionals and takes the time to discuss all options with the patient. For instance, if one steroid doesn't work, the doctor should inform her patient that a different steroid might be prescribed.

Hydrocortisone crosses the placenta quickly, but most of it is converted to inactive cortisone by fetal enzymes.[97] This is a comfort to those who are anxious about the effects of medicine on their unborn child. Oral prednisolone is another option. The placenta largely metabolizes the prednisolone; the vast majority of the active drug never even reaches the baby.[98] Once the drug slowly weaves its way through the filtering placenta about 10% of the mother's blood level of active drug reaches the baby.[99] Methylprednisolone differs from prednisolone in that it exerts more of an anti-inflammatory effect and retains less sodium.

In the sixteenth week of my fourth pregnancy I myself was on prednisone, thirty milligrams a day, with tapering beginning on the ninth day. Within three days of my initial dose, I went from eating nothing to taking in one thousand, two hundred calories orally. On the sixth day of treatment I was eating filet mignon. Would I use steroids again? In a heartbeat.

Corticosteroid Concerns

Some physicians find it acceptable to only consider steroid use in severe cases of HG that have lasted for more than four weeks,[100] as steroids have a certain systemic potency. There has been some evidence that steroids cause cleft palate (a correctible condition) in gestating rabbits, and at least one study has shown a correlation between first trimester use and an increased risk of oral cleft in humans.[101] However, in other studies steroid use has not been found to cause congenital anomalies in the first,[102] second or third trimester.[103]

Many doctors don't like to use corticosteroids for longer than six weeks. This is because long-term use can cause maternal issues such as: [104]

- femoral head necrosis (a degeneration of the hipbone)
- increased risk of infection
- reduced glucose tolerance (i.e., an increased risk of gestational diabetes)

Although several reviews of steroid treatment have concluded that there is little to no teratogenic risk to the baby,[105] some will choose to forego steroids until twelve weeks of pregnancy when all the baby's organs are formed. Actually, this may be an excellent time to begin, as at least one comprehensive review found that 99% of HG cases resolved by twenty weeks.[106] This means one could get relief from steroids and then potentially coast into a resolution. How perfect! One woman who had severe HG almost aborted her daughter because no one told her about corticosteroids and she sorely needed that option. When she found out about this drug therapy (from another woman on the Internet) her doctor refused to prescribe it, opting instead to allow her to endure an unwanted termination. At the last minute, she found a doctor who would prescribe corticosteroids and immediately switched her care over to him.

Treatment was started at around fourteen weeks, corticosteroids provided incredible relief, tapering the drug caused a relapse, and the course of corticosteroids was restarted. The entire treatment lasted around a month. When she tapered for the second time, she was in the eighteenth week where she resolved enough to complete and, at times, even enjoy the remainder of the pregnancy. Her baby was born without any anomaly whatsoever, and her personal story appears in this book.

The drawback of getting this type of significant relief too prematurely is that a woman will probably have to discontinue usage at a certain point to avoid maternal side affects. If her HG is not on the verge of its own resolution then she could be thrust back into extreme nausea, vomiting and the inability to eat again. This can be *very* depressing. Conversely, any relief may be welcome no matter how short-lived.

Tapering can cause headaches and be unpleasant, but it is vital that a woman does taper as directed by her physician, because the use of corticosteroids can suppress the body's natural production of corticosteroids. When you taper off of the meds, the body incrementally revs production back up.

Stopping the medication abruptly can cause a corticosteroid deficiency that can adversely affect blood sugar levels, mineral and water content and the immune system. Make sure you taper off as directed or there could be some real problems.

Corticosteroids can cause insomnia, dizziness, stomach upset, increased blood glucose levels for those on TPN, problems with diabetes control, etc. Unlike drugs such as Phenergan and Reglan, corticosteroids are not necessarily known for causing extrapyramidal effects.

Extrapyramidal Effects
These side effects can be pretty distressing and make you want to stop taking a drug that might otherwise be beneficial, so it is imperative that the effects be reduced. Extrapyramidal effects consist of any of the following:

Akathisia - a feeling of restlessness that compels a person to move their legs or feel like they need to pace or walk around in spite of having no real destination. Commonly misdiagnosed as anxiety or some other behavioral disturbance, akathisia is actually a side effect of a drug and not a mental problem.

Dystonia - a slow, sustained, uncomfortable and sometimes painful muscle spasm that can cause a part of your body to move involuntarily.

Parkinsonism - an extrapyramidal effect that can cause muscle stiffness and can make parts of the body tremor or shake.

Tardive Dyskinesia (TD) - involves involuntary muscle movements that are usually seen in the face or around the mouth. Sometimes TD affects the arms, legs and body.

Psychotropic Effects

Another type of drug-induced side effect is the psychotropic symptom. Antiemetics can make you feel depressed, anxious, euphoric, frustrated, etc.

Varying amounts of an antihistamine such as Benadryl can be given along with other drugs to decrease or eliminate extrapyramidal and psychotropic effects. If drug reactions persist after such administration increasing the dosage of the antihistamine may help to eliminate them.

If you are on medication, and experiencing peculiar reactions, don't let your doctors immediately attribute these to unresolved emotional issues. Ask for a written review of any extrapyramidal or psychotropic effects the drug may commonly cause. Not only might this help you get the care you need, but it may also help the next mother treated by the same physician. Information is your right. You will have to decide which drugs are ultimately working and which side effects you are willing to accept.

Heartburn

HG, having so much to do with repeated esophageal exposure to stomach acid, can precipitate some pretty hefty bouts of heartburn. The discomfort of this can cause vomiting, so it makes sense to reduce the symptoms. Agents like Pepcid AC may help and can even be added directly to TPN feedings for patients. However, acid blockers such as Protonix may be more effective. Protonix comes in pill and IV forms but can't be mixed directly into TPN. If you are having trouble with heartburn, ask your doctor about treatments.

Awesome Algorithm

Dr. Koren, author of many a professional paper on HG, and Director of Canada's Motherisk program, has come up with a wonderful treatment algorithm that gives us an idea of what drugs might be prescribed for the treatment of HG and when they might be prescribed in the course of the illness. You may have more pharmaceutical options than you know of, and the algorithm serves as an important visual reminder of this.

Treatment algorithm for nausea and vomiting of pregnancy: *If no improvement, proceed to next step.*

STEP 1: Give 10 mg of doxylamine combined with 10 mg of pyridoxine (Diclectin,* delayed release) up to four tablets a day (ie, two at bedtime, one in the morning, and one in the afternoon). Adjust schedule and dose according to severity of symptoms.

STEP 2: Add dimenhydrinate (eg, Gravol) 50 to 100 mg q4-6h by mouth (po) or suppository (pr) (up to 200 mg/d when taking four Diclectin tablets/d) or promethazine (Phenergan), 5 to 10 mg q6-8h po or pr.

(If no dehydration see step 3a. If dehydration see step 3b.)

STEP 3a: If not dehydrated, add any of the following (in order of proof of fetal safety):
- chlorpromazine (eg, Largactil), 10 to 25 mg q4-6h po or intramuscular injection (im), or 50 to 100 mg q6-8 pr ↻
- prochlorperazine (eg, Stemetil), 5 to 10 mg q6-8h im or po or pr ↻
- promethazine (Phenergan), 12.5 to 25 mg q4-6h im or po ↻
- metoclopramide (eg, Reglan), 5 to 10 mg q8h im or po
- ondansetron (Zofran), 8 mg q12h po

(If step 3a is ineffective proceed to step 3b.)

STEP 3b: If dehydrated, start rehydration treatment:
- intravenous (IV) fluid replacement ✓ (per local protocol)
- multivitamin IV supplementation
- dimenhydrinate, 50 mg (in 50 mL of saline, over 20 min) q4-6h IV

STEP 4: Add any of the following (in order of proof of fetal safety):
- chlorpromazine (eg, Largactil), 25 to 50 mg q4-6h IV ☚
- prochlorperazine (eg, Stemetil), 5 to 10 mg q6-8h IV ☚
- promethazine (Phenergan), 12.5 to 25 mg q4-6h IV ☚
- metoclopramide (eg, Reglan), 5 to 10 mg q8h IV

STEP 5: Add methylprednisolone ◄ (Solu-Medrol), 15 to 20 mg q8h IV or ondansetron (Zofran), 8 mg over 15 min q12h IV or 1mg/h continuously up to 24 hours.

Note:
Use of this algorithm assumes that other causes of nausea and vomiting of pregnancy have been ruled out. At any step, when indicated, consider total parenteral nutrition.

At any time you may add any or all of the following:
- pyridoxine, 25 mg, every 8 hours (q8h) po
- ginger, ♦ 250 mg q6h po
- acupressure or acupuncture at P6

---

* Only product of its kind available in Canada. New evidence indicates safety of doses up to 8 tablets a day.
☚ Phenothiazines listed in alphabetical order.
✓ No study has compared various fluid replacements for nausea and vomiting during pregnancy.
◄ Steroids not recommended during first 10 weeks of pregnancy because of possible increased risk of oral clefts.
♦ Safety of dose >1000 mg/d not yet determined for pregnancy

Thanks to Dr. Koren, Director of the Motherisk program, for permission to reprint this algorithm.

Patty's Story

I'm forty-four, married and currently suffering from HG. I've had Stage IV endometriosis since I was fourteen. The endometriosis caused me to become infertile, and I began IVF (invitro fertilization) attempts about nine years ago. I have a heart condition that I had elective surgery for because I wanted pregnancy to be as safe as I could make it. I really want a child. I have been pregnant three times. Every time I've had terrible nausea. My second pregnancy was a twin pregnancy, and the nausea was pretty bad but not quite as bad as my current pregnancy. Unfortunately, my first two pregnancies ended in miscarriage.

After the loss of my twins my husband and I were devastated. We waited another two and a half years to use our remaining ten frozen embryos. I asked the doctor to thaw all ten because I did not want to be tempted into doing another cycle if this one failed. I had been on this IVF roller coaster long enough. As it turned out, the majority of our ten embryos did not continue to divide after the thaw, but two of them did, so we had them transferred. Both of them stuck! I suspected that my hCG levels were very high because a day before I was scheduled for a pregnancy blood test I tested positive using a home pregnancy test. This was very early for such a distinct line to appear on the home pregnancy test.

About three weeks post-transfer, I began experiencing severe nausea. Absolutely everything made me sick. I could not work on the computer or read because I became dizzy. I couldn't watch my beloved cooking shows because I would vomit at the mere sight of food. Even food commercials made me vomit. I couldn't open my window because the outside scent of the Night Jasmine made me vomit. Dry, electric heat (oven, toaster, electric stovetop burners) sent me running to the bathroom. I banned my husband from making toast with his cereal in the morning. He thought he'd try and pull a fast one on me by making it very early in the morning while I was still sleeping, but the nose knows. I was deathly ill for two days because I simply could not get the smell of toast out of my system. I can't even turn on the burner to heat water because I become so sick. Everything has this sickening sweet-trashy smell to it. I used to love taking a shower, but now I have to psych myself up for hours just to be able to get in, because I can smell the pipes and every metallic, earthy thing in them. The steam and moisture make me gag.

One day I vomited every half hour from five in the morning until eleven at night. As a result of the vomiting, I developed this terrible burning pain just below my breastbone, but above my bellybutton. It was so bad that I could not even sip water without doubling over in severe pain. Aside from the nausea, the pain in my stomach alone made me vomit. At first I thought this pain was just the normal indigestion that pregnant women experience. I finally couldn't stand it anymore and had my husband take me to the emergency room. A very sympathetic nurse admitted me (she herself had been hospitalized with HG for three weeks during her third pregnancy). I was hooked up to an IV and given Phenergan through the line. I was told that I could have a tear in my esophagus from the severe vomiting and was given Carafate to drink. (Carafate coats the esophagus and stomach providing a "seal" over the irritated areas.) As it turned out, I had developed a very bad stomach ulcer. After about four hours I was sent home with a prescription for Phenergan pills and Carafate.

The nausea and pain continued. My fertility doctor referred me to a gastroenterologist for the stomach pain and to a perinatologist for the remainder of the pregnancy. The gastroenterologist prescribed Pepcid. The perinatologist prescribed 8 mg of Zofran three times a day. (The Phenergan knocked me out. By the time I would awaken, the effects of the medication had worn off and I was nauseous again.) I have to tell you, I was very leery about taking anything. I am a legal secretary and worked for a law firm in Los Angeles that tried thalidomide cases. I saw children come into the office who had full mental capacity but no limbs. In any event, I was so desperate that I really felt I had no choice but to try the medications or terminate the pregnancy.

I am feeling better by about 50% (which is still no picnic, believe me). I still have great difficulty getting fluids down and have absolutely no appetite, which is a far cry from my non-pregnant state. I always tell my husband that I refuse to throw up my twenty-seven-dollar-a-pill Zofran. (Luckily, insurance pays for most of it.) I am living on Sprite, watermelon, Ensure, yogurt, and water with honey in it. I still can't move around too much because stimulation makes me more nauseous. My husband keeps telling me to get out of the house and go for a walk. I would love to, but I just can't right now.

I have recently found out that one of my twins didn't make it. No heartbeat. The other has a nice, strong heartbeat. At my first ultrasound, we were told that one of the twins had no heartbeat, but that it just might be too early to see one and to return in a week. During my second ultrasound I was praying that there would be no heartbeat for that twin so that my hCG levels might drop and I could start to feel better. My husband and I have spent thousands and thousands of dollars over many years trying to have children. I must tell you though that I seriously considered terminating this pregnancy. I knew for a fact that I could not go on one more day without some kind of intervention. When I expressed my feeling to my best friend (who had mild nausea in her pregnancy) she laughed and said, "Do you think you're the only woman who has ever been nauseous from pregnancy?" When I explained HG to her she became very sympathetic, however, and said she had never heard of such a thing. I am very grateful for her sensitivity.

I am still very early in my pregnancy (six weeks). With my history of miscarriage, I am taking this one day at a time. I am very thankful for the information I am finding on the Internet. Talking with other women who have gone through HG and losses has been so helpful. I appreciate the fact that they do not try to offer explanations for my losses or tell me that "everything will be OK" with this pregnancy. As helpful as people intend to be, those types of statements often make me feel angry and resentful.

Had I not already used up all of my frozen embryos and decided not to do another IVF cycle, this experience with HG would have convinced me never to try pregnancy again. I will forever be sympathetic towards women who suffer from this dreaded condition.

SEVEN
IV Hydration

Thank God for IVs! Many of us wouldn't be here without them. If you have ever been dehydrated to the point where you needed to receive an IV, then you know how amazing and effective they are.

Dehydration

Most people think that a human can survive for around two weeks without eating. We know this isn't the case, because ten Irish protesters went on a fatal hunger strike in 1981. On the average, it took around sixty-two days to perish.[107] They lasted as long as they did because they were still drinking water. In contrast, as the nation learned from Terri Schiavo's ordeal, a bedridden person can only survive for a little over ten days without fluids. (An active person would probably expend more fluid and therefore not last as long.)

Vomiting brings about a loss of precious fluid. If this fluid cannot be replaced, due to the inability to take it in or keep it down, one becomes dehydrated. Without enough fluid, a person's body doesn't function properly, the thought processes are affected, and one feels pasty and dry like jerky served on melba toast. The skin becomes drawn and scaly, the eyes sunken, the urine dark and scant, the mouth dry, lips may chap, crack and bleed, and other problems can arise.

Hypotension

The lack of fluid lowers blood pressure (hypotension) because it eventually takes the plasma (fluid part) out of the blood. Less blood equals less pressure. The symptoms of low blood pressure include dizziness, light-headedness, headaches and blurred vision.

Fever

Human beings sweat constantly to regulate body temperature. When you become significantly dehydrated, sweating decreases and may stop altogether, thereby raising body temperature. Dehydration may also affect the centers in the brain that regulate body temperature, and this can contribute to an overall elevation of temperature.

Kidney Exertion

Prolonged dehydration reduces and thickens the blood. The body then tries to reserve precious fluid for the most important body functions. Urinary output becomes scant and dense with the waste that accumulates in the body. This taxes the kidneys which have to work extra hard to filter out all the waste.

Benefits of Fluid Regulation

Fluid is vital to your health and overall level of comfort. Vomiting causes a loss of fluid, which causes dehydration, which causes nausea and vomiting, which causes a loss of fluid. This nasty cycle can be corrected with intravenous hydration.

The better you control the dehydration, the more chance you have of avoiding exacerbated suffering. Proper hydration also maximizes blood flow to the placenta, which increases the baby's nourishment and prevents the baby from becoming dehydrated also. In addition, fluid maintenance can help to alleviate electrolyte imbalance.

IVs

Dehydration increases the severity of nausea and vomiting. In IV hydration, the patient is given fluids intravenously to replace fluids lost through repeated vomiting and inability to consume liquids. Many times the replacement hydration contains electrolytes (i.e., sodium, potassium, chloride) and/or sugars, and may be all that is needed to stop a particular vomiting jag. If the HG hasn't reached the point of resolution, the vomiting will eventually return, causing more dehydration and the need for more rehydration. IVs can be given on an outpatient basis over the course of a couple of hours, an in-patient basis over a period of days or an in-home setting over the course of several months if need be.

Out-Patient IVs

I like to call the outpatient IV the "impatient" IV because it seems some doctors can't get you and your pesky HG out of their office soon enough. You are in and out within two to three hours of lightning fast fluid replacement. Often the vomiting begins again within a period of hours after the IV. The authors of one study conclude:

> "Intractable [HG] cases are best treated with hospitalization and parenteral medication."[108]

It is my general opinion that HG patients who are sick enough to need IVs are sick enough to warrant *at least* 48-hours of the physical respite that continuous fluids can offer.

In-patient IVs

Some physicians recommend that women with dehydration, weight loss, ketones in the urine, or high urine specific gravity (concentrated, waste-laden urine) be managed as in-patients.[109] Hospitalizations shouldn't be too short, because relapses are frequent. Lengthy terms of intense suffering need to be broken up by periods of some type of relief. If a hyperemetic is not hospitalized when necessary, her treatment is inadequate. While some doctors and managed health care groups may work together to refuse expensive in-patient treatment, there is a suitable alternative: home IVs.

Home IVs

It would be great if all HG patients could get continuous fluids until they were able to, on a regular basis, drink the recommended six to eight cups of fluid per day without vomiting them up. Some may deem this "too expensive," but continuous fluid replacement is often the best option for patients with intractable HG, because it corrects and prevents dehydration for an extended period and gives patients a break from exacerbated symptoms caused by ongoing fluid loss. Also, from a financial standpoint, if HG is treated earlier and better, this could potentially prevent the disease from progressing to a point requiring more aggressive and expensive treatments.

One cost-effective solution for those needing frequent or longer IV support is home health care, and many moms prefer to receive treatment in the home setting. Home IVs require a nurse to come to the home periodically to change IV sites or otherwise manage lines. Nurse visits usually do not last long and therefore pose a minimum of inconvenience and intrusion.

In my fourth pregnancy I had home IVs, and they made all the difference. I could not drink anything. The more I tried, the more I vomited, and the worse I felt. IVs allowed me to bypass the dysfunction and futility of that battle and simply focus on getting through each day. Fluid management was monitored by my home health care agency and predominantly maintained by my husband and me. In truth, it was quite a shock to suddenly be thrust into the medical field where we were handling tubings, valves, bags, syringes, IV medicines, etc. However, HG is what it is, we did what we had to do to get through it, and ultimately, we managed our homecare responsibilities successfully.

Home IVs kept me from completely succumbing to my very severe HG, and I was glad to get them. A few times, some in the medical field threatened to discontinue my IVs to "see how I would do." I knew I wasn't physically ready, and I let them know unquestionably that I was not going to be a guinea pig. I protected my life with my fluids and my fluids with my life!

Line Types

One unfortunate problem with peripheral or regular IVs is that the site needs to be changed every four or so days to avoid infection. Some say seven days between site changes is fine, but let's stick with four to be safe. Another problem is that the veins tend to rupture pretty easily with this kind of line. There were nights when it took my home health care nurses seven sticks to find a vein only to have the vein blow the very next day. In less than two weeks I had no sites left but still needed fluids. Luckily there are line options that can help alleviate this.

Aside from the short line option of the peripheral IV, there is a longer line called a midline. This type of IV catheter can last up to fourteen days before needing to be changed. Still, for those requiring fairly long-term fluid management, a better bet may be a Peripherally Inserted Central Catheter (PICC). This is what I opted for, because it can last for a year or longer without ever needing to be changed. Also, I knew I was headed for TPN and would eventually need a PICC anyway.

The line is generally quite long. Make sure your tech uses Lidocane or something to numb the insertion area. The line goes in at the elbow bend or upper arm, is fed up the interior of the arm, around the shoulder and into the chest approximately two inches from the opening of the heart. The technicians will then X-ray the chest to check for proper placement before introducing fluids/nutrition. It sounds awfully scary and horrible, but it's really no big deal. Just turn your head and "find a happy place." You're going to make it through this.

I had three PICC lines in ten days! This is very atypical, but I was allergic to the silicone in the first two Groshong catheters. I got horrible phlebitis (see: PICC Problems) at the sites, and they had to pull the first and second PICCs. My third PICC line was silicone-free and lasted for over a month until I got a staph infection in the line and had to have it pulled. Several bags of antibiotics later, the fourth PICC line held until my HG resolved and I didn't need fluid/nutrition support anymore!

If I ever need a PICC line for fluid or TPN management again, I will ask:

- my IV therapist for at least a four french sized line (so blood can be drawn from it)
- that the line be inserted above the elbow bend (so I can bend my arm without an occlusion alarm going off)
- that a line with a double lumen be placed

A double lumen is a fancy way of referring to a line with dual ports. One port is for TPN/fluid and the second port can be used for other medications or blood draws. Having an extra lumen can prevent you from having a PICC in one arm and a peripheral IV (for medication) in the other arm, and it can save you multiple needle sticks for myriad blood draws. If you are on something like a Zofran pump, you can hook the pump up to your lumen instead of stabbing yourself in the leg with it every other day. Joy!

All my lines were single lumens except for my last line, and I was so sorry I hadn't had a double lumen right from the start! Although you can do a blood draw and even administer IV medicines through a single lumen, you normally have to disconnect from one tube to go to another tube or syringe. The goal is to disconnect a PICC line as infrequently as possible, thereby reducing the chances that any type of infection will be introduced into the line and body. Also, if you are receiving TPN, it is best if this administration remains constant.

With a regular IV, fluids can be delivered sufficiently via a gravity drip, but it is best to use a pump with a PICC line, as a gravity drip or dial-regulated flow may slow down in such a case causing dehydration or other problems.

Living with Pumps

PICC lines can be placed when a physician anticipates the necessity for fluid administration over an extended period of time. This means the person with a PICC will be living with a pump for a while. People who have not lived with a pump may underestimate the psychological impact of simply hearing the constant droning of a mechanical pulse for months.

When I got my first pump, I did fine for a week or so. After a while, however, the unending moan of the pump became disturbing. I developed a new appreciation for Poe's Tell-Tale Heart. Lying there feeling horrible for eons was depressing enough, and the pump only reminded me that my life had been altered in a significantly negative way. I was no longer normal but attached to a machine that became a part of me, and I was not allowed to forget. A month passed and the confounded pump would not shut up! I wept bitterly over the mental torture of the ever-present cadence when suddenly I realized that this was not the sound of torment but actually the music of life! Without such a device, death is certain for those of us who need life-sustaining fluid/nutrition. The pump became a bearable component of my altered life, although I had to remind myself daily that it was a life-preserving gift!

I've talked to other women with pump experience and was surprised to discover many with similar perspectives. One individual would pile clothes and blankets on top of her portable pump, hoping to stifle the emanating sounds. The never-ending hum became the bane of her daily existence. She was not able to reframe the situation and find the silver lining, and this added to her suffering.

Your pump is your friend. Remember that, and you'll be better for it.

PICC Maintenance

For the most part, in the home setting, you will maintain your PICC. You will keep it kink-free and clean between tubing changes but, once a week, your home health care nurse will come out and change your PICC dressing. *This is a sterile procedure!* I learned the hard way after an inept home health care nurse removed my dressing and *touched all around my unprotected site with her bare hand!* This is a huge no-no!

When your nurse changes your PICC dressing:
She should:
- Wash her hands
- Wear a mask
- Wear clean gloves just to remove the dressing
- Wear *sterile* gloves once the dressing is off
- *Remain sterile* until the new dressing is in place

You should:
- Wear a mask

If you trust your home health care nurse, it would not be a bad idea if you kept your head turned away from the site during the dressing change. However, as long as your mask is on, it is safe to keep your head toward the site so you can monitor your home health care nurse during the procedure.

If there is anything about your home health care nurse that makes you uneasy or distrustful, you may want to request that she not come out to your house anymore. I have had to do this. I have refused to let certain home health care nurses carry out PICC line procedures that they drove thirty minutes to undertake, because it was obvious that they didn't know what they were doing. I have even changed home health care companies (more than once) because I was repeatedly dissatisfied and had the option. I didn't like doing it, but I did what I had to do, and I'm not sorry.

Your best chance at a more comfortable pregnancy is to speak up for yourself and your baby. Invariably, you will probably make some people mad. Who cares. It's not about them, it's about you and your baby and your health. That takes precedence over peoples' feelings, and if they are not doing their job correctly, *they need to go!*

PICC Problems

In addition to the line complications listed in the section on TPN, PICC lines can cause allergic reactions, grow fibrin flaps or even push on heart valves. When a patient is allergic to the tubing material, this can cause a painful swelling known as phlebitis. If the phlebitis is severe enough, the line will need to be removed. PICC lines can also grow fibrin over the end. This really has no bearing on fluid/nutrition delivery as the fibrin flap can act like a valve that allows fluid to pass into the body but nothing to pass out. If a fibrin flap grows over the end of your catheter, you will probably not be able to do blood draws from your PICC. If inserted a little too deeply PICC lines can press on the heart valve causing heart palpitations. In this case, the catheter is just slightly extracted. I could be wrong, but I suspect that even if the line looks great on X-ray, it can sneakily crawl towards the heart depending on your position. For example, I sleep all curled up on my left side where my last PICC was placed. If I slept on my right side I had no problems, but every time I slept on my left side, I would get heart palpitations. My doctor ordered an X-ray to check placement, which was fine. However, X-ray was done with me sitting up straight, tall and perfectly still. Who knows? Maybe the rate of flow just didn't mesh with my system. My doctor couldn't explain the palpitations, but after they pulled the line I never got them again.

A Minimum of Suffering

If you are in need of constant fluid replacement, ask your physician about line options. Whatever procedure a patient and physician agree upon, hydration is extremely important. Fluid maintenance is crucial not only for survival but also for minimizing the level of discomfort. Every positive effort should be made to ensure that the mother and growing child are protected from unnecessary suffering.

Wren's Story

My husband and I started trying to conceive in 1997. A couple months later we found out we were pregnant. I was so happy, because I really wanted to have a baby. I was four weeks along and started to feel a little sick to my stomach when I would eat. A week later, I miscarried. We tried again as soon as possible. After eight long months of disappointment we finally conceived. I was so happy to be pregnant, but I admit I was somewhat afraid of miscarrying again.

At five weeks I was feeling a little nauseous whenever I would eat. At six weeks we got an ultrasound and were able to see a tiny dot and a little beating heart. It was so neat, and I was so happy to know that I was pregnant again. The very next day the morning sickness hit. My husband was out golfing, and I was at the grocery store when I started to feel nauseous. When I got home I quickly put away the groceries and made myself some lunch, thinking I would feel better if I just got some food in me. I tried to gag a turkey sandwich down but couldn't finish it. I just felt more horrible as the day went on. I tried to eat some leftover chicken for dinner but couldn't stomach more than a few bites before throwing it in the trash. My husband called and I told him how horrible and nauseous I was feeling and that I had not been able to eat or drink much.

The next day things were worse, and I ate and drank even less. My husband called the doctor's after-hours service, and a doctor called back prescribing vitamin B6 and Sea-Bands. Neither of these things worked. The next morning I called my doctor and said I was having trouble eating and drinking though I had not vomited at all. He prescribed Phenergan. It didn't help. Two days later I finally threw up for the first time. I called my doctor the next day and told him I was really feeling terrible and that the Phenergan wasn't helping. He told me to come in, and the urine sample they took had ketones in it. They told me I was dehydrated and that ketones can harm the baby, so I started to worry. I had also lost four pounds in six days. My doctor called labor and delivery and told them I was being admitted to the hospital for IV therapy for the treatment of hyperemesis gravidarum. This was the first time we had ever heard of the disease.

They gave me IV Phenergan in the hospital. It seemed to help a little but it made me really drowsy, and it wore off quickly, so they gave it to me about every three hours. I was also given ice pops and ice chips to eat. After being told I would spend the night, a nurse came in and said I could go home. We went through the task of packing everything up and ambling very slowly to the elevator when another nurse came running up to tell me I could stay the night. I went back to my room exhausted. In the morning they unhooked me from the IV and said I could go home.

At home, my husband tried to get me to eat, but all I could get down were gelatin and ice pops, and as the day wore on I started to feel very nauseous again. I had only vomited the one time, but the nausea was preventing me from getting adequate nutrition and fluid, so I called the doctor and told him how I was feeling. He prescribed IV therapy via home health care. The nurse and pharmacist got there in the evening and hooked me up to a 24-hour IV drip with something called

Zofran in it. The next day a nurse would come, change the bag, and check the IV site.

My doctor hadn't said anything about the Zofran, so I was a little anxious about what it might do to the baby. At that point, however, I was so sick that I was willing to try anything. My husband looked the drug up on the Internet and read many positive stories posted by Zofran advocates who had suffered from HG, taken Zofran, and had healthy children. This eased my fears.

At home I began to worry about using up all of my sick leave and vacation time. My doctor said I could go to work, so I went to work attached to my pole. Everyone was completely amazed that I had come to work hooked up to an IV. I pushed my pole around and everyone got the message of how sick I was. I stayed a full day, but my IV infiltrated, and after that my husband and I just decided it just wasn't worth going to work as sick as I was. When my sick and vacation time ran out, I went on short-term disability.

My husband learned to change the bags on the IV, and the home health care nurse would check on me and change my IV site every three days. The Zofran seemed to help, but I still couldn't eat much. Some of the foods I could eat were gelatin, scrambled eggs, frozen waffles with syrup and baked potatoes, but nothing tasted good. I couldn't drink anything except Gatorade, and it was difficult to get that down. My doctor decided he wanted me to try to go off the IV and take oral Zofran, so we did that, but I wasn't getting enough fluids and became terribly constipated. The doctor said to try an enema, but enemas don't work on impacted stools! When I told the doctor, he said to try Dulcolax. After several hours, it worked, but going to the bathroom was a very painful experience. I was told to continue oral Phenergan but to stop oral Zofran while I waited for the nurse to come back out and hook me up to an IV with Zofran again. Evidently, IV Zofran doesn't make you as constipated. I vomited twice before the nurse arrived. When she hooked me up she told me to take a stool softener every night before bed. I guess that helped a little, but really, when you're not eating and drinking much, you're not going to be able to go to the bathroom that easily.

In three weeks I gained back one of four lost pounds, and my doctor was satisfied that I was no longer losing weight. He continued the home IV and Zofran therapy. We consulted a hospital dietician who gave me ideas to try, but I couldn't do most of it, because I was still too nauseous and nothing tasted good. After about three weeks on Zofran, I began to notice that it wasn't as effective as it had been initially. My husband told me to call the doctor, and they scheduled an appointment. Needless to say, when I walked into the office my doctor took one look at me and told me that it was time to try something different. He admitted me in-patient and gave me IV Zofran and Reglan. This seemed to help a little, but it still didn't feel like enough.

My doctor consulted a perinatologist, and he recommended a Droperidol protocol. This consisted of IV Droperidol and Benadryl given several times over a period of forty-eight hours. I really didn't like it, because it made me feel drowsy and "out of it" and didn't help. The nurses didn't seem to have clear communication with the doctor, and they were giving me smoothies and ice pops for the first twenty-four hours of the therapy when the protocol called for fasting for the first twenty-four hours and then only clear liquids for the next twenty-four hours. Because the protocol had not been followed accurately, I was given the option to start over and try it again. I didn't like the way it made me feel, so I opted not to do it and just went back to the IV with Zofran. I was also on Reglan.

When I began to run out of IV sites, my doctor had a gastroenterologist (GE) see me because there was a possibility I was going to need a PICC line. The GE told me I could get a PICC or a nasogastric tube. My preference was for the PICC, but the GE told me he really wanted to try the nasogastric tube first, because the PICC carried more risk for infection which could be harmful to my baby and me. I consented to the nasogastric feeding tube.

They put the tube in, and I just couldn't stand it. I tried but it was *awful*. I couldn't stand the gagging feeling of the tube, and I could taste the liquid food that was being put through it. Horrible. I told my husband I wanted it OUT. He got the nurse, she called the GE, and the GE told me I was keeping it in until the next day and hung up on me. I was furious that he had the nerve to hang up on me and did not respect my choice to remove a tube that was making me feel sicker. My husband believed what the doctor had said about the tube being the best thing for the baby and me and tried to convince me that it would be OK to keep a hose in my face. However, they had turned the feeding solution off because they wanted to do an ultrasound on my stomach and gallbladder the next morning. So here I was with this horrible thing in my nose and throat, and it wasn't even feeding me! I tried to sleep, but I was so upset. As a patient, I thought I had rights to refuse certain treatments. I was so angry. At one point I looked over at my healthy husband who didn't know the misery of HG *or* a nasogastric tube and who was able to eat just fine. He was sleeping lightly on the cot next to my bed, and I just got really angry and blurted out that I hated him. I didn't mean it, but I really had to have that tube out, and it was making me very upset. My husband called the nurse and she refused to call the GE at two AM. She told me if I wanted the tube out I'd have to take it out myself. That really burned me up!

The next morning, after all tests had come back fine, I had had it. I told the nurse to call the doctor to come and take the tube out and that I didn't want to argue about it. The GE came and tried to convince me to leave it in, but I absolutely refused. He asked me what alternative I wanted to try. I wanted the PICC, but he still didn't want to do it, so my only real option was to try and eat. When I promised that I would force myself to eat, he took the NG tube out. They brought me a ground beef patty and noodles with gravy. I tried to eat all of it like a "good little girl," but of course it all came back up half an hour later. I felt horrible, but I was determined to keep trying.

The dietician came to see me, and we worked out a plan of snacks that I could eat so I could get enough calories to be able to go home. Three times a day I drank Resource or a protein shake and ate peanut butter crackers or cookies in between meals. It was very difficult, but I was finally able to get in about two thousand calories per day and was switched to the oral Zofran again. Five days after the ordeal with the nasogastric tube, I was sent home at around twelve weeks pregnant. For several weeks I continued working on the dietary plan we had made in the hospital. Mainly I lived on Resource, ice chips and ice pops.

A month later I went back to work part-time. I would often feel light-headed and almost fainted a few times in the car while driving to work. That really scared me, and I decided to quit my job at a legal firm rather than continue to risk the lives of my baby, myself and others.

I was able to eat and drink more the farther along I got, although nothing ever tasted good. I had problems with cooking smells, and my husband had to do all the food preparation. The nausea never went away, but by the last month or two it became quite mild. I found that if I kept something in my stomach I would feel better, but this was not possible in the first few months.

I continued taking Zofran until the end of pregnancy despite my doctor's attempts to get me off of it. He knew I was feeling bad and finally abandoned the idea. He told me that if all looked well he would induce at thirty-eight weeks to spare me two more weeks of nausea. I agreed, and my perfect, healthy little boy was born weighing eight pounds and four ounces. I still felt nauseous the day after I delivered, but after one more dose of Zofran I never felt sick again!

Throughout my pregnancy my husband was absolutely supportive and wonderful! He took the best care of me. He cooked, cleaned, did laundry, even gave me baths while I was at home hooked up to the IV. So many times I wished I would miscarry just so I wouldn't feel so sick anymore. He told me to hang in there, that it would eventually go away. When I told him that I was thinking of terminating the pregnancy, he had me focus on how I would feel a month later when the abortion had been done and our baby was gone forever.

My obstetrician was great! He was very compassionate and understanding. He really wanted to do what he could to help me feel better. He supported me, encouraged me, and offered me positive options.

My family, friends and co-workers were caring but had never known anyone with HG. I guess they couldn't believe that someone could be so sick while pregnant. My mom was never sick when she was pregnant, so she couldn't relate. In fact, when I was in the hospital once she asked me, "What is *wrong* with you, Wren?" The way she asked made me feel like it was my fault and that I was causing it to happen. I had anorexia when I was thirteen, and I got the feeling she thought HG was related. Let me tell you I have had anorexia, so I know what that is. Anorexia is having the ability to eat food but willfully refusing to do so. With HG you have all the will in the world to eat and none of the ability. It's the exact opposite of anorexia. In my pregnancy I eventually gained thirty-five pounds. Those were the most beautiful, welcomed thirty-five pounds of my life!

My HG was atypical in that I only vomited a handful of times. I realize that I did not have the severe vomiting that many women have, but the nausea was so intense that it disrupted my nutritional status, my job and my life in general. It was not "morning sickness." It was debilitating. It took my joy away from being pregnant, and it affected our family-building plans. Though my husband and I would like more children, at this time I can't say that I will ever be willing to do it again.

EIGHT
Nasogastric Enteral Feeding

Sometimes, when HG is *severe*, the inability to consume nourishment and fluid continues to cause malnutrition, dehydration and weight loss. Certain authors suggest an association between losing more than 5% of one's body weight during the second and third trimester and an increased risk of fetal complication and death.[110] My guess is that most women lose more than 5% early on and are still rebounding in later trimesters. Even so, the majority of HG women have healthy babies. However a more aggressive nutritional intervention is certainly justified at times, and experiencing fluid and electrolyte imbalances along with a total body weight loss of greater than or equal to 5% can be an indication of that necessity.[111-112] This intervention may take the form of nasogastric enteral feeding (NGEF).

How It Works

The NGEF method suspends the need for oral intake of food and fluid. For those whose nausea and vomiting are particularly triggered by attempts to eat or drink, this method is an answered prayer if tolerated. The tube supplies hydration and nutrition, and there is absolutely no pressure to take anything orally. It's cost effective[113] and can be managed at home.[114] Positive physical results can be seen in twenty-four hours.[115]

Physiologically, the body begins to receive much-needed nutrients and fluid. This begins to correct unstable body functioning. Psychologically, it's a huge relief knowing the baby is receiving nourishment. One woman was so satisfied with the physical and psychological results of NGEF that she remained on the tube for one hundred seventy-four days until it became dislodged.[116] That's more than half of her pregnancy! A properly irrigated (rinsed) tube can stay in place for months.

Procedure

NGEF provides fluids and nutrients via a tube placed through the nose and down into the stomach. This allows formula to pass through the stomach and intestines. First, a naso-numbing agent should be applied so insertion is more tolerable. The tube will be around six to eight french which means it will resemble a long, thin spaghetti noodle. Physicians feed the "spaghetti noodle" down your nose, into your throat and finally into your stomach. Proper placement is confirmed by sucking out a little stomach fluid and by hearing the appropriate bubbling sound after pushing some air down the tube and into the stomach.

Once in place, the tube delivers a feeding solution into the stomach. This milky looking formula is your food for as long as you require and tolerate it. Enteral alternatives to NGEF are nasoduodenal and nasojejunal feedings. These are similar to NGEF except that nasoduodenal feedings involve the insertion of the tube *past* the stomach and into the duodenum (first length of the small intestines). In nasojejunal feedings, the tube goes past the duodenum into the jejunum (first two-fifths of the small intestine past the duodenum). Many texts recommend X-ray confirmation of placement for the duodenal and jejunal procedures, but nasojejunal placement has been successfully carried out without X-ray and has virtually the same benefits and risks as NGEF.[117]

Benefits

Other methods of supplemental nutrition, such as needle methods, carry greater potential for risks and are much more expensive than NGEF. Since there is no needle with NGEF, it doesn't carry the risks of bleeding and blood clots. This method also provides a physiologic feeding that is more natural to the way your body processes nutrients. "Enteral" means the intestines will be used at some point in the delivery of nourishment. In NGEF your stomach still gets to digest and distribute food to the intestines and rest of the body in the usual way. This keeps the cells of the gastrointestinal tract active and therefore functioning normally.

Complications

The rate of risk is low. Complications include tube obstruction, tube dislodgment, aspiration, irritated throat, hyperglycemia, diarrhea and vomiting.

Tube Obstruction - One mechanical problem is a clogged NG tube. In one study, a recurrence of HG symptoms alerted physicians to the fact that the tube became clogged.[118] When the tube was unclogged the symptoms were corrected. Immaculate care and cleaning of the tube can help safeguard against obstruction.

Tube Dislodgment - Another mechanical complication is tube dislodgment. The tube itself can become displaced after coughing, vomiting, falling, etc. This requires reinsertion.

Taping the tube securely in place and frequently using a stethoscope to check placement (especially before beginning a feeding) can minimize displacement.

Aspiration - If the feeding tube becomes displaced, solution can creep into the lungs. You will probably know something is wrong because the fluid is irritating and you'll cough. When this fluid enters the lungs it can become a medium for bacterial growth, which can cause pneumonia.

Tube displacement isn't the only thing that can cause liquid to come up out of the stomach. Sometimes a person's gastrointestinal tract doesn't have the capacity to absorb all the feeding solution as quickly as necessary and a sort of "spillover" occurs. Other times the person's position during feedings can allow the fluid to creep out of the stomach.

Lastly, some people have a fistula, an abnormal hole, between their esophagus and trachea. If there's a hole between the esophagus and trachea, fluid can get in the lungs just by vomiting. A fistula is rare and has usually been diagnosed before adulthood.

Raising the head of the bed by thirty to forty-five degrees during feeding, and keeping the bed that way for an hour after the feeding, can reduce the risk of aspiration. If, however, a person continues to have trouble with aspiration, the NG tube can be placed past the pylorus (the outlet of the stomach) to try and minimize the condition, but such placement usually requires X-ray confirmation. This X-ray will not harm the baby at all.[119] Technicians should place a lead apron over the womb just to be extra safe.

Esophageal Erosion - In this uncomfortable condition, the tube irritates the throat. If the tube repeatedly moves in the throat or has to be reinserted time and again this can cause wear and tear on delicate tissues. Minimizing the number of insertions and keeping the NG tube as immobile as possible might reduce or prevent rawness of the throat.

Hyperglycemia - NG tube feeding may result in glucose intolerance especially since pregnancy already predisposes a patient to insulin resistance. Therefore, blood sugar needs monitoring to prevent hyperglycemia.

Diarrhea - The feeding formula can cause gastrointestinal complications such as diarrhea. However, drugs like Reglan can also cause this particular ailment. If feeding formula is identified as the actual problem, it can be changed to prevent diarrhea.

Vomiting - One reference contraindicates the nasogastric method in cases of intractable vomiting.[120] Some people cannot tolerate something that slides down their nose and throat and hangs there, because a gag reflex makes them vomit. Remember that malnutrition and dehydration worsen the severity of HG. People who are dehydrated and malnourished have a heightened sense of nausea. Correcting dehydration and electrolyte imbalance *before* initiating NG tube feedings may increase a patient's tolerance. Once nutrition can be restored, nausea and vomiting may be reduced even further.

While the tube has been shown to reduce symptoms, it is only a method of feeding, not the cure for HG. Many women repeatedly vomit the tube up, making placement futile.

Therefore, this method may be best for those whose vomiting is primarily triggered by oral intake of food and fluid.[121]

Indications for NGEF

When a woman can't stop vomiting, continues to have ketones in her urine, has lost more than 5% of her total body weight, has electrolyte imbalance, and continues to be malnourished, the literature says she is a candidate for supplemental feedings. This is true for those in the first trimester and particularly important for those in the second or third.

When NGEF Is Contraindicated

The American Gastroenterological Association prefers using an NG tube for short-term alternative nutrition needs that last less than thirty days.[122] When an HG patient cannot tolerate nasogastric enteral feedings, other enteral methods such as PEG and PEJ have been successful in studies of patients with HG.

Eve's Story

My husband and I had been married for seven years when we found out I was seven weeks pregnant. This was a planned pregnancy, and I was very excited, somewhat scared and in complete awe of the prospect of having a child. My due date was July 19, 2001. My husband and I decided to tell the whole family right away.

One week later, at eight weeks, I started throwing up all day and decided this could not be normal. I called my doctor, and He said it was "morning sickness." It didn't sound right to me, but he said, "Some women have it worse than others." He prescribed Zofran and told me to drink lots of fluids by taking baby sips all day. I tried to follow this advice for four days until I just had to concede that it wasn't working. I was in bad shape, so I went back to the doctor and he admitted me to the hospital because I was so dehydrated and had ketones and protein in my urine. In the hospital I got IV fluids and a shot of Phenergan and was sent home two days later. I was still being told it was just morning sickness.

Christmas day was completely awful. I started throwing up and just couldn't stop. My husband called the doctor, and I was admitted into the hospital again for IV fluids. I was discharged a week later on New Year's day. This is how it would go for weeks on end. Admitted and discharged, admitted and discharged.

On top of everything I got ptyalism. I started noticing that my mouth produced way too much saliva and I had to spit it out constantly. It was totally aggravating, and I had it for the rest of the pregnancy. At the end of January, my doctors decided that my gallbladder was making me sick. At sixteen weeks I underwent gallbladder surgery. That was supposed to stop the vomiting, but it didn't. This is when the doctors diagnosed me with severe HG. My doctors prescribed Thorazine, and I went three entire weeks without throwing up at all. For some reason though, at the end of February, the Thorazine stopped working for me. I was put back in the hospital because I was dehydrated again. This time I was discharged with IVs and home health care.

At home I received IV fluids around the clock, but I still could not eat, and I started passing out. On two occasions I was in my bathroom and lost consciousness attempting to get back to bed. I woke up on the floor not knowing how I got there. One night I was talking to my mother and grandmother in the den. At one point I tried to get up to go to the bathroom, and the next thing I remember I was in the ER. I had passed out again and my husband had to call 911 because no one could wake me this time. My doctors kept telling me that passing out didn't make any sense. Since they couldn't figure it out, they just accused my family and me of making it up.

By March I had lost thirty pounds, and my doctors decided it was time for an NG tube. The placement of the feeding tube was extremely painful. The tube stayed in five days until I threw up one day and some of the tube came out of my mouth! I began to choke. I pushed the nurse call button, but I couldn't say anything because I was choking. All I could do was bang on the speaker. Finally a nurse came, and I had managed to pull the tube out further so I could get some air. The nurse freaked. They had to get a nurse from the cancer floor because no one on the prenatal floor knew what to do about all this NG business. The cancer nurse took the rest of the tube out and said the doctors were going to put another one down. I refused. Instead of recording the fact that I puked the tube up and was trying to get it out of my throat due to choking, my doctor only documented that I pulled it out myself. The therapy didn't work and I felt blamed.

Next my doctors decided to put a PICC line in my left upper arm. In this one site I was able to get total parenteral nutrition (TPN), my IV medicines, and they could draw blood. I was attached to TPN and the doctors were telling me to wear Sea-Bands (used for motion sickness)! Unbelievable. Two cardiologists saw me and said I had a heart murmur. A gastroenterologist saw me and said I had an esophageal ulcer from vomiting too much. This is when the insulting questions began.

My doctors started hounding my mother in the hallway outside of my room asking her if I had been mentally or sexually abused as a child. I was not abused as a child in any way. They would also ask me constantly if my husband abused me and if the baby was wanted. No, my husband did not abuse me, and yes, this baby was very much wanted. I felt totally harassed. I was sick as a dog and having to defend my family and my childhood took a lot of energy. This was energy that I needed to get through each day. At the beginning of April my doctors told my husband and me that there was nothing medically wrong with me and that I needed to be placed in a medical psychiatric ward. However, they said they wouldn't force me to go. I didn't know about HG and had no idea what was wrong with me. Medical professionals who had studied medicine for decades were telling me that I was not physically sick and needed mental health care. At the time, I believed that my doctors ultimately knew what was best for my baby and me. And honestly, if the psychiatric ward was going to make me stop throwing up, I was all for it.

When I was admitted to the mental ward, my depression got very bad for two reasons:

1. In addition to the hell that I had already been suffering, my husband could only see me for three hours a day (whereas before, on the prenatal floor, he could stay with me as long as he wanted).

2. My physicians were treating me as though I did not have a real illness. I was so puking sick that I was hooked up to feeding tubes, and my doctors were telling me that I was not really sick! Nothing in my life ever prepared me for that.

I stayed in the psychiatric ward for two weeks. I had no phone, no television, and I was locked in, which prevented me from leaving the psychiatric ward. Some days I would cry for hours in my room alone. If I couldn't get physical comfort, I wanted at least emotional comfort, but my time with my husband was severely limited. The mental ward is also a scary place to be. The people who stayed in the rooms beside me and across the hall from me were true mental cases. One girl would cut her arms with anything that had a sharp edge, one girl tried to kill herself, and the other girl was from the county jail. And what was my "crime?" I was six months pregnant and sick as a dog. I went there because my doctors told me to. They were doctors, demigods. I trusted their advice, because I wanted to get well. Being in the psychiatric ward, however, was *not* making me well. It only scared and depressed me, and I was still puking my guts up. Finally I had enough and demanded to be released.

I was discharged and given home health care again. Five days later I was back in the hospital for a week and then discharged again. Finally, I was admitted and would stay until my baby was born. At the beginning of my pregnancy I weighed two hundred sixty-two pounds and lost sixty-three pounds by the end. This was probably the only time in my life I was glad to be fat. If I hadn't had all my fat to burn, I sometimes wonder what would have happened. I was scared that my son was not going to make it, and I was worried that if he did make it he would be severely disabled due to the rash of drugs I had taken. I was on Zofran, Phenergan, Thorazine, Reglan, Pepcid, Prevacid, Zoloft, Paxil, Atarax, Benadryl, Carafate and others that I can't even remember. These might work for someone else, but none of it worked for me. I got paranoid that the HG might not end even after my son was born. I asked my doctors if the mysterious and terrible illness would go away after the birth, and they didn't know, which terrified me.

Months after delivery I decided to get copies of my medical records from the hospital where I was treated during my pregnancy. At one point, my HG is attributed to Post-Traumatic Stress Disorder (PTSD), but this is usually diagnosed in people who have been in a war or seen something very traumatic like a murder. My HG may have caused PTSD, but not the other way around. In some of the nurses' notes it was documented that I was very "flat," that I had very little facial expression or wasn't talkative. What they were expecting from someone with severe HG? Cartwheels? They also documented that I did not look clean. Well I did the best I could, and when I could amble to the shower I did. A shower every other day was all I could muster, and I literally had to wait until my husband could get to the hospital, because I was so weak that he had to stand right there in the bathroom as I showered. The nurses' aid refused to do that. When I asked for help to take a shower, I was told: "That's what the call button is for." My medical records also state that I did not ask about my baby and didn't seem excited about him. One nurse even documented that, when she came in to check the fetal heart tones, I looked away.

All of these impressions and insinuations are based on opinions, yet the lies on my medical record are left to stand as a representation of who I am as a patient and as a person. To an outsider leafing through, I might appear to be a mental case with no clear desire or concern for my own child. How will the next person reading over my records know that the ONLY thing that kept me going was hearing my baby's heartbeat twice a day? How will they know that the constant reminder of my son's life is what enabled me to endure severe HG? I fought so hard for my baby, but *that's* not in the records!

Because of severe HG, having a baby was the most difficult thing I've ever done in my entire life. However, two very simple things could have happened to make it much easier for my family and me:

1. Doctors could have acknowledged that this is a physical illness and not a mental health problem.

2. Talking to an actual former sufferer (who had been through HG and survived) would have helped to validate my suffering and ease my fears. I didn't need a ticket to the mental ward. I needed good medical care, validation and hope. Isn't that what you're supposed to get when you're sick?

The only personal regret I have is that I did not question my doctors more. After my ordeal, I realize doctors don't know everything and are just human beings like the rest of us. I wish I had stood up for myself and insisted that I was sick and not crazy. I should have simply refused to entertain any accusations. But I was trying to get well, and they were my doctors. I did what they told me to do. It's all I knew. I just hope that somehow I can help the next woman get through this traumatic illness. HG is a *real* sickness that has a name, and it will end. My healthy son was born in July. He weighed five pounds and five ounces, and I haven't thrown up since.

NINE
Percutaneous Endoscopic Gastrostomy/ Jejunostomy

PEG

Percutaneous (through the skin) endoscopic (lighted viewing tube) gastrostomy (hole in the stomach), or PEG, is a surgical procedure that consists of placing a tube in the stomach from the outside of the abdomen.

Procedure

PEG can be placed during an overnight hospital stay or in an outpatient surgical facility. More than likely you will be awake during the procedure. First your throat will be numbed with a spray so experts can pass an endoscope down the esophagus and into the stomach. An endoscope is a flexible viewing tube with a light on the end of it. It allows the physician to see exactly where the feeding tube needs to be placed in the stomach. Then a doctor will administer a local anesthetic and make a small incision in your abdomen through which an IV tube will be inserted directly into the stomach. After the tube is properly situated, the doctor will sew it into place. The feeding solution can be administered directly into your stomach without having to deal with a tube down your throat or the triggers associated with eating.

Benefits

PEG may reduce some major vomiting triggers by bypassing oral intake of nutrients. It also delivers nourishment the normal way, via the digestive system, enabling the cells of the gastrointestinal tract to remain active and healthy. Administration involves less time, less money and less risk than a classic surgical gastrostomy. PEG is easily removed, and the fistula (hole) it leaves behind closes in twenty-four to forty-eight hours.

PEJ

PEG is not suitable for all patients. For some, holding anything in the stomach exacerbates vomiting. Other patients may have problems with gastroesophageal reflux (heartburn), which increases the risk of aspiration and related pneumonia. When there is a problem that requires bypassing the stomach, a patient may receive alternative enteral nutrition via percutaneous endoscopic jejunostomy (PEJ).

PEJ is placed very similarly to PEG except the tube does not go into the stomach but into the jejunum, which is the first two-fifths of the small intestine just after the duodenum. The small intestine is the last stop for nutrients before they go into the blood.

Benefits

PEJ basically carries the same benefits as PEG in that the feeding method is more natural than receiving nutrition directly into the bloodstream.[123] However, PEJ may actually be better for HG sufferers than PEG, because it tends to reduce emesis-related formula loss.[124] The formula goes right into the jejunum, the stomach is completely bypassed, and there's nothing of any nutritional value to throw up. Still, some doctors believe that PEG should come before PEJ, because PEJ is generally more difficult to place and maintain, has a greater tendency to migrate out of position, and nutrition has to be run at a slower rate.

Complications of PEG/PEJ

PEG/PEJ nutrition has been associated with a variety of risks ranging from moderate to severe. The four main types of complications are:

- *Mechanical problems* – when the tube becomes dislodged, clogged or when it migrates to a different place internally (when, for example, a jejunostomy tube moves into the stomach)
- *Gastrointestinal complications* – from the feeding solution itself; can involve diarrhea, abdominal distention (bloating), constipation, nausea and vomiting.
- *Infectious complications* – due to contamination of the site or feeding solution; can result in sepsis (blood infection). Aspiration pneumonia can occur if the feeding solution leaks out of jejunum and accidentally gets sucked into the lungs.
- *metabolic complications* - such as hyperglycemia (elevated sugar levels) and fluid and electrolyte imbalances.

These complications are usually due to nutrient selections that are incompatible with individual needs, poor management of the mixture and inadequate clinical care.

Enteral vs. Parenteral Feedings

Enteral feedings have three distinct advantages over parenteral feedings. First, enteral feedings distribute nutrients in a more natural way that helps to keep the digestive tract active. Next, enteral feedings cause fewer metabolic and technical complications. Lastly, enteral feedings have been described as "relatively cheap" [125] and can be less expensive than parenteral feedings.[126] Some experts suggest considering enteral feedings before moving on to the riskier parenteral methods.[127-128]

Tawny's Story

I married in my early twenties and shortly thereafter became pregnant. At the time we were living in Europe, and it didn't appear to me that the doctors had a good understanding of what was happening to me. My well-meaning mother would constantly supply home-cooked meals and encourage me to "eat an apple a day."

By the time I ended up in the hospital I was totally dehydrated and fainting. I didn't care any longer. I just wanted to get better. My mother was very worried, and my husband came to visit all the time. I tried, but I just could not take the suffering one more day. I was young and no one counseled me. An abortion was performed right there in the hospital. I was released home and went back to work.

At night, I would have nightmares about my baby descending from heaven asking me why she wasn't allowed to live. I would wake up crying, unable to go back to sleep. I felt so guilty. I took my child's life, and I felt like a murderer. I was Catholic and felt like a hypocrite returning to church. I never went to confession after the termination. It was awful.

I no longer felt like I could have sex with my husband. At first, I was afraid that the abortion had physically damaged me and that sex would be harmful. I also began to view sex as the reason for my bad experience; I eventually lost all interest. We had a good marriage, and my husband was very understanding, so we hung in there. But after ten years, I guess he just couldn't take it anymore, and he left me.

It was a few years before I recovered from the divorce; I took it pretty hard. However, I met a wonderful man and we married. We are in our late thirties and both of us felt the biological clock ticking away right from the start. I hoped things would be different. Both of us wanted a family and children very badly. So much time had passed. Pregnancy couldn't have been as bad as I thought it was when I was in my early twenties. I was older, wiser and stronger. I could make it this time.

I got pregnant and it wasn't long before the hyperemesis kicked in. I begged my OB/GYN to help me. He gave me vitamin B and Unisom and cited that his wife was sick all the time and just "endured it" through the whole pregnancy. He went on a two-week vacation, and the hyperemesis got so bad that I could no longer work and was admitted to the hospital. After a brief stay for hydration, I was released to home IV treatments. The people from the home nursing company who oversaw my PICC line appeared rather disinterested and unknowledgeable about my HG. The nurse misread the dosage instructions of the antiemetic medication and gave me half the dose ordered by the doctor. We had no idea. She noticed after about a week and a half. All the while the hyperemesis was getting worse and worse. At the same time I was expected to learn how to manage my own IV line, which appeared fairly ancient. There were procedures with syringes and different sequences of pharmaceutical solutions to remember-*without written instructions*! I was expected to learn in one day what nurses go to nursing school for years to learn, and I was expected to do it while I was terribly sick! To top it all off, each nurse who visited had her own idea of how it should be done, so I was hearing that I needed to manage my PICC differently every time! I eventually lost hope.

After two weeks of weariness and total frustration with no improvement, I gave up. My husband tried in vain to obtain written instructions for maintaining the PICC line, but it seemed no one could help.* My husband was supportive hoping it would get better, but he felt very helpless.

My OB/GYN never followed up on how I was doing after the PICC. While I am usually quite capable of standing up for myself, I just felt too weak and defeated to fight anymore. After everything I'd been through, I picked up the phone book and made an appointment with an abortion clinic. My husband was devastated, but he said he would stand by me no matter what. I had no idea how abortion clinics operate. My God, it was awful. There was no counseling, only a video for a mass viewing of twenty people. Some of these girls looked like little kids.

The actual room was dark and non-ventilated. I noticed a fly in the area of the instruments. I was horrified. We had an appointment but ended up having to wait all day for the doctor to appear. They told us he was performing abortions in other locations and flying in and out of state on a continual basis. I wanted to get better *desperately* and was not going to leave, but are there no regulations for these doctors and clinics? It was appalling. If only I hadn't been so desperate. I kept throwing up in the waiting room.

Finally the doctor appeared. This is when it became clear to me that there were not going to be any anesthetics! Two nurses held me down while the doctor suctioned out my baby. They kept telling me to hold still and to calm down, but I was just crying uncontrollably. Afterwards I was told to get up and go to a waiting area, so the doctor could be with the next patient. I told them I couldn't get up, so they jerked me up and I blacked out immediately. I awakened to smelling salts and was shouldered by two nurses to a waiting area until my husband was allowed in.

I am still shocked at the procedure. What a horrible process! Another baby gone. I killed another one of my children! As my body healed the reality started to set in again. I kept picturing what it must have been like for my baby to be peaceful and warm one moment and then violently torn and sucked out of me the next. She was my child, entrusted to me. She was a little soul that I loved and was supposed to shield from harm. I just wanted to die.

I tried to forget; it was the only way to survive. I began to research HG. I wanted to know why my life had ended up this way, what caused HG and how to treat it. My husband and I went to a specialist to get more insight and educate ourselves. The Internet turned out to be an invaluable resource. After a year, I promised my husband and myself that I would try one more time, and then we would pursue adoption.

I got pregnant and changed my doctor to a practice of three OB/GYNs who specialized in high-risk pregnancies. At the first series of days of vomiting and constant nausea I went to the hospital. I was admitted and remained there for two months. My husband refused to have me released early to home care unless I was visibly better and ready. I had taken Unisom, vitamin B, Phenergan suppositories and Pepcid. I had numerous IV sites on my hands and arms. I continued to vomit and lose weight, and finally, they gave me a PICC line with round-the-clock fluids, TPN, lipids, and the highest dose of continuous Zofran I could take. I was also given Phenergan, which knocked me out, via IV at the closest intervals possible. At long last they decided to give me steroids. This really helped and got me into my fourth month!

I am now at home with a PICC line. My husband has learned all the ins and outs of managing my PICC line and has been home with me for several weeks since my release. I get better every day. I can even eat and drink now! I have occasional nausea, but I don't vomit! The company I work for is sensitive to my needs, and my health insurance is good and has paid for nearly everything.

I am halfway there and so encouraged! I am crocheting little baby shoes, sweaters and blankets. Slowly but surely I feel like a person again, and I can't wait to hold my little one in my arms. This time I will protect my child like a mother should, like I wanted to all along.

Hyperemesis can have a seriously negative impact on a woman physically, emotionally, socially and financially. She needs help, and there should be no short supply of it. Knowledge is power. Learn all you can so you can make sure you get the care you need. Demand to be taken seriously by health care professionals. If you can, stay in the hospital on fluids and medications until YOU are physically ready to leave. Take things slowly. Don't try to be Super Woman. Ask for help, and *never give up.*

❧

*At the writing of this book, a page on PICC dressing changes and management procedures can be found on the Internet at:

- http://www.horizonhealthcareservices.com/resources/ picc_dressing.pdf

Also, a very efficient overview of PICC line management can be found here:

- http://www.cancerbacup.org.uk/Treatments/ Chemotherapy/ManagingaPICCline

TEN
Total Parenteral Nutrition

If a patient is not doing well with, cannot tolerate, or opts out of enteral feedings, parenteral feedings, which bypass the intestine, can be established. Total parenteral nutrition (TPN) consists of delivering a feeding solution directly into the blood stream by way of a tube placed deeply in a vein via a needle. The tube is often referred to as a catheter or line. Again, when there are fluid and electrolyte imbalances and a total body weight loss of 5% or more, this is justification for alternative nutritional support.[129]

Types and Procedures

In *centrally* placed TPN a needle is inserted into the neck or shoulder area and a catheter is snaked into a large vein where a nutritive solution is delivered directly into the bloodstream. After placement, an X-ray is taken to make sure the catheter is in the lower superior vena cava, which is one of the two largest veins in the body that leads right to the heart. Once proper placement is confirmed, the feeding solution can be administered. Central line insertion can be tricky. It can collapse a patient's lung, requiring a very un-fun chest tube. Central insertion isn't usually the first choice for a central line. Peripherally inserted central catheters have less potential for complications than centrally inserted central catheters;[130] therefore peripherally placed parenteral nutrition may be preferable to central parenteral nutrition.[131]

In *peripherally* placed TPN, the line is typically inserted into the inner arm somewhere near the elbow bend. Unlike central TPN, the tube does not go as close to the heart. *Peripheral TPN is considered to be safer than central TPN* because it is not a likely source of catheter sepsis or thrombotic (blood clotting) complication.[132] Although the risks are reduced with peripherally placed central lines, there can be a drawback, because caloric intake is limited.[133]

X-Rays in Pregnancy

It is very important to ensure proper placement of the line, and X-ray exposure from a single diagnostic procedure doesn't harm the baby at all.[134] Even CT scans, are OK in pregnancy. It actually takes a huge amount of radiation to affect the baby. I had six chest X-rays in my fourth pregnancy, four of them in the first trimester, and my daughter was born perfectly normal. A trusted OB/GYN advised me that I could have 100 chest X-rays before he would even blink an eye and remarked that the abdominal shield is used just to be "extra safe."

Benefits of TPN

TPN ensures an appropriate caloric intake and balances electrolytes.[135] It can be managed at home and has the potential to keep you and your baby fed and alive for as long as you need it.

Sometimes medical professionals can scare you with the list of risks that they may be legally behoved to provide. One woman's home health care nurse repeatedly warned her that the longer the PICC was in, the higher the risk of complication. This was very frightening, and there was nothing the otherwise capable HG sufferer could do to speed her recovery for PICC removal. The nurse's risk fixation was unhelpful. If you encounter such a fixated health care professional, remember that there are many patients with cancer, AIDS, short bowel syndrome and other illnesses who have benefited greatly from TPN for over a year.[136]

Complications

TPN, while only somewhat invasive, carries potentially serious risks. This is why some doctors prefer trying different methods of enteral nutrition before moving to TPN.[137] Catheter sepsis, thrombosis, and air embolism are among possible complications of TPN.

Catheter Sepsis

Catheter sepsis occurs when bacteria or fungus enters the bloodstream through the needle or tubing. This complication can be avoided by inserting the catheter under very sterile conditions after proper skin preparation. Regularly cleansing and dressing the catheter site can also help minimize the risk of sepsis. *All care associated with the bare catheter site should be carried out under sterile conditions.* Do not let anyone remotely near your bare site without sterile gloves and a facemask. Specially trained medical technicians should handle these responsibilities. Risk of sepsis can be reduced to less than 2%-3% if those who are specially trained to do so manage the TPN site.

If your insertion site becomes red, tender and you notice any pus, call your doctor. Also, if you experience spiking fevers, changes in vital signs, or malaise (a vague sense of ill-being) beyond the HG, contact a physician. These can all be signs of catheter sepsis. Your doctor can determine if these symptoms are caused by catheter sepsis or something less troublesome.

If sepsis occurs, the doctor will likely remove the PICC line and treat the patient with antibiotics and peripheral IVs until the infection clears. If the infection takes too long to clear and the woman can not go without nutrition any longer a centrally inserted line may be placed to deliver antibiotics and TPN. My own wonderful gastroenterologist related that on many occasions this works just fine.

Catheter sepsis can be very serious.[138] I personally know a woman who developed a dangerous case of infection that affected her heart. Faced with the real possibility of her demise termination became an issue. (Her story appears in this book.) This stresses the need for handling a catheter site with the utmost sterile care. Bacteria and fungus must be prevented from breaching the site. As serious as it is, sepsis is not always the end of the world. I got a staph infection in my line, and unlike my poor friend, several bags of antibiotics cleared it right up and saved the day. I have also heard from fortunate others for whom this was the case.

Thrombosis

A thrombotic complication arises when a blood clot forms (usually around the TPN tubing). A clot is more likely to form if the catheter has not been inserted into the proper location or where insertion has been handled roughly and tissue has been traumatized. Taking time to insert the catheter with gentle and accurate skill can minimize risks.

If you notice swelling in the hand on the side where the TPN is inserted, call your doctor. The swelling might mean a clot is blocking blood that is trying to return to the heart for circulation. If a clot is discovered, it should be managed and resolved *before* removing the tube so as not to dislodge the clot. If the tube were to dislodge it, the clot could travel and become serious. Heparin or other clot busting drugs can disperse a clot before this happens.

Air Embolism

The risks for air embolism only occur when inserting or removing TPN and during manipulatory sessions when tubings or caps are changed. During these times the risk increases with coughing, sneezing, crying, etc. It is best to try and remain calm when medical professionals are servicing tubings. (To prevent a sneeze, stick your finger on the space between your two front teeth, slide it up to the gum as far as it will go, and press the spot underneath your lip. It looks silly, but it works.) During insertion or removal, I always sang a Third Day song in my head and tried my best to pretend I wasn't really there.

On the bright side, air embolism is not a constant risk, and a health care professional will be present during risk times because she will be the one manipulating tubing. She knows techniques, like Valsalva's maneuver, that will help reduce complications. (In Valsalva's maneuver the patient tries to slowly but forcefully exhale while holding her nose and mouth shut and preventing herself from breathing out.)

Breathing difficulties, increased heart rate, turning blue or purplish, sudden low blood pressure and a change in your level of consciousness will alert your caregiver to suspect air embolism and offer treatment promptly. Treatment is fairly simple and involves laying the patient on the left side and withdrawing the air.

Blood Glucose Level Fluctuations

Being on TPN means treating yourself like a diabetic. In the hospital setting, your health care professionals will constantly bombard you with finger sticks for blood tests. My glucose levels were checked every four hours. In the home setting you should receive a blood glucose monitor complete with everything you need to check your own levels. My monitor consisted of a blood-drawing "pen" and a small electronic unit that spat out test strips, which sucked my blood up and tested it. The "pen" is virtually painless, and you might actually want to keep it with you in the hospital as it hurts less than the nurses' "clicks."

If my blood glucose levels got too low I'd "bottom out." "Bottoming out" consists of feeling odd, heavy breathing, rapid heart rate, sweating, etc. This only happened to me once because I received too much insulin initially. Glucose tablets (that taste like orange-flavored candy) resolve the issue quickly, but I was told that jellybeans or any sugar candy also work well.

When blood glucose levels climb too high, some notice a satiated feeling, buzzing sensations in the body, confusion, headaches, trembling hands, etc. However, when my blood glucose levels climbed too high (over one hundred thirty) I didn't really have any symptoms. Most people don't, which is why it is important to check blood glucose levels often. Insulin injections lower blood glucose levels. I had to jab myself in the thigh or stomach with two units of insulin. If it sounds horrible, just remember the four-year-old diabetic who told a thirty-year old newly diabetic patient (who was hesitating during her first self-administered insulin shot): "Hey, Lady, I do it all the time, and if I can do it, you can do it." Out of the mouths of babes. And the kid is right. It's no big deal.

HG is what it is and you do what you have to do. You *can* get through it! Such an attitude will also make your weekly injections of vitamin K (pregnancy category C) more bearable! Needles, needles, needles!

TPN Checklist
To reduce anxiety and other suffering that can arise due to home health care scheduling blunders, you should probably schedule a TPN orientation visit with your home health care nurse *before* you leave the hospital on TPN.

Before going home, learn how to:
- work your pump
- respond to pump alarms
- change tubings and bags
- reduce risk of infection via clean procedures, etc.

You should also be equipped with:
- a glucose monitor (and taught how to use it)
- glucose tablets (though jellybeans will do the job and taste better)
- syringes
- insulin (which, prior to leaving the hospital, you should practice injecting via a benign saline solution that *you* measure out)

NGEF & PEG/PEJ vs. TPN
TPN is more invasive than NGEF, less physiologic than both NGEF and PEG/PEJ, and the risks are generally more

serious. TPN has other drawbacks. Since TPN bypasses the stomach and intestine, this can lead to gallbladder problems. Also, when TPN lasts a few months, the cells of the intestine can atrophy and become temporarily dysfunctional.[139] For me this spelled bowel troubles. After TPN cessation it took me two painful weeks to have regular bowel movements again. The powerful constipated cramping and multiple fruitless trips to the bathroom were quite unpleasant. If I never drink prune juice again it will be too soon. Be that as it may, *the rate of TPN complication is relatively low.* In one study of twenty-one women on TPN, four developed infections, two experienced blood clots, and *no one died.* Were it not for TPN, many of these women and their children might have developed severe HG complications which could have led to death. Although studies are quite clear about the benefits and complications of each feeding method, I am inclined to think that most doctors rely on TPN rather than NGEF and PEG/PEJ. My gastroenterologist preferred it for whatever reason, and I was happy just to get it. For women with severe, intractable HG, the benefits of TPN likely outweigh the risks.

YOU CAN DO THIS!

Tell yourself again and again that HG is what it is, and you do what you have to do to get through it. The procedures are not fun, but they are not the end of the world, and YOU CAN DO IT!

Having adequate information can be comforting, but knowing too much can sometimes cause a lot of anxiety. Try to keep things in perspective. Death due to HG is very nearly unheard of today, and you are fighting for a beautiful growing child who will be a source of joy for the rest of your life.

If you would like to know more about the risks and benefits of any HG treatment, contact your doctor. She may have pamphlets or procedure-teaching videos, which you can borrow or purchase. For those who would like to see a procedure before having it done, training videos can also be found on the Internet but are often very expensive to order.

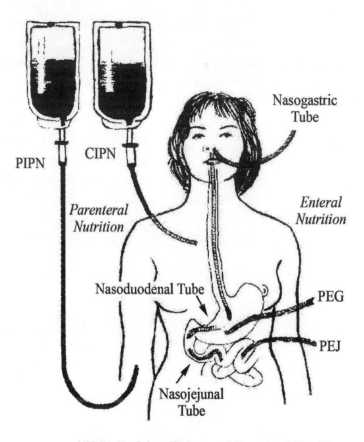

PIPN: Peripherally Inserted Parenteral Nutrition
CIPN: Centrally Inserted Parenteral Nutrition
PEG: Percutaneous Endoscopic Gastrostomy
PEJ: Percutaneous Endoscopic Jejunostomy

Fiona's Story

Post-Traumatic Stress Disorder (PTSD) rears its ugly head in many forms and fashions. My daughter's birth was a miracle in so many ways, but I hardly remember the events that led up to it. I wonder where the secret compartment I built during those long seven months has gone...surrounded and wrapped like a present with fear, sadness, anger, betrayal, pain, guilt and resentment. I was in an ugly place that should have been beautiful country. Pregnancy should have been a glowing time of respite and relief, joy and contentment, learning and sharing. It pains me to know that my child grew in darkness alone, in a place I grew to despise. I spent hated days unable to share in her beauty, yearning for her to not be a part of me, wanting it over more than wanting her life.

July 6, 1999. I felt out of sorts all weekend and even rejected my favorite food because of a strange bout of nausea. Here it was, Monday; I should have stayed home. I remember the very first time I threw up. I knelt retching on the cold, white tile floor at work. The flu turned out to be a baby.

The pregnancy began in turmoil as I was bleeding from a surgery I'd had six weeks prior. An ultrasound was performed to check for fetal viability. I lay on the table holding my husband's hand, wondering what was wrong and worrying that there was no way a child could be growing safely if I was bleeding. The cold paddle was placed on my stomach and the nurse found the pumping heart, but the doctor was fearful the baby wouldn't survive. The detachment I felt for the "thing" growing inside me began that day. Mustn't get too close.

The very next day I was admitted to the hospital due to severe vomiting. This was the first of many times I would be treated as a human pin cushion for the purpose of shoving electrolytes and fluids into my body. The next seven weeks were a struggle between fighting and giving up.

At first there was hope that the nausea would abate. This idea ended with the realization that I could not keep down the anti-nausea medication. I remember thinking: "How does this medication work if I can't even keep it down? Something must be really wrong." In-home treatment was ordered the next week as my doctor's office could sense that I would need several sessions. A nurse came to my home with an IV stand and all the medical supplies necessary to start the fluid and medication transfer.

The nightmare began when I received my first IV push of Phenergan. Unbelievable burning coursed through my veins. This later led to a Reglan push being added to my bag of foul smelling, yellow-colored electrolyte solution that my husband had to concoct everyday. Time passed, hope waned. The sickness got worse with each course of treatment. The medication was not effective even though it was being given intravenously. My body was giving up... along with my heart and my determination to complete the pregnancy. I kept hoping that each course of fluid and medication would stabilize my condition so I could resume my life, but it always ended in uncontrollable episodes of violent vomiting.

I'm a fighter; nothing beats me. However, I was falling deeper and deeper into a pit that I could not claw my way out of. There was no light at the end of the tunnel, only darkness for me to fall more deeply into. The nurse that often came to my home could see that I was becoming thoroughly depressed. When I began talking in euphemisms about "not wanting to be sick anymore" she suggested that I see a counselor. This nurse would listen to me and comfort me when no one else would. It was a lonely time. My friends disappeared and my family was in disbelief. I held onto the light that appeared in my husband's eyes when I told him he was going to be a father. I kept fighting; I did not want to let him down.

After one month of on-again-off-again IV treatment a different nurse came to the house to start a new intravenous line. (This occurred when my veins would collapse two to three times per week.) He had been out before and had some difficulties starting the line, but this was a totally different experience. He tried seven times to find a vein that would take an IV and seven times my veins collapsed. My arms eventually looked like a junkie's; black and blue marks covered them. He finally gave up as I was in hysterics crying trying to figure out how I was going to survive without my "supply." He gave up, yelled at me, and called my normal nurse. She came out to the house and sat down with me. We talked about my options. She said if I wanted to fight, the only option was a long-term IV that ran in a vein from the inside of my arm up into my chest and right outside my heart. It was called a peripherally inserted central catheter (PICC). I wept in her arms. I trusted this woman with my life and agreed to it. She called the doctor from my home, and he ordered the procedure that day.

With the PICC line installed and my eight hundred-dollar-a-day liquid steak and lobster dinner (TPN) running, I was able to have medication pushed through my line. This lasted about two days before I said I would rather vomit all day than go through the side effects of a pushed medicine. The illness reached its plateau, and I was vomiting between eight and twenty times per day. My husband and I finally made an appointment with the counselor to discuss our options, but I had already made up my mind. This "thing" was not going to beat me, and I wanted it to end. Abortion became the answer.

I was tired, the PICC line ran on a 24-hour pump, and I had to keep my arm straight *all day and all night* or the alarm would sound. I swear, to this day I can still hear the sound of the pump undulating in my head. I was alone; my friends had deserted me and left me to suffer without their valuable support. I was sick; I had not eaten a meal in weeks. I was ready for this to be over, ready to live again.

The most difficult part of my choice to abort was telling my husband. He had been a saint. He had always been there for me no matter what was happening. The pregnancy was about to end; I was destroyed for him. We were in counseling when I told him that I was going to abort. He was devastated but so very understanding. It shattered him to watch me suffer existing in so much agony.

At twelve weeks, Monday, August sixteenth, I had little time to make a decision. I called my doctor to ask if he would perform the abortion. His nurse got angry with me and told me that he would not end the pregnancy; however, she did make an appointment for me to talk with him. During the interim I called another doctor for a second opinion. After listening to my story and reviewing the treatment I was receiving, he told me there was nothing else that could be done for me. That was it. I made the appointment at a local abortion clinic. My child would die on Sunday.

There was an ounce of determination still hidden somewhere in my body. I decided to get on the Internet (something I hadn't been able to do in six weeks). I guess I wanted answers that my doctor was unwilling to give me. There had to be other options. Through the darkness I found the Web site of a woman that had been sick with HG. She was writing a book and had done research and listed alternative treatments for the illness. I seemed to be at the end of my rope, but I found kinship in her words; she had aborted her first child. I could barely sit up, but I felt the need to write her. I guess it was a desperate cry for help, a search for someone who could understand me and commiserate after the abortion.

Fate opened a door.

This woman became my child's savior. She wrote me back and asked me to call her. She said there were other alternatives and that I would get through this even though I felt like I was dying. I called her, and ironically, she only lived thirty minutes away. We talked about my doctor, about my abortion appointment and alternatives. She begged me to meet with her doctor and said she would set up an appointment with him. I agreed.

My husband, my mother and I met with my doctor one last time. I had lost seventeen pounds in six weeks. The doctor was ambivalent about the new alternatives I presented him with and said it was up to me whether I could endure this sickness. He stated that there were no other options for treatment, and he was not willing to look at any studies. He gave me no hope, and I left his office a shattered fragment of the person I had been before.

I returned home to find that a consultation with the new doctor had been scheduled. This appointment was for the day after my abortion appointment. This caused a lot of anxiety, because Sunday was the last day the abortion clinic in my area would perform the abortion due to their thirteen-week limitation. One day over, and I would have to travel five hours away for the abortion to be performed at the very same clinic where my new computer friend lost her first baby because of HG. I was worried, but my "virtual" pal begged me to meet with the doctor and try to find other alternatives. She said she would do whatever it took to help me through this process, and she did! My mother and I went to meet with the new doctor and he said he would also do whatever it took to get me through the pregnancy, and he did!

Within two weeks I began corticosteroid treatment (Solu-Medrol aka methylprednisolone sodium succinate). I remember eating my first tomato and weeping with gratitude; I had not eaten anything for over five weeks. I called my new friend and we celebrated such an awesome moment! I remember having the PICC line removed from my arm, taking a shower alone for the first time in months and just crying as I scrubbed the dead skin from the area where the PICC line had been.

It wasn't easy. At week twenty-nine I was still puking. I remember getting bronchitis, vomiting blood for hours, and being sent to the hospital for three days while my husband was away on business. I never felt good or cured, and I threw up almost every day for seven months, but it was nothing like it had been in the beginning, and I could manage it.

I vomited throughout labor, and just before my daughter was born I threw up for the last time. I remember looking into her eyes. It was over, and she had been worth it all.

For me, pregnancy was an incredible nightmare that I could not have continued without my husband, my friend and my nurse. It was a horrible nightmare, and I have done my best to distance myself from the experience. I try to focus on the good things. My daughter is three-years-old. She is happy and healthy and so full of life. I cannot imagine what life would have been like if I had aborted her.

ELEVEN
Mental Health Care

HG is devastating emotionally. It's no wonder that some HG sufferers seek mental health care as part of their treatment.

HG Negativity:
1. Depression (when you lose health and autonomy)
2. Inability to focus, care, or derive joy from anything due to constant suffering
3. Isolation (when you can't leave your room/house)
4. Neglect (when your needs are not met)
5. Invalidation/alienation (when HG is not taken seriously by others who *think* they know what you're going through)
6. Anger and confusion (when others offer offensive advice/observations)
7. Jealousy (when others are pregnant, happy and well)
8. Guilt (when debilitating illness negatively affects family and job responsibilities)
9. Hopelessness (when it feels like the illness will never end)
10. Fear (of severe morbidity and/or death of self and/or baby)

Mental/Emotional Help

Psychotherapy and hypnosis are associated with the treatment of HG. These treat the depression caused by HG and can be immensely helpful in learning to accept the illness, necessary treatments and all that is required to move positively through the ordeal. Private psychotherapy, group psychotherapy, "peer psychotherapy" and hypnosis are a few different options.

Private Psychotherapy

Psychotherapy usually involves talking to a professional therapist, one-on-one, about the physical and mental effects of HG. Many people are more comfortable talking to a neutral personality, because they can express sentiments that they are hesitant to reveal to others. Sufferers have secretly admitted that they often pray to miscarry or consider abortion as a way out of the illness. These are things they may feel they can never tell anyone close to them for fear of inflicting pain or being judged. Psychotherapy won't cure the HG, because HG is a physical illness. However, thoughts and feelings can be explored, and many women are truly relieved to know that they are not horrible or abnormal and that the avoidance of pain and will to survive only confirm that they are human.

Group Psychotherapy

In group therapy a number of people get together to discuss feelings under the guidance of at least one trained professional. Currently, I know of no non-online support groups specifically for women actively suffering from HG although there is certainly a demand. One sufferer's mother asked physicians about the availability of such a group:

"They looked at us like we were crazy. 'Gee, why would anyone need a support group for throwing up twenty times a day?' Before this started I guess I would have thought it was crazy too. But not any more."

Even if a support group existed, I'm not sure HG moms would be able to attend during peak symptoms. Even so, for those who could attend, it would be a great resource.

Another great group would be one consisting of those who at one point suffered from HG, because many experience lingering, negative emotional effects. Like soldiers of war, veterans of significant illness have fought a battle that was often debilitating, isolating, alienating and beyond the realm of usual human experience. Guided by a trusted counselor, a group of post-HG sufferers could meet and explore common facets of having had HG. These women could help each other cope with additional issues such as the effects of HG on personal relationships, methods of family building, etc. If any advocates or current sufferers *were* able to attend such a meeting, the veterans could potentially offer support of endless value. In the very least, veterans could provide local phone support.

"Peer Psychotherapy"
It is difficult to watch a family member suffer so intensely for months without respite. There's a sense of powerlessness and failure that witnesses feel. It is natural to want to avoid these feelings; therefore HG sufferers are often unconsciously avoided. For the sufferer, the isolation and alienation of HG can be the hardest to deal with emotionally.

Previous and current sufferers who have Internet access can always find and talk to others who are in similar situations. This is a casual, unprofessional form of psychotherapy that often works wonders. There are entire web sites, some with message boards, devoted to HG and a few are listed in Appendix B of this book.

No one can ever completely understand the unique experience of another individual, but fellow sufferers probably come closer than anyone else. Although most of them are not professional psychoanalysts and cannot give professional advice, they hold something of an "honorary degree" in HG counsel. A fellow sufferer can offer the one thing no one else can: commiseration. I can honestly say that relating to others is one of the things that helps me the most. With this "lay psychotherapy" comes the realization that I am not alone. As the vast majority of the gravid female population sits fat and happy with the warm glow of a healthy pregnancy, other sufferers enable me to see that I'm not the only one with problems, and I spend a little less time dwelling in self-pity.

Hypnosis
Hypnosis is not some sort of involuntary coma but a natural state akin to daydreaming. In simple terms, it is a focused period of intense concentration. You can't get stuck in a trance or be made to act contrary to your will. In fact, hypnosis is not something done *to* you but something you do to *yourself* under suggestion. It's very safe and can even be achieved without an office visit. Relaxation tapes, for instance, elicit focus and are actually tools of self-hypnosis.

Focusing

When a person focuses intensely on certain things, she may temporarily suspend critical judgment and possess an ability to change things that are usually inaccessible to psychological influence. Here's an example, *if you do not have HG and if you are able to do so safely*, close your eyes and stand on one foot for sixty seconds. Chances are, the more you try to remain still the more you wobble and have to start over. Now try it again, but this time, think only of squishing bread dough through your hands. Think of the softness of the dough. Feel the sensation of powdery flour moving gently between your fingers. Think of the silky smooth surface of the dough as you roll it into a ball. Is there a dimple in the ball? Roll it around and around until the ball is perfectly smooth like the skin of a dolphin. Feel the weight of the soft, warm orb in your hands. Now feel the tender resistance as you firmly squeeze it all over again in your hands. Before you know it, you've stood on one foot, without wobbling, for a lot longer than you did when you were concentrating on standing still. By focusing mentally on something totally unrelated, you have just brought about a physical change, an ability that wasn't there previous to the self-hypnosis.

Imagery

Imagery is a type of informal hypnosis. Sometimes, when I was in significant misery, I would close my eyes, lie very still, and try to fixate on my feet. I would see them in my mind's eye and focus all of my attention on them. I would see the bones, the toenails, and the fine, blonde hair on the tops of my feet. Concentrating on the image of my feet, I would remind myself that they were not nauseous, that they were a part of me that was not influenced by HG. I concentrated on the fact that no matter what was happening to the rest of my body, my feet were still normal, unchanged, something I had control over. It may sound a bit silly, but just knowing I was still "me" somewhere, even if only in my feet, was a little empowering. I still had HG, I was still violently ill, but I do believe the imagery was periodically some consolation though very brief.

Guided Imagery

Before I got pregnant the second time, I bought a hypnosis tape for managing general pain, which featured a man's deep, monotone voice. I listened to it before I became pregnant, and practiced the techniques while I was not sick and while my ability to focus on outside stimulus was better. When I did get sick, I had already become familiar with the technique and was able to use the tape more efficiently as it took me on a tour of my own pain circuitry. After guiding me through familiar relaxation techniques, the voice told me to view my body as a machine I could somewhat control.

Example of Guided Imagery

Suppose I shrink myself down and travel to the inside of my body. I walk up my vertebrae like stairs until I climb into my head. In my head there is a long wooden table. On the table are a number of glasses that represent pain receptors in different areas of my body. The glasses are filled with clear liquid, which represents health and comfort. As soon as I start to perceive discomfort in any part of my body, the corresponding glass begins to turn cloudy and dark. In order to rid myself of the pain, I must dump the contents of the glass into a bottomless bucket underneath the table, return the glass, and refill it with clean, clear liquid. I am to do this as often as necessary. This is imagery I might focus on at necessary intervals.

Guided imagery didn't really take a significant amount of my nausea away, but it gave me something to do at a time when I felt powerless to do anything. Other individuals might have a higher level of suggestibility and therefore hypnosis might be more effective for them. In the very least, guided imagery is a brief distraction.

Paying for Hypnotherapy

Sometimes HMOs won't pay for hypnotherapy in particular, even though it has been reported as beneficial for HG sufferers. If this is your situation, ask an advocate to dig up as many medical journal articles related to hypnotherapy and HG as they can find. Some are listed in the Consulted Works section at the end of this book. This way, you can cite the medically studied beneficial effects as concrete evidence justifying your request of the HMO. Also, if your HMO doesn't have anyone trained in hypnotherapy or just has a standard policy of not paying anyone billing herself as a hypnotherapist, then you can possibly ethically circumvent this by finding a counselor who is also trained in hypnotherapy. She will offer you psychotherapy and hypnosis, but it all falls under "counseling" and that is how it can be billed.

The American Society of Clinical Hypnosis (ASCH) certifies practitioners and can provide referrals to experienced and qualified hypnotherapists. If you have problems finding a certified hypnosis practitioner, you will find contact information for the ASCH in Appendix B of this book.

Assuming every beneficial treatment option is available to you, and assuming you can get out of bed and stop vomiting long enough to talk to someone, there is the choice of an office visit with a professional trained in psychotherapy and/ or hypnosis technique. But how do you find the right one for you?

Choosing a Professional Right for You

As with any profession, simply holding a degree does not make a person good at what they do. A particular psychotherapist may not know beans about treating the HG sufferer. I do not believe that the right kind of HG counsel includes antidepressant drugs and a refusal to acknowledge that the HG is the primary disease. Anyone who talks Prozac and wants to get to the root of HG by delving into an HG sufferer's relationship with her mother may be in need of some serious psychotherapy herself. Just being professionally qualified in the mental health field isn't enough. If possible, ask around to see whom others liked and didn't like.

Word of Mouth

Sometimes a physician or friend will suggest a few sessions with someone in the mental health field. Even if you adore the one suggesting, her recommendation is not a guarantee that the therapist will be helpful. You might be able to superficially research the recommended professional by examining any available ads in sources such as the Yellow Pages of the phone book, but you must look beyond the flashiness of the ads.

If you are ambulatory (up and able to walk around), the best way to find a good counselor is to visit a few. However, many women with HG are unable to get out of bed without becoming ill. (Please see appendix D for information on bed rest.) Some therapists are willing to offer their services over the phone. Talk to a few if you are able. If you get the feeling that the person just doesn't "get it," drop them like a bad habit, no explanation necessary. If you are personally insulted, secondarily victimized, or just not helped, then make a beeline for the door and don't look back.

Searching for a therapist that clicks with your personality and way of thinking and communicating can be pretty difficult for anyone, much less someone suffering a staggering illness. Also, at a time when finances are low due to inability to work, loss of employment and mounting medical bills, professional psychotherapy may be impossible. Do not lose hope!

Surfing Sufferers Unite

Many current and former sufferers are dedicated and eager to help other victims of HG. The illness is as old as time but the movement of women who are outraged at poor treatment is coming forward and gaining momentum. At this time, the best way to find HG peers is on the Internet. No one is more qualified to talk about the personal suffering experienced in HG than someone who has been there. Particularly encouraging are the stories of those that have suffered severely and had successful pregnancy outcomes. At a time when we feel we are drowning, peer support can give us something to hold onto. In their success, we can find new hope.

Physical Treatment

This one is listed last, but physical treatment is THE most successful psychological treatment. Alleviate the suffering, and the related emotional crisis will wane. There is more than one way to try and achieve this, and this book is filled with positive options. You may be surprised at the choices you didn't know you had!

Nani's Story

My husband and I are planners and we thought very long and hard before deciding to bring a child into this world. We tried to get pregnant for six months. I guess I still feel the need to express just how much we wanted our daughter, because I received so much abuse from medical personnel who claimed I had HG because I had maternal issues and wasn't really sure that I wanted to be pregnant. How dare they!

This is how it went: I threw up for the first time on a Thursday, stayed home from work on Friday, was sick to my stomach all weekend and assumed I had the flu. I threw up again on Sunday night. Monday I went to work and got a pregnancy test on my lunch break. Boom! Positive. I shook with excitement. I called my family practitioner and told her that I was pregnant and feeling very sick. She told me that I probably just had the flu, because I was too early to be so sick. Then it really started; I was vomiting all the time. One week after my first vomiting episode I called my doctor's office and told them that I had been throwing up all week, urinating less, not eating anything and asked them if it was normal. They told me it wasn't normal and asked me to come in immediately. I drove up to the city with my puke bucket in hand.

I was dehydrated and sent to the ER for rehydration and Phenergan. I left there feeling great! Heck, I could do this once a week and go through the pregnancy with no problem! No such luck. The Phenergan worked for one week only. I was able to work, but I am really stubborn and had a bad case of the "but we need the money." My first hospitalization was a week before Thanksgiving. I went to the doctor's office with my husband and my sister to ask them to terminate the pregnancy. I am unable to use the term "abort," because in my mind, abortion is a choice and termination is something one is physically forced to do because of an illness. My mother says it is all the same, but it isn't the same to me.

When my doctor asked me if termination was what I really wanted, I told her, "No, but I just don't think I can do this. The Phenergan isn't working. I'm just too sick; I can't stand it anymore." She told me that we hadn't tried all of the possibilities. She asked me if I wanted to try other options. Of course I did! She admitted me. I was on IV fluids for four days and released on the fifth. A nurse suggested they try Kytril.

Total hospitalizations from November to February were seven. I am unable to count the number of ER visits I had for rehydration. During one of my hospitalizations I was given Compazine. This stopped the vomiting but sent me to the ER again because of a bad reaction. The doctor at the ER advised me to take a Compazine-Benadryl cocktail. This worked, but I was so worried that my baby was going to be harmed because of all these drugs. During this entire time I was struggling with terminating the pregnancy. If only it had been possible to terminate the pregnancy but keep the baby... if we had the technology to take the baby out and grow her in a jar I would have done it in a heartbeat. I didn't want her to die, but how much can anyone take?

I survived on water. I was told that this would be OK for the baby until twenty weeks and then we would need to worry. All smells bothered me but the worst was the smell of the baby, which smelled like my husband coming through my skin. I know that sounds crazy, and I am sure that only an HG patient would know what I mean. Everyone thinks I'm nuts when I describe it, but I know exactly what I smelled. The scent of my husband still bothers me because of that pregnancy.

In January I decided to get a new doctor who admitted me to the hospital and pulled me off all my medications. She told me that they were all too dangerous for the baby and that the number of medications I was on was "ridiculous." On my second stay, I was throwing up blood and begging for Pepcid because the burning was so bad. Finally, the doctor brought in this purple liquid that smelled like sour grapes. She said that she takes this stuff for heartburn and it works great so I should try it. It tasted like battery acid and hurt so bad that I immediately puked it up. On my third visit I called her up and told her that I was pseudo-suicidal. I promised I was not going to kill myself but told her that I was obsessed with thoughts of dying so the pain would finally end. She admitted me so that I had people around me at all times. This is when the "professional" opinions began.

They claimed that if I just "embraced my vomiting" it would stop. They said I needed to look deep within myself and find out why my body was rejecting the pregnancy. They also thought it would be best if I was admitted to a mental institution. I reminded them that I was not crazy but pregnant and sick. I will never understand how people so smart could not grasp that suffering taxes a person mentally and that I was only this way *because* of all the vomiting.

I had enough. I screamed, "THAT'S IT! TAKE IT OUT! I CAN NOT DO THIS ANYMORE!" The doctor got instantly nasty with me and said that I was too far along in the pregnancy and that there are laws, and I wouldn't find a doctor who would terminate. Thankfully, I didn't know any better and believed her. At this time we tried acupuncture. It didn't help. I threw up while the attendant was taking the needles out of my wrists and legs.

My doctor would not give up. Every time I would talk termination she would admit me. Insurance got fed up with all of the hospital stays, so they assigned a nurse to come to my home three days a week. This was emotionally hard for me, because "keeping up appearances" is something I value. However, I could no longer keep the house spotless; it was a mess and I was pretty embarrassed about it. The nurse was great, but this was just one more indignity, one more area of my life that I had lost control over. Depressing.

As twenty weeks approached, I was not getting any better. I had lost close to thirty pounds, was eating nothing and throwing up at least five to ten times an hour. The nurse came to administer IV fluids and, after seeing my condition, she phoned the doctor and said I needed to be admitted immediately. My mom drove me up there with my puke bucket in hand, full of blood, bile and vomit. I have to say that this was the worst point for my husband and me.

I paged the doctor on duty and demanded that they take the baby out of me and put an end to all of this madness. I was told that a termination could only be done the next day. The next day my doctor came in, told us the baby was healthy, and asked me what I wanted to do. My husband and I cried and cried. We wanted our daughter so bad. We planned for her. Damn the HG!

My dad got on the computer and pulled some info about what others did for the treatment of HG. One lady mentioned a PICC line for TPN and how it saved her life and her baby's. I asked my doctor about it and she researched it. I was her first HG patient. They came in and installed the PICC line in my arm, ran it through one of the main vessels and fed us through my veins. I was in the hospital for over a week, but it was because of the PICC line that we are both alive today.

Someone needed to be with me constantly, so my sister moved just down the road from me. The nurse came in every day to draw blood, weigh me, and take vital signs. I had to have someone flush out my tubes several times a day to prevent clogging. Every day I would get out all my equipment and switch my bag while sitting there crying. I knew it was saving me and helping the baby, but it was so depressing and scary to have to be my own medical "professional." I didn't have a degree in nursing and believe that someone more qualified should have been managing my PICC. It was all so depressing, so they put me on Prozac. I was still throwing up with the TPN but there was less stress and fear knowing that we were getting nutrition.

I stayed on TPN for six weeks, which got me to the last trimester of the pregnancy. I weighed less than I did when I got pregnant. I still threw up every day, but I was able to eat small amounts and stop losing weight. At full-term, I delivered a nearly seven pound baby girl. I threw up through the entire delivery, but it was finally over! She is alive and well and a true miracle. I have never loved anyone so much. She is perfect. Very intelligent and maybe even advanced. It is so comforting to know that all of those medications didn't harm her.

When I had been sick with HG, I was forced to take a leave of absence from work. I didn't believe we could do it with our finances, but we did. That leave of absence helped me get through my HG and even showed me that I could be a stay-at-home mom. I fought too hard for my daughter; I'm not going to miss one minute of her precious life!

ADVOCACY

TWELVE
Psychology and Self-Advocacy

When doctors refuse to recognize a real, physical, medical condition, a patient is at risk. Women have literally died due to such dereliction. HG has been assigned an official numerical disease rating (ICD 643)[140] and has been presented as a disease in studies and a major professional conference on pregnancy-related nausea and vomiting.[141] Even so, one paper boldly reminds the reader that "HG is not a disease."[142] It goes on to suggest that younger women or those with first pregnancies may not be able to cope as well with pregnancy as older, "more experienced" women. The "blame game" ensures the elusion of a cure, promotes suffering, causes the deaths of women and children, and hinders or puts an end to family building in those who don't want to risk a recurrence.

HG is so debilitating that a sufferer may find it difficult, if not impossible, to carry out even the most basic of daily tasks such as brushing her teeth, bathing, getting out of bed, or even raising her head to attempt to take a pill. Some women are too sick to talk on the phone. One woman endured nine months of HG only to be too weak to give birth. The doctors delivered her baby via C-section. Shortly thereafter I read an article in a nursing magazine that spoke of another patient who ended her pregnancy as soon as it was possible to do so without harming the baby.[143] She elected to have a cesarean section nearly a month early, and doctors consented, as she was too physically weak to give birth. Think about that.

Emotional Effects of HG

Many physicians underestimate the long-term physical and psychological effects of weeks of eating very little or nothing at all. Women abort children they *want* because of this disease. Others, after giving birth to their first child, consent to sterilization because of it! Many women have lost their jobs and/or their marriages due to the increased demands of HG or residual issues that HG introduced.[144] HG is anything but a normal component of pregnancy.

We've all been eating since the day we were born, and it's disturbing to suddenly lose the ability. An HG sufferer can feel herself literally starving, but she can do nothing about it aside from accepting alternative methods of feeding if her doctor gives her that option. This, coupled with the unpleasant side effects of drug treatments, can certainly precipitate depression.

Depression does not cause HG, but the depression HG causes can increase the physical suffering. For example, if starvation, hyper-vomiting, and concerns about her child's health upset a woman to the point of tears, she may cry. Stomach contractions, nasal secretions, the taste of tears, and other physical components of crying can be enough to initiate a vomiting cycle, and this exacerbates suffering.

Busy professionals who view patients in brief sessions must understand that the HG sufferer is not going to be able to accurately represent herself as the functioning person she and her family knew *before* the illness. Anyone in the throes of such an illness is going to be upset, confused, depressed and in a fair amount of physical and emotional distress. It is unconscionable to make a personality judgment at such a time. Instead, the professional must assume that the emotional state is a result of the illness and not vice versa.

One in four women is depressed.[145] Five in one thousand women get HG. The ratio of women who suffer from emotional issues does not correlate with the number of HG sufferers.

Every high school has a number of troubled girls who engage in premarital sex and have children in their teens. Most of these moms skate through their decidedly un hyperemetic pregnancies. In fact, one study showed that psychiatric conditions actually lowered the incidence of pregnancy-related vomiting![146]

Consider the following real situations and see if you can guess the one thing all the women have in common:

1. "Blair's" biological father sexually molested her repeatedly from the time she was in diapers until her seventeenth year of life. She was not a happy camper and was so plagued by negative emotional issues that she was unable to nurse her children because she couldn't stand the thought of anything involving her breasts.

2. "Daisy," who was in her third trimester had obviously resolved to have and keep her baby. However, she expressed that she didn't want to be pregnant at all, didn't want another baby, and very much resented her unplanned pregnancy.

3. "Leigh," a chronic alcoholic, made headlines by trying to drink her unborn baby to death. She consumed alcohol like a flame and was drunk in the delivery room when she gave birth to a little girl who was severely and permanently disabled due to fetal alcohol syndrome.

What's the one thing these women have in common? All of them had serious emotional issues but none of them ever had HG.

The Blame Game
Friends, family, and even doctors may blame HG on immature personalities or psychological conflict. This attitude kicks us when we are down and inflicts unjustified guilt and emotional pain. The two most common charges healthy people make against those with HG are that they don't really want their baby or that they are just trying to get attention.

Baby Rejection
Some people make unfeeling assertions that the sufferer is unconsciously making herself ill because she is ambiguous about wanting her baby (especially if the baby was a surprise). It is particularly offensive and bewildering when a learned physician suggests this. No doctor would suggest that an oncology patient gave herself cancer because she didn't really want to live.

Kaltenbach seems to have started this whole "HG as a neurosis" mess in 1891. In 1968 a frustrated Fairweather concurred and published a study that was shamefully uncontrolled and obviously biased.[147] He hypothesized that women with HG had mental issues that basically caused psychosomatic illness. Certain objective personality tests were administered only to women with HG, so the study was uncontrolled. Also, the psychologists who conducted the personal interviews knew that the women had HG. If they were aware of the psychogenic theory, which they probably were, their own bias could have affected results. Nothing was done to prevent bias. Lastly, the one objective personality test that was administered to both women with HG and pregnant women without HG showed no significant differences. *Interestingly*, Fairweather claimed otherwise, and his conclusions were left to stand. Even more concerning is the fact that this study is commonly quoted in medical textbooks and other professional literature today.

The constant influence of such a paper on the modern doctor is baffling, especially since there have been a smattering of newer, more controlled studies that conclude there is absolutely no evidence which supports the psychosomatic angle. In one study, three physicians address the misconception put forth by older literature that HG manifests out of a rejection of pregnancy.[148] They reason, "This view is not supported by evidence and is utterly rejected by our study showing women ready to endure immense suffering before giving up wanted pregnancies." Many authors agree, and I believe we are finally beginning to see a shift away from the punitive insinuation of neurosis. (For great articles on this issue, see the S. Munch and Tichener-Bogen papers in the Consulted Works section.)

In published research one hundred five married women were studied for social and psychological differences; women with HG were compared to asymptomatic women.[149] There were no differences regarding planned and unplanned pregnancies and positive feelings about the baby at the beginning and by the seventh month of pregnancy. *Differences only appeared during the period of HG* and were due to the illness itself and the non-supportive way folks chose to deal with the sufferer. Still, many physicians incorrectly attribute HG and even the varying degrees of HG to an array of psychological aspects.

If a pregnancy was unplanned and the mother happens to suffer from HG, some will say she doesn't want the baby. If she argues that she *does* want the baby then she is suffering from an unconscious rejection. If she has problems with her mother then, absurdly, she is suspected of rejecting her mother through the baby. If the pregnancy *was* planned, problems at home or mental instability are said to be the cause of HG. And pity the ailing mother who actually did suffer from unrelated depression prior to HG! The fact is that many women experience HG before they even know they are pregnant, so how can they be rejecting a baby they don't even know exists?

One article describes a particular scenario in which a mother asserted that she wanted her unplanned child.[150] Even though her psychological tests all came back normal, the authors claim it was somehow "clear" that her HG symptoms had a significant emotional component. Although she said she was not ambivalent about having her baby, she made the "mistake" of expressing the common feelings of anxiety that concern most first time parents. She was concerned with her ability to properly care for a newborn, had fears about being a good mother, was vexed by her mother-in-law, and wondered sometimes if her husband wasn't more loyal to his own family than to her. Because she dared to address these very normal concerns, the authors came to the conclusion that, in fact, she *was* ambivalent about wanting the baby. She was given hypnotic suggestions "so that she did not need to continue to *make herself sick* over all of this" (emphasis mine). Eventually her HG resolved, and the authors considered hypnosis a success. What they don't discuss is what week the HG stopped or the other treatments the woman underwent during the time she received hypnosis. Other variables could have accounted for the resolution.

In another article, a severe HG sufferer was told her symptoms were psychosomatic.[151] Janet Tichener-Bogen confides,

> "It was my first realization of being classified as a 'nut', blamed for my disease, my symptoms viewed as a weakness of character. More specifically, I was accused of rejecting my unborn child [subconsciously trying] to rid myself of my baby."

Three times this woman had HG severe enough to necessitate TPN via a centrally placed catheter. *Three times* she endured this for babies doctors claimed she didn't want.

Roughly four thousand, five hundred pregnant women terminate every single day in America.[152] If not wanting your baby makes you sick then a significant number, if not all, of these women, should have HG, and they don't. In fact, over 95% of all abortions are for social reasons and not maternal illness.[153] We live in an era in which a woman's access to abortion is easier and faster than access to the Internet. If a gal doesn't want her baby, she is *not* going to fight her way through even a day, much less months of HG's debilitation, victimization and humiliation. The psychogenic theory just doesn't add up.

Having a baby is an enormous step in a person's life, and any pregnancy authority will tell you that it's quite normal to experience stress and/or doubt concerning pregnancy and one's parenting capabilities. To say this equates rejecting pregnancy or that it causes HG is irresponsible, punitive and dangerous.

A United Kingdom Report on Confidential Enquiries into Maternal Deaths between 1991 and 1993 describes three fatalities due to HG.[154] In this day and age death due to HG is always suspicious, because, with all of the medical advances we have made, it really ought not to happen. A closer look into the UK deaths reveals that two of the women were diagnosed with psychosis when in fact they were suffering from Wernicke's encephalopathy due to substandard treatment of HG. In Wernicke's parts of the brain basically begin to atrophy due to malnutrition, specifically thiamine depletion, and it's relatively easy to prevent. If the HG had been validated as physical, if physicians had cared to learn more about the disease and proper treatment methods, if the sufferers had not been secondarily victimized by their healers, perhaps there would be six happy people alive today. Their treatment was archaic.

Attention-Seeking
Some friends, family members and even physicians mistakenly believe that HG is just regular morning sickness that the sufferer misrepresents. They hold one person to the measure of another. They can't help comparing the hyperemetic pregnancy to their own or someone else's normal pregnancy. The logic is that it was easy for one and so for all. These personalities secretly, and sometimes openly, have a very low opinion of HG sufferers, believing that they are big whiney babies who simply blow things way out of proportion in an effort to be pampered, showered with attention, or to get out

of work. It is not unusual to hear healthy people complain that a woman's HG is just a ploy for attention. It's irrational. There are *much* easier ways of getting attention. Wrestling alligators comes to mind.

Secondary Victimization

In the 1930's one abusive approach was to prevent HG patients from having any contact with their families for the first two days in the hospital.[155] These patients were also not given receptacles to throw up in and were forced to vomit all over themselves in bed. Nurses were then instructed to let patients sit in the emesis for a while before changing the bed linens and cleaning them up. This was supposed to "teach them a lesson" thereby encouraging them to "cut it out." Another method of therapy was to administer painfully harsh treatments to terrify the hyperemetic mother in hopes that she would stop vomiting in order to avoid further medical abuse.

Patients still report incidents such as medical staff making them empty their own vomit basins and engaging in intimidation. During my fourth pregnancy, the weekend rotation gastroenterologist came into my hospital room and started spouting off about how terribly dangerous my TPN was and how I really needed to "*try harder*" to eat in order to get off the TPN and reduce the "very real risk of something dreadful happening." Being no sort of rookie to this kind of thing I let him know in no uncertain terms just how much fun not eating and being on TPN was and told him that my body would darn well eat when it was ready. After I began to resolve the doctor came for another visit and patted himself on the back quipping that his "fear therapy" had worked. Don't think for a minute that I let him get away with it.

In yet another unpleasant episode in my fourth pregnancy, I was readmitted to the hospital for the millionth time due to a staph infection in my PICC line. I also had what resembled a massive bladder infection, a fever of one hundred three, and was puking up a fair amount of blood. My nurse came in to change my sheets and sat me in a chair where I puked, peed and had glycerin diarrhea all over myself. She stood me up to clean me off, and I told her I was going to pass out if I didn't sit back down immediately. After being told that there was "no physical reason" why I would be passing out, I crawled into the bed. The nurse stood over me annoyed with my "behavior" before finally shaking her head in genuine disgust. "Ashli, Ashli, Ashli," she started with disdain, "Pregnancy is a normal part of life." I was completely dumbfounded. "Do you think I am doing this to myself?!" I asked incredulously. "I didn't say that," she retorted. "I just think you're getting yourself all worked up." Some people just don't get it.

In contrast, no one accuses a patient of causing her cancer in an effort to get attention or the day off. Fortunately, the oncology patient does not feel the need to defend her mental health like the hyperemetic pregnant woman does. HG involves a certain bias that simply doesn't exist in other physical diseases that are better understood.

Folks may offer any number of offensive explanations regarding HG. Some have religious reasons for the illness, some have psychological reasons. These people have a lot in common with Job's comforters.

Rabbi Kushner, author of the book <u>When Bad Things Happen to Good People</u>, chronicles the events of the book of Job[156] and the explanations Job's buddies gave him for all of his suffering. His "comforters" conveyed various punitive rationales in order to placate Job and most importantly, in order to reassure themselves that suffering makes sense and is therefore truly avoidable. Times may change but people do not.

Behaving Badly: The Rationale

Most people mean well, and it is human nature to try and make order of chaos. For some people there simply has to be a reason for everything, and these reasons can be pretty painful. Surprisingly, most of these awful comments are *intended* to soothe, to help you identify what you are doing wrong, so that you can correct your behavior and resolve the illness. If only it were that easy! Those who are on the outside looking in can afford to make judgments, because life still makes sense to them; they can eat and drink and take care of themselves and their children, and they don't have to be around you for long stretches of time. Perhaps confidently assessing your situation makes *them* feel better. If they know why you are sick and what you can do to get better then they are able to maintain the comforting illusion that they are in complete control over their own lives, and nothing of this nature can ever happen to them. Fortunately, the majority will live out their lives without ever getting HG, and they will never have to wonder for a moment that they might have been wrong about us.

Physicians go to school for almost two decades to learn their trade; their specialty is knowledge. Knowing what is wrong with you and why, knowing what to expect if treatment is or is not initiated, knowing what remedy to prescribe, knowing what the odds are... *Knowing* is the cornerstone of a physician's ability. When you take this component away from someone who relies that heavily on knowledge, it can make her uncomfortable. For some, it's easier to have an answer even if they have to invent one. This is human, but it's wrong. As Tichener-Bogen puts it, "...medicine's tendency to scapegoat diagnoses to neuroticism is a huge barrier to the advancement of medical knowledge – particularly for women."[157]

Weathering Insults

Defending yourself against judgment, misinformation and unhelpful advice requires a lot of energy when energy is at an all time low. Choose your battles wisely reserving what little energy you do have for those who need it the most: you and your tiny tummy tot. Yes, it is difficult to ignore the insensitive comments, particularly when coming from caregivers or those most important to us. It is very common to feel abandoned by those whom we have loved the most. Reading this book may help you understand the motivations of well-meaning people, but understanding does not necessarily make it hurt any less. Know that you're not alone.

If you have a good friend who avoids the pitfalls of explaining why HG happened to you or how you can feel better, make her your designated advocate. If you find a good doctor go online to hyperemesis.org and list the name and geographical area of the terrific professional who afforded you and your child excellent health care and treated you with dignity and respect. Help another mother and child beat HG.

June's Story

At thirty years of age I eagerly planned my pregnancy and was thrilled when I finally got pregnant after two very early miscarriages (at five weeks). The horror of HG started in week five of my pregnancy. I was put on stronger and progressively "riskier" drugs to no benefit. In fact my reaction to the drugs was very negative. By the time I was fourteen weeks along, I had been in the hospital twice, lost thirty-five pounds, and was vomiting an orange mixture of bile and blood three times an hour. I had not eaten anything in two weeks and was unable to bear even the smell or taste of water for the last week. It may sound dramatic to anyone who hasn't been there, but I begged for death. I started going into convulsions while in the hospital and developed a high fever. I developed terrible acidosis. An ultrasound showed that the single fetus was small but strong;; however, I miscarried in the fourteenth week.

I cannot even begin to explain the emotional turmoil, which was very much complicated by the lack of understanding from my family and friends. The lack of support during that time remains a source of pain even today. Thank God I have a loving and supportive husband who has always stood by me.

We do not have any living children and have sadly decided that the risk is too great to attempt another pregnancy. I consulted with several doctors and specialists, and without exception, found them to be incredibly ignorant and completely insensitive. I've stopped going to doctors, and I've stopped talking to others about this, as most of their "supportive" comments only hurt my feelings.

Through all of this I got to see my family and friends for who they really are: people who abandoned me when I needed them the most. I no longer maintain contact with the majority of them.

HG is not a problem that lasts a few months and then vanishes. In cases of severe HG, the results can have an impact on the rest of your life.

THIRTEEN
How to Care for a Person with HG

H G is something the vast majority of people never experience. While we can be thankful for this, a lack of experience can lead to difficulties when dealing with those suffering from the disease. Trouble may arise when caregivers try to help by doling out advice. While this advice may make perfect sense generally, it may be unhelpful or even harmful in the specific instance of HG. Many sufferers relate that ineffective advice often involves:

- taking a walk outside
- taking Emetrol
- employing various home remedies
- opening a window
- eating crackers, peppermint candy or several small meals a day; forcing yourself to eat
- sipping ginger ale
- applying cold washcloths
- thinking more about the baby; having a positive mental attitude, etc.

None of these suggestions is a remedy for HG. In fact, depending upon the severity of HG, most of them can actually exacerbate vomiting. Movements, inside/outside scents, flavors, oral consumption, thermal extremes, etc., have all been known to over-stimulate and cause vomiting. Also, for the record, happy thoughts don't cure cancer, and they won't cure HG. That being said, certain individuals may respond to some of the above advice, and that's just dandy. However, these suggestions are typically beneficial for easing the effects of normal "morning sickness," and HG goes beyond morning sickness. Women should not be pressured to try things that they don't feel will be helpful. Also, women should consult their physicians before following anyone's advice.

Help for Helpers

(This section is available in the form of a free pamphlet designed to educate concerned parties efficiently. See Appendix E.)

If you are interested in helping a hyperemetic but don't know where to begin, you might try any of the following:

- Offer to clean the house of someone suffering from HG. Pay particular attention to the bathroom. The sufferer may be horrified for you to go in there, because there may be lingering traces of vomit. This is precisely the reason why this room must be cleaned. Try to reassure her that the vomit will not bother you, but if you sense that the idea is causing her significant anxiety you may want to abandon it. If you can convince her to let you clean the bathroom, consider using unscented cleaners such as baking soda, salt and water.

- Offer to change the bed sheets if she feels comfortable with that and can get out of bed for a moment. When one spends a lot of time in bed with HG the sheets can become sullied with body oils, sweat and sometimes traces of vomit or other unpleasant elements. The smell of these sheets can exacerbate vomiting, and they really should be changed every day.

- Offer to prepare meals for the spouse of a hyperemetic woman. Many times a large casserole can be frozen and will last the spouse several days. It is helpful to enlist other people to cook/deliver a meal at least one night a week. In this way a variety of meals can be prepared for the spouse throughout the week. The availability of fast food may seem to trivialize the issue of meal donation, yet this is one of the easiest and most helpful things one can do. The spouse rarely has time to cook for himself (and can't risk the smell of food cooking anyway) and tires quickly of fast food and TV dinners. If there are children in the household they need meals that are both tasty and nutritious during what can be a very traumatic time for them. Surprisingly, the person who can benefit the most from meal donation is the hyperemetic woman, because she no longer has to worry about her family or feel guilty over not being able to fulfill what may have been her previous roles as menu planner and chef.

- The hyperemetic woman often suffers from hyperolfaction, which basically means she has the nose of a Bloodhound. Any scent can cause vomiting and can make it impossible to eat anything for long periods of time. If available, offer to lend a small microwave oven (and a long extension cord) to the family you are helping. This will enable the spouse to prepare meals far away from the sufferer such as in the garage.

- If you are wearing perfume or are a smoker, be cautious when entering the house of a hyperemetic woman. Scents can precipitate violent vomiting cycles, which can cause a trip to the hospital. Likewise, you may want to refrain from entering the house with a cup of coffee. It is another noxious smell that is wonderful when one is not suffering from hyperolfaction but "deadly" when one is. Scented hairsprays, soaps, detergents, etc., can cause pungent odors others may not be aware of. Try to be conscious of any aroma, and avoid it like the plague. Not all women with HG suffer from hyperolfaction, but it never hurts to assume that the person you are helping does.

- Unless specifically asked, use caution when turning on the radio, TV, bright lights, etc. Any stimulation can cause vomiting.

- Offer to keep the pet of someone with HG.

- Offer to tend the yard. However, if windows are open or the jalousie type, you may want to refrain from using gas-powered implements close to the home. These items give off a smelly exhaust that can cause vomiting.

- Offer to wash the car.

- Offer to baby-sit the children, and do something fun with them when they are with you. Mother's illness can be very scary and depressing to them. A mental respite is crucial. Likewise, guys can invite the spouse to a movie, ball game, dinner or a night of cards, etc. He may feel helpless, guilty and worried about his wife and growing child. Breaks are absolutely necessary for those who witness constant suffering.

- Offer to attend medical appointments (particularly if the woman is single). Often the woman feels too vulnerable to question medical staff because she has placed her trust and life in their hands. Also, she may be too sick to fully absorb and remember her doctor's advice. You can be a second set of ears. If you feel the woman isn't getting adequate medical treatment, discuss this with her. Perhaps she will come to the same conclusion and seek a second opinion from a different doctor in a different practice.

- If the woman is able to watch TV and wants to, see if you can lend her a TV or VCR, set it up in her room, and maybe even check out videos from the library. She might also be able to read books and play hand-held games, though many will only feel well enough to watch a little TV at best.

- One of the best things you can do is learn about the illness. This will help you help others. For example, if a woman has difficulties with odors, you will recognize hyperolfaction and can offer scent-reducing suggestions. If she complains that even saliva is making her vomit, research can tell you that ptyalism can be problematic in HG. You can relate that it's relatively common in HG and offer suggestions and so forth. Good sources of information on HG are in medical libraries, and a few good sites can be found on the Internet.

Dos and Don'ts

- Do listen if the sick mother wants to talk. Let her know that, although you don't know exactly what she is going through, you will assist her in any way you can.

- *Do follow through on all offers to help.*

- Do be sensitive and reconsider impractical advice. For example, you may think a nice walk in "fresh air" will be just the thing to revitalize the HG sufferer. Realistically, she may be unable to walk to the living room without throwing up. Try and respect her ability to know best what she can handle.

- Don't pressure the woman to eat. HG is not an "eating disorder." The mom sorely wants to eat but can't. She will eat as soon as she is physically able. Forcing herself to eat can cause vomiting, and while pressuring her won't help her eat, it will increase her stress. This can:

  a) isolate her by reinforcing her belief that no one understands that she is sick and not trying to be difficult

  b) increase her feelings of failure when she is not able to perform so basic a task

    c)   ultimately make you unavailable to her if she wants to avoid you

- Don't comment that her vomiting and inability to eat are bad for the baby. She knows it can't be good. Reminding her only causes more anxiety about the health of her baby and makes her feel like a bad mother. It is quite comforting to know that studies do not show babies of hyperemetic mothers to be at an increased risk for congenital abnormalities despite the mother's compromised nutritional status and antiemetic drug use.[158-160]

- Be especially helpful to single women who are hyperemetic and have no one to assist them at home. They are at particular risk for therapeutic termination and desperately need your help. This is especially true if they have other children to care for.

Marney's Story

My HG story began with my first pregnancy when I was on a plane to Australia. It was about three to four days since conception and I had no idea I was pregnant. The plane began descending for landing, and I said to the person next to me that I really did not feel too well. I was overwhelmed with nausea. I got myself off the plane but had to be ferried through customs and immigration by wheelchair. They took me up to see a doctor, but I refused and lay down for about fifteen minutes until I felt well enough to leave the airport on my own. I got myself into bed and slept all day.

I was OK until eight days later when I woke up feeling nauseous. For the first time I thought I might be pregnant. Five days after that, I tested positive within seconds. Doctors count weeks of pregnancy from the first day of the last menstrual period, so I was about five weeks pregnant and feeling sick 24-hours a day. This continued for the rest of the pregnancy. I vomited occasionally, and spent as much time as possible lying down. I needed to stay in a silent room and had to put sheets over all the windows in the house. Twenty-five days after the plane ride, I began to vomit several times a day. I was losing weight and telling people how awful I felt, and everyone reassured me that this was what pregnancy is like.

I began my month in bed where I couldn't even watch TV because the images would add to the nausea. After losing seven pounds in ten days I called the doctor. She suggested I take B6 and Bonine and call her if I got worse. It didn't help. I couldn't even drink water. I called the doctor again and she prescribed Compazine suppositories. The next day I woke up feeling some relief from the nausea, but I was still very shaky. I felt like I couldn't wait until my next doctor's appointment, so I called the office. They told me to drink fluids and come in at the scheduled appointment. When I was leaving to go to the appointment my tongue started to push slowly out of my mouth out of my control. Shortly after getting to the office my teeth started to clench together causing intense pain. I tried my hardest to keep my mouth open, but I couldn't. I asked to be seen immediately and broke down in tears. The doctor came in and asked all these questions and didn't tell me what was going on. I moaned loudly because of the pain, and she yelled at me before giving me a shot of Benadryl to counteract the reaction. Just before the shot, my neck started painfully going backwards out of my control while my teeth were still clenching up. It was scary, but I got the shot and had relief in about fifteen very long minutes. The doctor came in and said I appeared dehydrated and sent me to the ER for IV fluids. Before I left, she explained that the reaction might return and told me to ask for IV Benadryl.

I got to the hospital and sat in a chair waiting for a bed for nearly two hours. Shortly after getting the bed I had the dystonic reaction again and told a nurse who just ignored me. I finally asked another nurse about the intensity of the pain and got the doctor immediately. Five minutes after receiving the IV Benadryl the symptoms were still there, so they gave me more Benadryl until I slowly got better. I got my fluids and was sent home with instructions to discard the Compazine. Soon enough I was terribly sick again and vomiting six times a day. I called the doctor and she sent me back to the ER for fluids and an ultrasound. She finally told me I had HG.

They catheterized me and filled up my bladder and did an ultrasound and heard a heartbeat. I was in so much pain from the procedure I couldn't even look at my baby. I asked them to remove the catheter when they were done and they said no one was available. I was in a lot of pain and just did not need the catheter on top of it all. I threatened to pull it out myself, and magically someone appeared and removed it. I was sent home on Tigan suppositories and Benadryl to counteract a possible dystonic reaction. I still vomited some and felt nauseous 24-hours a day.

Each time I took a suppository I would have a bowel movement which popped the thing back out. A few days later at the doctor's office I asked for oral Tigan and found some relief. I was still confined to my bed and very tired. I had to eat something every half an hour, and if it was the right thing I wouldn't get nauseous or vomit; otherwise I would. Starting at eleven weeks I slowly got out of bed for an hour a day. During the previous month I had been working from home primarily making phone calls. I was so bored. My mind was still very active even though my body was not. I couldn't sleep well. At twelve weeks I actually went to work a few times. My breasts shrunk and so did my abdomen, and I felt a little better.

I miscarried my baby in the thirteenth week. My body felt alive again, but my heart was broken. My daughter was fully formed. I delivered her at home. She was perfect and beautiful, and I counted all her fingers and toes.

I still struggle with it, wondering why I was put through so much physical pain only to experience such intense emotional pain. I was surprised to miscarry because so many people said the sickness was a sign of a healthy pregnancy. They were wrong. I am going to try again someday.

FOURTEEN
Tips for Sufferers

Quick List

1. See Appendix E for a free educational pamphlet that you may reproduce and distribute to family and friends who are looking for real ways to help you.

2. If prenatal vitamins make you vomit, ask your doctor if you can take Flintstones Complete chewable children's vitamins.

3. If you are constantly dehydrated ask your doctor about home IVs.

4. If your family needs food but you can't physically shop, see if your market offers a grocery delivery service. They can deliver prepared meals from the deli or the frozen food section.

5. If you are cold use a blanket instead of heaters. Heaters can exacerbate dehydration. If you are hot, use air conditioning to prevent the loss of precious fluids through sweating.

6. Drink what you can and never assume. I thought I would surely die if I tried a milk product, but in one pregnancy I found that for one week, I could drink

chocolate milk, and chocolate milk only, without throwing it right back up. (The same principle applies to food: Eat what you can, avoid eating what you can't, and don't feel guilty.)

7. If you aren't on IVs, monitor and record your fluid intake religiously. If you eat any morsel of food record that as well, so that you can give your physicians an exact representation of your nutritional status. If monitoring and recording is too strenuous for you, try to enlist someone else's help.

8. Keep a solution of baking soda and water near the toilet so you can quickly rinse out your mouth after vomiting. This solution is a base that will help to neutralize stomach acid and prevent dental damage.

9. Buy test strips and monitor ketones in your urine so that you can personally convey your status to your physician and get the care you need as soon as you need it.

10. Suffering from feelings of isolation/alienation? Find a compatible "HG buddy" online by visiting some of the URLs listed in Appendix B of this book.

Expanded List
1. *Learn about ptyalism and management methods.* Ptyalism is the sense that one is producing too much saliva. Saliva levels may not actually be increased, but the act of swallowing liquid can create such nausea that it heightens awareness of saliva production and swallowing. This new awareness can make it

seem like there is excess saliva, and nausea may prevent you from swallowing it. Ptyalism can last for months. The only thing to do is suffer through. As with many of us, the simple solution is to live with a disposable spit cup in hand. Conversely, you may buy an aspirator and continuously suck it out, but that may be too involved. Some find that they can suck on hard candy and swallow the flavored saliva without throwing up. Ptyalism is aggravating and gross, but time will cure it.

2. *Learn about hyperolfaction and management methods.*

Hyperolfaction is a heightened sense of smell. In fact, odor perception is so grossly amplified that it becomes problematic. Formerly pleasant aromas can make a hyperemetic vomit. Also, generally imperceptible scents may become unbearable. Unfortunately, this can make the sufferer look crazy or exaggeratory.

Common Offenders
- Food/refrigerator scents
- Flowers (which people tend to deliver when you're sick)
- Perfume/cologne/samples in magazines
- Soap/detergent/fabric softener
- Room fresheners/disinfectants
- Coffee/coffee breath
- Dirty diapers
- Cigarettes/ashtrays/cigarette breath
- Body odors (including one's own): vomit, gas, sweat, elimination
- Burning trash/leaves/wood/etc.
- Trash cans

Theories

The cause of hyperolfaction is unknown. Some theorized culprits are: hormones, vestiges, and built-in fail-safes.

Estrogen is a hormone that seems to affect the vascularity of the respiratory tract. Since pregnant women have more estrogen, perhaps the vascularity increases, which results in being more able to detect odors.

Perhaps hyperolfaction is a leftover from prehistory, a vestige which evolutionists theorize hasn't quite been eradicated in some. In days of yore a pregnant woman may have needed to be able to detect dangerous animals from far distances so that she could get a head start when fleeing with a huge, heavy belly.[161] A heightened perception of smell might facilitate this.

Another theory reasons that unclean places have a tendency to smell. Perhaps hyperolfaction prompts the woman to seek a cleaner environment, which would be especially important in pregnancy.

Maybe hyperolfaction is only a way to keep us from eating spoiled food. While suffering from HG, I could smell the items in our closed refrigerator two rooms away from behind a door with towels stuffed in the crack. I could not even attempt to eat. What did it mean?

From the beginning of pregnancy up until around twelve weeks the baby is rapidly developing all her major organs and physical features. Because she is not fully developed, and because the development is so dramatic during this time, the baby is at her highest risk for environmentally caused malformations.

Ingesting toxins could be especially devastating. One might draw the obvious conclusion that a heightened sense of olfactory ability is actually beneficial in a normal pregnancy.

Despite all these theories, no one really knows what causes hyperolfaction. We do know that it's enough to precipitate some bad vomiting spells, and since HG consists of vomiting, and vomit usually smells bad, we've got a cyclical combination.

No-Nos the Nose Knows

Odors are everywhere; they invade all environmental spaces. Previously innocuous sources can be terribly bothersome when you have hyperolfaction. What was once a clean, good-smelling home can be transformed into a nauseating nightmare. Food preparation, bathrooms, your body, the bodies of others, pets, the mail and even "fresh" air can increase suffering and trigger vomiting spells that result in a hospital stay. However, there are options for combating troublesome odors.

Kitchen Odors

Other people in the household will continue to need food, and they will often offend you physically (and even psychologically) by eating it. Meal preparation can be a hyperolfactory nightmare. At such a time, the odor of food cooking reminds me of the old cartoon where the scent of a pie baking in the oven sends its long, diaphanous arm through the twists and turns of the house seeking out inhabitants to entice. With HG however, the arm grabs and throttles the sufferer. This extremely heightened sense of smell can be one of the worst vomit-inducing factors. Runners up are sight, texture and taste of food and the mechanical act of swallowing. Whereas food can technically be avoided, totally avoiding food aromas is tricky. The easiest thing to do is to stuff a rolled up towel in the crack of the door that divides you from the rest of the house. If that doesn't work there are other options. My husband got a small, portable microwave and an extension cord and "nuked" the food outside. If the dish was particularly noxious smelling he would even *eat* it outside. When it rained there were obviously electrocution issues with the microwave, and he would eat a sandwich or simply dine out.

Bathroom Odors

If your bathroom is connected to your room, you might be able to smell the water dripping out of the metallic faucet into the ceramic sink. You might smell the dank shower drain and all the hair and soap nestled moistly in it. If you can, enlist the aid of others who can attempt to rid soiled bathrooms of telltale foul odors. Remind your support team that using chemicals with noxious fumes might trigger vomiting episodes. Request odorless cleaning agents such as baking soda and water. Lemon juice and salt are also good cleaning agents, but the aroma of fresh citrus may be intolerable.

Your Own Odors

Another offensive home-related scent could actually be you! Unscented deodorant can work to prevent at least one offensive odor, but I can't tell you how many times my own gas sent me puking to the toilet. I can laugh about it now, but at the time it was terrible. When you're this sick, you may not even have the strength to clean up your own vomit. It can splatter on the floor, bed, sweaty sheets and/or clothes that haven't been changed in a couple of days. Even if you somehow manage to avoid the splatters, just the smell of your own body odor on your clothes, sheets or hair can be enough to set you off.

Hot, humid climates can speed up the loss of fluid from the body and enhance odors. However, no matter where you live, often you may be cold due to weight loss. Lying in front of a ceramic heater may seem like the thing to do, but the dry heat will cause you to dehydrate more quickly and could precipitate a smelly vomiting cycle. It is better to wrap yourself in clean blankets.

Every other day or so, helpers should change your bed linens. In addition, your sheets and clothes should be washed in unscented detergent/fabric softener. Bathe every day if at all possible. You may need help. In my most severe pregnancy, I was given sponge baths for weeks at a time, and some days my husband had to hold my head up for my weekly shampoo. Support is integral.

Unscented shampoo, conditioner, soaps and lotions can be purchased at your local health food market even if the market has to special-order it. Beware: contrary to the label, many of these products do have an odd, unpleasant odor. Try different brands until you find one that is least offensive to you. Eventually, I used a lightly scented salon shampoo that could have been labeled "Sweet Stink." It was awful, but it was better than the weird smelling "unscented" shampoo I tried initially.

I learned a lot from my first pregnancy, and the next time I got pregnant I opted for a very short haircut. Vanity be damned! It was worth the freedom from the hassle and odor of clinging vomit. And in a way my shearing was symbolic. After all, one of the first things issued a new soldier is a short coiffure.

Others' Odors

Hopefully you do not live alone. If there are others at home they are often big stinkers. One mother swears her hyperolfaction was so severe that she could actually smell her unborn baby! When I suggested that it might have been the scent of a pregnancy hormone, she assured me that it was not and added that, years later, "He still smells the same way."

Others' good hygiene can become an issue. Folks slather the body with aromatic soaps, saturate hair with scented shampoos, coat underarms with odiferous deodorants, brush teeth with pungent smelling pastes and then douse mouths with scented, alcoholic mouthwash. Heads are drenched with smelly gels and hairsprays, and scented powders and even scented cosmetics are applied elsewhere. If that isn't enough, clothes are washed in perfumed detergents and softened with scented solutions all while the immaculately clean person munches away on a pungent stick of cinnamon gum. The craziest part is that all of these tactics don't even prevent the occasional case of bad breath or body odor! It's a winning combination for a plethora of emetic episodes.

Mornings can be especially difficult. Morning breath and stale body odors are a bit of a rude awakening for the hyperemetic. Later in the day, smelly foods and beverages can transform annoying, minty fresh breath into a nightmarish fog. If the alcohol or coffee-drinker is a mere annoyance, the cigarette smoker is "death on a stick." The foul stench of soured breath and burnt tobacco oozes from every pore of a smoker. There is no way to scrub it off or cover it up. It's a second skin that can gag a hyperemetic all the way to the toilet if not the hospital.

To combat these things, ask people oh so nicely to stop smoking, put a moratorium on perfuming, and take other actions to make the environment scent-free for you and your growing baby. Hand them this book, marked to this section, and hope that they'll put their preferences aside and be eager to help you survive your crisis.

Pet Odors

During the long, lonely period of HG, it helps to have a constant companion, and no one is going to stick by your side like your pet, but when you have hyperolfaction pet odor can be stomach turning. Your furry little darling may reek you right into the hospital, and something will have to be done. See if a family member or friend will board your paw pal for a while, send her to a kennel until you are well enough to tolerate her, or contact a church or a crisis pregnancy center and explain your situation to someone who claims to care. They may be able to take her for an extended vacation until you are well. It will be sad to see your pet go, but foul scents must be reduced. Remember, your pet will come back, and she'll more than likely have a new little friend to play with!

Mail-Order Odors

Certain magazines contain paper inserts laced with perfume samples. To the hyperemetic, these inserts can mean insta-vomit. Some magazines will mail issues without perfumed inserts if you notify them with this preference. Of course, perfumed inserts are no problem if you are too sick to read magazines!

Outside Odors

HG can be so severe that it limits mobility significantly. This can have you cooped up in bed for weeks or months. The imprisonment adds to the depression of the illness. Others may want to cheer you and may suggest that you go outside or open a window and get some "fresh air." However, the moist pile of dog poop baking in the neighbor's yard smells like a wooly mammoth plop and is hardly soothing. Also, if it's the fall season, people are out avidly burning trash and leaves, which is akin to the refreshing scent of smoldering oil tanks topped with hot roofing tar. Even when windows are closed, outside aromas can be a problem. Scents are evil and have a way of stealthily slithering in.

Sometimes one can reason with an offending neighbor, but if that doesn't work, caulks and tapes may seal up gaps and cracks blocking pesky odors. If, however, the smell of caulks and tapes send you to the toilet, you might try wearing a swimmer's pincher on your nose. It's certainly an option, although I must admit that when I tried this I felt and looked more than a little silly, and the constant pressure of the pincher hurt my nose and made me vomit anyway. Foiled again.

Additional Odor-Reducing Tips

Carpet deodorizer, smelly paint or other persistent scents may be difficult or impossible to get rid of. If closing the door or moving to a different room doesn't help, you can try masking the odor.

Some women use peppermint or citrus to mask other odors. When an offensive smell threatens, they whip out their lemons and snort like fiends. For me lemon and peppermint were as bad as any other offensive odor. If masking doesn't work, one may have to resort to drastic measures.

When the scents in your home really become a significant problem, you might try staying at someone else's house. Hopefully friends and family will be supportive and will assist you in efforts to limit your suffering and stay out of the hospital. However once all the above suggestions have failed to alleviate an aroma-related vomiting cycle, a trip to the hospital may be the only thing that helps. Rehydration can reduce nausea and so can escaping from a house that reeks of an offensive odor. However, hospitals themselves can be full of odors that trigger vomiting.

Hospital Odors

An extended period of hydration may work wonders on the body but it does nothing for hyperolfaction. Aside from the aseptic, "mediciney" smell, hospitals can also reek of a number of other offensive elements including hot beverages, food and other people.

Nurses' Station

In my first HG pregnancy, I was put in a hospital room right next to the nurses' station where coffee brewed all day, often boiling down and creating a viscid, scalding sludge that only I seemed able to smell. When I complained about the odor making me vomit, I was laughed at, considered a nuisance, and not moved! That's because others couldn't smell the offensive odors or else considered them pleasant. Physicians continued to enter my room with steaming coffee, nurses continued to torment me with their perfume (despite clear hospital policy prohibiting perfumed staff), and I still continued to vomit.

I should have demanded excellent health care; it doesn't take much effort to move a hyperemetic to a room away from a coffeepot. Were I ever in such a situation again I would demand to be moved or I would call a lawyer.

3. *If you have to go to the hospital, get a private room.*

Hospital roommates can be a huge problem. If you have the funding to get a private room then by all means do so. This can cut down on vomiting triggers, as you won't have to suffer the fragrance of the other patient as she gobbles down aromatic hospital meals. Nor will you have to deal with the onslaught of her smelly, perfumed, coffee-drinking, loud-mouthed visitors or with the room temperature your "roomie" wants. One woman with HG complained that in her shared room experience, the other patient insisted on maintaining a room climate of eighty-nine degrees. For a hyperemetic, dry heat can equal dry heaves. Incessant chitchat and a blaring radio and television are other room-sharing complications that can trigger headaches and vomiting for the HG patient. In addition, a shared hospital room can compromise the dignity of the HG patient.

Extra Special Joys of the Communal Room

The symptoms of hyperemesis and treatment can be embarrassing. If you can't make it to the bathroom, vomiting in front of someone else can cause anxiety and tension, which can make the situation worse. Some antiemetics commonly cause diarrhea, and when you are on IVs and haven't eaten in a long time it can be very liquid and smelly. If you are so sick that it is hard to walk then they will put a toilet by the bed. Here you may hunker down, simultaneously vomiting, passing loud gas and squirting runny, foul-smelling stools while your roommate and her visitors sit completely horrified on the other side of a thin curtain a few short feet away. HG removes enough of your dignity without the addition of this unnecessary affront.

The Case for a Private Room

Miriam Erick, considered an authority on nausea and vomiting in pregnancy, says:

"A private room is the main ingredient, after hydration, for reducing nausea."[162]

I firmly believe that a private room is *necessary* for HG patients and that insurance should pay for this. Not only does it help maintain a level of human dignity, but it also reduces vomiting triggers. Reducing triggers potentially reduces the length of an expensive hospital stay, and it definitely reduces a fraction of suffering. In the case of HG, a private room should not be looked at as a convenience but as a *necessary component* of therapy. The better the quality of hospital care, the sooner the patient is out of the hospital.

4. *If you are still working, don't expect too much from co-workers.*

Co-workers might be pleasant at work, and you might be great pals when you're well, but too much time away from the job can increase their workload, and no one appreciates that. You may find that people at work aren't as happy to accommodate you as you thought they would be. First, like everyone else who never had HG, they have no clue as to what you're going through. Unfortunately, they may perceive you as a big whiney baby who can't deal with silly, old morning sickness. Second, if you are in a particularly competitive job, your tough luck can actually be beneficial to a co-worker. Your lack of attendance or your inability to perform duties with your usual efficiency can make them look good.

Co-workers are just that: people you work with. Understand their motivation. They are there to earn a paycheck, not to make sacrifices for your health. It would be one thing if HG lasted a week or two, but this stuff can go on for months. People who might have been there for you in the beginning may grow tired of it and have their own problems to deal with. Maybe you will be lucky, and your co-workers will take up all the slack, help to preserve your job, and support you in every way possible. I have heard from women for whom this was the case. Good people still exist.

5. If you are still working, consider taking time off.
Some people have mild HG and swear they can work around it. If you feel that you can work and your doctor agrees, then go for it. Hopefully you have the kind of job where you can stop and vomit any time you need to, a job where people respect your situation enough to support you by making small changes that ease your suffering or at least don't exacerbate it. If it doesn't work out, have your doctor confirm in writing that you need a leave of absence for health reasons. Your employer may grant it. In any case, take a work leave and realize that someday you will be able to return, if not to this job, then to another one. A job can be replaced, a child can't. Take care of yourself.

Possible Financial Options
Social Security has a uniform policy for everyone seeking disability, but to date, HG sufferers do not qualify. To qualify for disability, a person must either have a debilitating illness

that prevents her from working for twelve months or she must have a disability in which death is expected (i.e., terminal cancer). Since Social Security is a dead end, a woman might consult her employer. Her job may have an insurance package, or she may have independently purchased insurance that has its own disability policy. Some may offer short-term disability while others only offer long-term disability. See what your policy offers, and here's a tip: see it in writing. Don't take anyone's word for it. One woman's boss told her they didn't offer short-term disability, but after personally reviewing her policy she found out that they did!

Don't forget FMLA (Family Medical Leave Act). You or even your spouse may be entitled to up to 12 weeks of leave from work. If you do not qualify for FMLA or do not have financial backup options, you may be particularly frightened when you suspect your boss is trying to fire you because you are missing too much work. Sadly, this happens, and legally too. When one single mom lost her job due to HG, a local "pro-life" group came to her rescue, providing financial assistance and a place to stay. Whether you are married or not, contact your local crisis pregnancy center for any help they may be able to offer.

Covering the Cost of Medical Treatment

If you do lose your job due to HG and the inability to work, you can still receive medical treatment. Most women who had a job with medical benefits can maintain that insurance plan via the Consolidated Omnibus Budget Reconciliation Act (COBRA). If this option is available and feasible, you can remain on your plan with your same doctor for the remainder of your pregnancy. If keeping medical insurance through COBRA is not an option, you can still receive medical care via emergency Medicaid. It is against the law to withhold medical care from those who need it. Still, you may lose your current doctor and the standard of your care may suffer. A young woman told me that she lost her job and had no insurance. She applied for and received emergency Medicaid, but her new doctor wasn't willing to prescribe medication that he felt was "too expensive." This is a terrible shame.

In another case, a single woman on Medicaid determined she was receiving substandard treatment. Among other things, her doctor made insensitive comments that revealed to her that he neither understood nor cared about the extent of her suffering. He refused to order a test for helicobacter pylori even as she was suffering from an ulcer in the midst of her HG. He also dwelled on and repeatedly emphasized his opinion that she could die from the combination of her pregnancy and her hiatal hernia, and rather than try corticosteroids when other antiemetics had failed, he suggested she terminate. At the end of her rope, she felt she had to terminate the child she loved and wanted. Interestingly, on the way into the abortion facility she challenged some protestors who, surprisingly, agreed to cover all her financial needs and find her a new doctor who would treat her HG appropriately. After seeing the new physician a few times, she finally began to feel that she was getting the medical care and compassion she needed to continue the pregnancy. Months later, she delivered a healthy baby boy.

In order to have her son, this woman lost her job, her home, her car and her ability to financially care for herself during the course of a hellish nightmare pregnancy. The payoff was that after her baby was born, she was able to work again and rebuild her life. She shared that had she aborted her son, there would have been no way to rebuild him. As horrible as it is, HG is temporary, and this particular mom was not willing to accept the permanence of abortion.

Covering the Cost Of Living

Paying the rent, car payment and maintaining one's standard of living is difficult after losing a job due to HG. If everything starts to fall apart at the seams and you are in danger of losing your electricity, phone, house, transportation, medical insurance, daycare, food for your children, and so on, you may benefit from contacting local organizations such as churches and crisis pregnancy centers (CPCs). These groups claim to exemplify charity and compassion. Challenge them to deliver on those claims. Often they can help financially, emotionally, spiritually (if you are so inclined), and can even direct you to a doctor who regards your growing child as her patient too. Churches and CPCs can be found in the Yellow Pages. (CPCs are often listed under *Abortion Alternatives.*) When in doubt, keep things in perspective for those who claim to be "pro-lifers:" remind them that their involvement could mean the difference between life and death for your child. If whomever you talk to says they can't help, then ask them to direct you to someone who can. You may encounter *numerous* "do-nothings" before you find that one person who will snap into action. Don't let unmotivated hypocrites crush your spirit. ***Don't give up.***

In addition to local entities, national organizations exist that might be able to help. You might contact a social worker that specializes in children and families, and see if you can get assistance in obtaining emergency Medicaid and/or food stamps for your children already born. The government can also supply daycare, gas money, and other assistance. Consult government listings in your phone book. If talking makes you vomit, find someone who will help you make phone calls. Compassionate volunteers can also help with paper work, do the shopping, and transport children to and from school/daycare. For help in finding resources for basic needs, consult Appendix B.

6. *If someone makes an offensive comment, ignore it or educate the offender.*

I have heard from many women whose husbands think initially that their hyperemetic partner is crazy, weak, "faking it," looking for attention, or merely overreacting. Nothing could be further from the truth. Additionally, hyperemetics may be surprised that some of the most unsupportive people are other women. Since most women have glowing pregnancies, many of them can't understand why the hyperemetic's pregnancy is so different. This lack of understanding can lead to a lack of acceptance. Hyperemetics are often secondarily victimized.

Negative comments hyperemetics have heard:
- Don't you want the baby?
- You're just trying to get attention.
- You're overreacting.
- You're obsessing about the pregnancy.
- Are you making yourself sick?
- Other women get morning sickness and they don't act like you do!
- Eat a cracker (drink ginger ale/ apply a cold washcloth/ etc.).
- I/my wife/friend/sister/mother had morning sickness

worse than you and worked nearly sixty hours a week.

- I never behaved the way you're behaving.
- I know what you're going through; I couldn't eat bacon for my entire pregnancy.
- Lying on the couch all day is what's making you sick!
- I just got over a 24-hour stomach flu, and you have no idea what it is to vomit like I did. (Said to a hyperemetic who endured tube feedings.)
- You need to get up and do things!
- This perfume is sixty dollars an ounce; I won't stop wearing it for anybody!
- We're not going to stop baking potatoes in the lounge just because you don't happen to like the smell.
- Was this pregnancy planned?
- You're not sick-you're pregnant.
- Pregnancy is a normal part of life.
- Are you trying hard enough to eat?
- HG is not a real illness like pregnancy-related diabetes is.
- This is a hospital, not a hotel; your constant vomiting will only disturb patients with *real* illnesses.
- Don't you want to eat?
- You just have to *make* yourself eat.
- Why are you starving yourself?
- I wish I were lucky enough to get HG; I need to lose some weight!
- Your baby is going to die/be retarded/deformed if you don't eat.
- I work hard all day; the least you can do is clean up around here and make me dinner.

- Don't you care about your children? Get up and make dinner!
- This house is a sty! Get off your lazy butt and clean up!
- You don't love me anymore. (Said a husband to a wife.)
- You can't lose your job over this; MAKE yourself go to work!
- Why don't you just "take care" of this?
- You can't really think of it as a baby.
- Just abort.

If you hear these or similar comments, hand the offender a copy of the reproducible pamphlet mentioned in Appendix E. It might be helpful to tell them that you're looking for daily assistance and not advice. You may want to enlist a friendly advocate to be at your bedside if you are expecting a visitor. The advocate might be able to subdue the type of aforementioned verbal abuse.

Find a mantra that works and repeat it often, particularly during the roughest times. Depending on who you are, this can be anything from an encouraging Bible verse to a simple affirmation such as "I can get through this!"

Stormy's Story

I am a four-time survivor of HG. I could write a book about it, but I don't have the time what with raising four children! My most recent child was born with Down syndrome, and what a joy she is! My sister, my only sibling, has Down syndrome also. If I had the time, I could write a book about that too!

I suffered horribly with each pregnancy. The last one was the worst. I had so many weird complications with that pregnancy. For six moths I had ptyalism, which is extreme watering of the mouth. It was terrible. I soaked two or three dishtowels a day. I literally had to sleep with a towel under my mouth and lie on my side. Saliva just poured out of me, and at times it was hard to talk. They told me not to swallow it or it would make me throw up. I could have told them that! I never had ptyalism in any of my other HG pregnancies. I also had a Groshong PICC line put in during this last pregnancy. It's a feeding tube that goes into a large blood vessel near the heart. I had home IV therapy and had to start my own IVs at times, because my insurance company penalized me due to the fact that my husband is a physician. The problem with that was: *he's a physician*! Physicians are never home! His partner had just retired and he couldn't get a replacement due to the doctor shortage. Anyway, I'm a nurse, so I had to take care of myself.

After I had two children I had to get help with the kids. I tried calling nurse's aids from home health care agencies. Not one that I called had anyone they felt comfortable sending. That's just not what they do. I had to find someone. There are NO tax benefits or anything if you hire help for an illness.

We could afford it, but I worry about those who can't. What will happen to them? I had to hire my help and then treat her as a "household employee." This meant I had to file tax info, social security info, Worker's Compensation, etc. You name it, I had to fill it out. I was filing paperwork constantly like I was some big manufacturing company or something. All these government bureaus sent me tons of stuff to work on. I'd have to fill out the nanny's "time card," send it to my accountant, and get it back to where it needed to go before the deadline or they would FINE me and make me do it all over again! It was very unreasonable to expect me to do all this while I was suffering from HG. To make matters worse, I couldn't take a tax deduction on the children since I wasn't working! Isn't that something! I tried to avoid all this by hiring from an agency, but they want a year contract and usually take a couple of months to get you hooked up with a nanny. I needed one "yesterday," and couldn't wait *one week* much less two months. And the nannies usually required their own room and bathroom and often a car. They get paid vacation and sick time, and you have to pay a substantial "finder's fee" to the agency. Going through an agency would have been extremely expensive, and the nannies were quite limited in the duties they would perform. Many *only* took care of the kids. My nanny did laundry, grocery shopping, and errands...basically, she was me! It was very hard to see my one-year-old cry in my arms reaching out for *her* when she went home.

One of the worst parts of dealing with HG was the way people treated me. It was like no one could remember or comprehend my illness. Since there was no cast or scar, they just never could believe I was as sick as I was. People would say, "You need to get out; let's go to lunch!" I'd say, "I've been on the couch for three days in a row too sick to bathe or keep anything down, and I don't think I'll be going out to lunch today." Directly after telling them this, they would ask me if I was going to the fair! I'm a wiseacre so once I did show up to a holiday party...with my IV pole! That one act miraculously caused a sudden understanding. Even my own husband, a physician, wasn't as disturbed by it until he stayed home from work one day and witnessed my vomiting episodes. He said, "I can't stand to watch it any longer!" That's when he jumped on the Internet to try and help me. I know you've heard the cracker stories. We ALL have to hear about the wonders of eating crackers before you get out of bed. I'd say, "I've been in the hospital on IV drugs of every kind and I'm still throwing up. I don't think crackers are going to do the trick." One of my nursing friends gave me grief about not taking my prenatal vitamins. I said, "Would you feel better if I got up every day and threw one in the toilet? Because if I take it, that's where it will end up anyway!"

I tried the ReliefBand, drugs, drugs, and more drugs, and only one thing helped even a little: Zofran, a drug used to control nausea in cancer patients who are undergoing chemotherapy. It helped, but it turned my bowel movements into cement! I lived each day struggling to get through HG. I was depressed by the sickness and by the length of it. It is like having the worst stomach flu imaginable for nine months straight. People barely get that much jail time for *murder*!

My religion prevents me from using birth control. Thank God for answering my prayers by giving me a need for a hysterectomy after the fourth child. I had the surgery as soon as my doctor would let me after the last delivery. I did NOT want to get pregnant again, especially since I had three small boys to take care of and a daughter who needs a lot of therapy and tender loving care.

My OB said I was one of the worst cases he ever had. Luckily a friend of mine, a pharmacist, kept thinking of new things for me to try and researched them. None of them helped except the Zofran, but the many options gave me hope. I just kept trying to hang on.

I have two friends. One is a physician who had HG twice. She was extremely ill. She lived on hyperalimentation (TPN) with her second child. Another friend, a physician's wife, was pregnant with twins. She was very sick. Her sister-in-law told her, "Oh, just get out of bed, throw up, and get on with your day. Why do you have to make such a big deal out of it?" A big deal? This woman broke ribs vomiting and her hair fell out. She was so horribly ill that she couldn't take it anymore. The only "treatment" they offered her was therapeutic abortion. They did not consider the health of her twins or even her own emotional health. She thought she would die, so she underwent the termination. It has been eight years and she still can't forgive herself. She is tormented by her "weakness." She is crushed at the anniversary date, the due date and every time she sees twins. She still suffers terribly.

I know it's rare, but people still do die from this if not treated properly. I personally know of three women whose children lost their lives because of terminations due to HG. Usually the doctor hasn't done his job in helping the mother stay strong enough to fight. My husband is a physician and he agrees. He and I had to do a *lot* of my own care. Something needs to be done. There is no excuse for needless suffering and death.

FIFTEEN
Finding Dr. Right

When it comes to HG, some physicians are definitely better than others. You want a doctor who knows her stuff or is at least willing to learn. You want someone who will listen and respond positively, someone who will give you her time and personally observe your progress or decline. You require a doctor who will be an advocate, research for you, find positive options for you, inform you, work with you, believe you, validate you, and offer you the care you need without ever giving up. This is a tall order. How do you find this person?

Dr. Jekyll & Dr. Hyde

Many healthy women think their reliable ol' OB/GYN is just dandy until they are sick with HG and realize for the first time what a dud the doc is. If you are one of the very lucky people who ended up with a great doctor from the very beginning, drop down on your knees and thank God for your good fortune. For the rest of us, we've got some work to do to get the same kind of excellent health care.

Cheating on Your Doctor: An Extramedical Affair

When you are sick, it can be a disappointing blow to discover that your physician just isn't working for you. This person may have been your doctor for many years, and she may even have been the best, most helpful doctor in a previous medical situation. You may feel that you owe her your loyalty and that seeing another doctor would be unfriendly, ungrateful or even cheating. Try and remember that what is most important is getting excellent care in *this* pregnancy.

Even if you don't have such concerns, the thought of starting over with an entirely new doctor, who might possibly be as bad as or worse than the one you've got, may be very discouraging. It is depressing to find yourself stuck with an unhelpful doctor when you are so debilitated. At a time when making phone calls is physically challenging, you certainly lack the energy and ability to go running all over town interviewing doctors. It may be too much work but if you have a bad doctor, for the sake of your health, you must try and find a way. If at all possible, designate an advocate.

Simply put, an advocate is an able-bodied person who cares about you and wants to help. She can make phone calls for you and ask questions. She can accompany you to appointments, do most of the talking, and record doctors' comments. She is the type of person who does not make empty promises but follows through. Her hard work will be invaluable, as she can help you get better medical care and even a better doctor if need be.

Beginning the Process

Take full advantage of your HMO. You or your advocate can find out their policy on consultations. Some HMOs only allow three consultations. If your HMO limits this type of interview, then you will have to take steps to ensure the most bang for your buck. First, get out the phone book and call various doctors who seem promising. If you must rely solely on your HMO for financial reimbursement of medical care, then this will limit you to doctors who accept your HMO. In this case, the first thing you want to ask is if they take your HMO. If they don't, the elimination process has begun. If they do, you will want to know if the doctor is taking new patients. Cross her off the list if she isn't. If they accept your insurance and are taking new patients, then request to speak to the nurse. Here is a short list of questions you might ask her:

1. *How much experience does the doctor have with hyperemesis gravidarum?*
   If she doesn't know what you're talking about, make a note of it.

2. *How does the doctor typically treat the disease?*
   If psychotherapy is involved in her answer indicate that in your notes.

3. *Do severe HG patients usually receive home health care or are they normally treated with IVs in the hospital?*
   Home health care can be a plus.

4. *Do you know if the doctor has ever prescribed corticosteroids or parenteral nutrition for HG in the past?*
   Corticosteroids can be a plus, and TPN can save your life.

5. *Does the doctor carry medical malpractice insurance?*
   If she does not, she may not have certain hospital

privileges and may discharge you from her care should you become severe and need aggressive intervention. If that happens, you will have to start all over again in your search to find a new, good doctor. Is this really what you want during the worst point of illness?

6. *Can you think of any other doctors who might have much experience treating HG?*

If you see any names popping up repeatedly in these interviews, it may indicate that a certain doctor has more experience than others and is known for her success in treating HG.

After you or your advocate hangs up, jot down the overall feel of the conversation. Did the nurse take time to answer your questions or was she rude and short? Could she answer all of your questions? Was she extra helpful? Did she give you even more information than you asked for? Of course she isn't the one who will be treating you, but your conversation with her may help you in the elimination process. There is always a chance that a good doctor just happens to have a clueless, grumpy nurse. Do the best you can. This is not an exact science!

Once you have narrowed down your list to the number of consults you are allowed, make your appointments. Remember, if you have a trusted advocate, you need only worry about getting yourself out of bed and to all these appointments. Hopefully the first doctor you interview will have wings and a halo, and you can cancel your other consultations. If your introductory consultation takes place in the doctor's personal office, take note of the surroundings. What can you learn about her from her personal environment? Are there degrees and certificates on the wall or pictures of people? Are there plants, and are they alive? Are cartoons posted anywhere or just pharmaceutical premiums? Is there anything religious in the room, like a plaque or a mug or some other evidence of individual ethic that might be important to you? Your impression is just one small component to add to the total experience of the interview process.

When interviewing a prospective physician, start out with the fact that you have HG and are looking for a doctor who will offer excellent medical care in order to achieve well being and a positive pregnancy outcome. (If you are consulting pre-pregnancy, explain that you have experienced HG in the past and are planning for a future pregnancy. If the doctor reminds you that "Every pregnancy is different," and it feels patronizing or dismissive, make a note of it.) Have your list of questions ready and explain that you would like to tape-record the interview so that you don't forget anything after the session is over. This is especially important if you are sick and finding it difficult to concentrate. To be honest, most physicians will probably balk at the idea of being tape-recorded due to scattered instances of lawyers, insurance companies and TV shows sending fake patients to doctors for suspect reasons. Tell your physician that recording your visit wasn't your idea, that this book suggested it, and assure her that your purpose really is solely to have an accurate record of the conversation after leaving her office. If she will allow you to record her answers, this may indicate flexibility, sensitivity and particular helpfulness. Ask any questions you might have. Here are ten suggestions:

1. *Can you estimate the number of HG patients you've treated in the last five years?*

If the doctor has a lot of experience, this may mean she knows what she is doing and has lots of positive options to offer. It could also go the other way and mean that she *thinks* she knows it all, is set in her ways, and is unwilling to see you as anything but another number in the timeline of her ample experience. Older doctors may be uninterested in researching and trying newer treatments, especially if they are nearing retirement, while younger doctors may not know as much. Conversely, younger doctors may know newer, cutting-edge treatments and may be more excited about their profession and more open to your input.

2. *What is your standard treatment protocol?**
The doctor will probably talk about rehydration and antiemetics such as Phenergan, Reglan or even Zofran. If she mentions counseling or psychotherapy, pay close attention to what extent she relies on it as treatment. Is it complimentary treatment or primary treatment? Her comments may reveal a tendency to view HG as psychological in nature, and medical literature has demonstrated that this attitude can be dangerous. Merely incorporating counseling as a complimentary component of the overall treatment approach does not automatically equate substandard treatment. In fact it can be very helpful. Often people with debilitating diseases benefit from sharing their feelings about what they are going through. But *HG should never be viewed or treated as though it is a neurosis.*

3. *Would you consider prescribing Zofran? (Or if you are interested in the ReliefBand you might ask if she would consider prescribing it.)*

Zofran is extraordinarily expensive. If she is willing to prescribe it that may tell you that she cares more about you than keeping costs down for your medical insurance company. A willingness to prescribe the electrical stimulation band may show that she is open to newer, different ideas and will supply you with every possible option that you feel comfortable trying.

4. *Have you ever prescribed corticosteroids to treat HG?*
    If she says yes, this may show that she keeps current with medical literature on HG and that she is willing to try newer treatments for it. She might even consent to reading a study or trying a new treatment that you suggest. If she says that she has not had experience with corticosteroids for the treatment of HG, ask her why and if she would consider it, and mull over her answers.

5. *Are initial IVs administered in the office in a time frame of two or three hours or are they are administered slowly over a 24-hour period in a hospital setting? And do I have a choice?*
    It may be more beneficial to be placed in the hospital for at least a 24-hour slow drip, as your body gets constant hydration over a longer period of time, giving it a much needed rest from the onslaught of pronounced dehydration. Still it is not entirely unreasonable to have a few initial wham-bam IVs for the purpose of establishing the necessity of more aggressive treatment. However, if you have already gone through the initial, closely repeated IVs at another practice, you should not have to go through them again before receiving more dedicated treatment.

6. *What are indications for home health care IVs?*
Basically, this asks the question: "How sick do I have to get before you will finally help me?" This type of question *must* be answered, so you can justify the need for treatment when you are at that point. For instance, on your third rehydration trip to the ER in two days, you can remind your doctor that she told you that home health care would be indicated at this juncture. And legally speaking, it doesn't hurt that you will have it on tape.

7. *What are indications for alternative methods of nutrition such as enteral or parenteral feedings?*
Again, this is for your reference so you can help manage your health care. You will know what you need when you need it. And try not to let a doctor get away with obscure comments like, "We'll cross that bridge when we get there." That tells you nothing. Explain that you really must know something specific because it's part of your selection process. If she refuses to give you information, that tells you something right there. Antiemetics and repeat hospitalizations that are ineffective, along with the loss of greater than or equal to 5% of your total body weight, can justify par/enteral nutrition.[163-164] If the doctor says she has never prescribed such feedings for HG and isn't about to start, you may want to find another doctor who can offer you more options.

8. *Have you ever prescribed PEG or PEJ for HG?*
If she has then she gets bonus points for being super current and for her willingness to expand women's options for a positive outcome. *Don't forget to ask her when this treatment is indicated in HG.* If she says she has never prescribed it and

wouldn't, you might not necessarily deduct points. Many physicians are consulting with gastroenterologists who do not feel comfortable implementing these procedures during pregnancy. There are other feeding methods that are adequate and more commonly accepted.

9. *Whom will I see each time I make an office visit?*
If she gives you a number of people, ask if she is willing to make a special exception so that you may see her exclusively. It is best to see only *one* physician for HG office visits as it gives the physician a more linear representation of your disease process. If the person who saw you last time sees you the next time, she will have two consecutive images of you to compare, and will be better able to notice any decline. If you drop twenty pounds in two weeks she doesn't have the opportunity to notice if she doesn't even see you. If someone else records your rapid increments of weight loss, you simply can't count on it getting back to a doctor who is too busy to even see you much less keep up with your chart. Being seen by one or, *at the most,* two people will increase the chance that any physical decline will be noticed and treated.

10. *If I confer notarized patient status on my gestating child, and my own life is not in immediate danger, will you honor the conference and refuse to terminate the pregnancy even if, in desperation, I should resort to asking for it?*
This question may be especially meaningful to those who have, due to HG, terminated in the past, as many worry that they will repeat such an unwanted experience under extreme physical duress. It is an earnest request that cries, "Save me from myself!" Although it doesn't prevent you

from seeking termination elsewhere, symbolically, it can be very meaningful to you and can help you hang in there when the symptoms are at their peak. Also, it informs the doctor from the very beginning that you are not ambiguous about wanting to complete your pregnancy.

As with the nurse, if the doctor seems insensitive, unreasonably rushed, elusive, arrogant, unwilling, unaccommodating, grumpy, stodgy, terse, bored, irritated by your questions or just plain creepy, drop her to the end of the list. If, after all your consultations, you still don't like anyone, call your HMO and tell them you want to consult some more. It never hurts to ask. If they say no, you may want to shell out the money for additional consultations. After all, a good doctor is more than worth a few hundred bucks, and once you become a patient your HMO should resume payment if the doctor you choose is on their list.

❧

*The language of this question can establish that you are interested in your disease and treatment and have been gathering information. However, medical terminology can be tricky for laypersons. It can either make you look very smart or very stupid so be sure you know what you're doing, and use it with care!

DeWanna's Story

I always expected to be sick during pregnancy. My mother had five children and was progressively sicker with each one. I was fifteen during her last pregnancy. I watched her suffer and realized that I, like my mother and her mother before her, would be one of those women for whom pregnancy is not easy.

I was married in 1994, and conception came very easy to us. I was not sick yet but had been very tired and assumed it was due to the new house we were finishing up and the process of moving. The first time I threw up I actually was excited as it felt like a rite of passage, and I knew now that I was "really" pregnant. I also took it as a good sign because my mother had three miscarriages and was never sick with any of them. I understood that with my family history it would be all day sickness for me, rather than the understated "morning" type. I wasn't afraid of it.

Things got bad fast. I wasn't even scheduled to have my first OB appointment until twelve weeks, but two weeks after I found out I was pregnant I ended up in the ER for rehydration. I called my doctor that day, as I couldn't keep even a sip of water down. I talked to the nurse who told me that I should try Emetrol or Bonine, an over the counter drug for motion sickness. Neither worked. My husband took me to the ER where the doctor was wonderful and reassuring. He told me that soon I'd be feeling fine, and he gave me Benadryl and Phenergan along with two liters of fluids. I did *not* feel fine.

The Phenergan gave me a horrible feeling of anxiety, so I was pumped full of more Benadryl and sent home. I did feel better the next day, but it didn't last long. I was teaching fourth grade at the time, and six of us were pregnant. My co-workers gave me much advice and assured me that it would be over soon, but none of their suggestions worked, and it was getting very hard to teach. I felt nauseous all the time and constantly ran across the hall to vomit in the kids' bathroom. Thank God I taught at a year-round school and was able to go off-track by ten weeks. I was looking forward to the twelfth week because that is when everyone told me the nausea and vomiting would magically disappear. It didn't, of course, and although I was thrilled to hear the baby's heartbeat for the first time at twelve weeks, my never-ending vomiting overshadowed the joy.

I tried everything I could to feel better and keep food down. Some days frozen juice would stay down, and once fries and a shake did. Still, when I started to really lose weight I began to worry. In addition to the nausea and vomiting, I had the excessive saliva condition known as ptyalism. My spit cup went everywhere.

My home health nurse, who had been doing short term IV fluid therapy for me for a few weeks, convinced my very traditional doctor to let me try Zofran. I was told this was the strongest antiemetic drug on the market. It didn't do a thing. Aside from being a little sleepy, the so-called wonder drug had no effect whatsoever!

Soon my three-week break from school was up and it was time to go back to teaching. I started coming home at lunch most days and was not at all productive at work. At thirteen weeks I was admitted to the hospital. The night crew tried so hard to find something to ease my suffering, but I had tried everything they had in the hospital: Compazine, Phenergan, Inapsine (which like Phenergan gave me horrible anxiety attacks), Tigan, and of course Reglan and Zofran. Nothing helped in the slightest! Luckily I was in a good hospital, but the lead perinatologist decided that my thyroid was causing the problems and started me on medications for hyperthyroidism. I couldn't keep the pills down, so I was given Thorazine suppositories, which would nearly put me to sleep. Then I would be given thyroid medication, which would stay down. Once again, this drug theory did not help my HG, and my doctor threatened me with a PICC and TPN. He did mention that he had a "better option," a nasogastric feeding tube.

The NG tube procedure looks easy on medical shows on TV but is one of the worst procedures I've ever had. They numbed my nose and mouth with a spray and then stuck a tube down my nose into my stomach. It was done under X-ray to make sure it was placed correctly, and I had to swallow as they pushed it down. This would be bad enough for a person who *wasn't* nauseous, but it was horrible with my overactive gagging reflex. I barely made it back to my room when I violently coughed-sneezed-vomited the thing up! A nurse scolded me saying, "*Now* look what you've done! Oh well, they'll just have to put it back again!" I refused.

The combination of IV fluids and bed rest enabled me to drink liquids again, and I was able to go home. However I was not home for more than four days before my husband insisted I be admitted again. I vomited at least twice an hour and because I couldn't eat or drink anything without vomiting, I was now dry heaving or vomiting up blood and bile. At the hospital they inserted a PICC in my right arm and started me on TPN. It made a *wonderful* difference, and by Halloween I was back to teaching and feeling a lot better. I still could eat only select items and not a lot of fluids, but I started to believe my nightmare was almost over.

After being on TPN for about a week, my line was removed and I did OK for another month. We found out that the baby was a boy.

By Christmas I was very sick again and glad to be off-track. The vomiting, nausea and "spits" had returned with a vengeance and I quickly ended up back on IV fluids, once again not being able to put anything in my mouth. I begged for TPN, and after two weeks of my OB waiting to "see if it gets better on its own with time," I finally got it. This time the miracle did not happen and I was miserable. The holidays that year are a blur to me, as I stayed in bed too sick to read or watch TV.

I finally started my third trimester. I dreaded going back to teaching. I had long since used up my ten sick days and was paying for subs out of my paycheck, but I still tried to teach. One day, as I was leaving at lunch again, my principal asked me if I had considered quitting. I sensed it really wasn't a choice for me as she had my replacement all lined up! I cleaned out my classroom and went home to concentrate on surviving for three more months. It's hard to remember the two weeks following my dismissal from work, but I recall clearly the moment I realized that my baby hadn't moved in a couple of days.

At thirty-two weeks I went to the doctor's, was taken to my regular ultrasound room, and laid down on the table. Within seconds the dreaded news came: "I'm sorry, but this baby has passed away." I was in a state of shock, and I just started bawling. After eighteen hours of hard labor our beautiful boy was stillborn. It changed me forever.

I left the hospital the next day at a loss of what to do with my life. All I'd ever wanted to do was to be a mother and a teacher. I'd lost my teaching job two weeks before the death, and now I had no child to mother. All I knew was that I wanted another baby so much and even though I dreaded it, I had to be pregnant again soon. We were advised not to try again both because my body was too weak and because my thyroid was still acting up. Surgery and radiation treatments were discussed. I refused to listen and when my thyroid problems "mysteriously" disappeared, I was determined to try and conceive immediately.

After only one period, I discovered I was pregnant again. I used my same OB again, because I naively thought that since he knew my history, things would be easier. And of course with my HMO, I would use the same perinatologist team including the doctor who casually told us our son was dead. At six weeks, I was getting rehydrated at the doctor's office. The HG returned with a vengeance and my poor, weak body had no strength to fight. I quit my job again and was put back on TPN and Thorazine. The TPN kept my body alive and the Thorazine helped me survive the endless days and nights of eternal nausea and vomiting. As bad as I thought I had it the first time, it was much worse this time. The months passed in a fog as the Thorazine kept me too doped up to do anything. I remember hearing people talk around me, but could not answer them. I spent a lot of time at my parents now because of my husband's shift work. I had enough energy to change my IV bags when I absolutely had to do it myself, but could do nothing else without help.

My husband washed and brushed my hair and even my teeth for me when I could stand it. He cleaned up after me when I lost control of my bodily functions and held me while the waves of nausea crashed over me. He dressed and undressed me, as I could not physically do it myself. Day after day this living hell dragged on. I don't remember hearing this baby's heartbeat for the first time, but I do remember learning she was a girl. Somehow it didn't matter as much this time around. I did not consider this thing inside me a baby. It was an alien force that had stolen my health. I could not get excited for her to come, as the due date seemed beyond my reach. I did not know how I would survive until then. I never worried about the baby because she *wasn't* a baby to me. I was not scared of losing her, because I did not even believe I could have a living child.

I was at my parents' house when I felt funny twitches in my pelvic and vaginal area, but did not realize what they were. I was also coughing and wheezing heavily. My mother recognized that something was wrong and we called the on-call OB. I was told that my sensations were normal, and not too worry unless they got worse. Minutes later during a coughing fit, my water broke. My parents put a towel between my legs and rushed me to the hospital. My husband called their home only to be told by my youngest brother that I was at the ER. I was rushed to a back room and examined right away. I was alone when they told me my temperature was one hundred four, and my pulse was skyrocketing as well. I remember hearing the words uterine infection and: "If it is, the baby will have to go." I was soon in a labor and delivery room with my parents when the "casual" doctor walked in. Matter-of-factly, he told me that my baby was still alive but wouldn't be for long. Because my temperature and pulse were so high they did not want to risk my health by waiting for the baby to be delivered naturally. My husband arrived just in time to help me sign papers for the termination that would take my dying baby from me but hopefully save my life.

I had no idea how serious the situation was. All I knew was that it was happening again. All at once she became a baby to me. My baby. I can still hear myself telling my husband, "We're losing our little girl!" My parents went home and we were left alone in a very dark room. I suddenly had the urge to go to the bathroom, and as I sat down on the toilet my baby fell out into my hands. I screamed, "She's here!" and struggled back to the bed still carrying her between my legs. I do not remember if she was alive or dead and only have a very fuzzy memory of a tiny baby. I was eighteen weeks along.

In recovery they discovered how sick I really was. My uterine infection was most likely caused by a contaminated PICC line. This also led to a heart valve infection called endocarditis. I was also found to have a case of bacterial pneumonia. That alone could have killed me if left untreated. I obviously had no idea that I had all these conditions on top of the HG. No one did. I had been too sick too long to notice any change, even a bad one.

After three weeks of recovery, which included fluid drains from my back and a chest tube to clear the fluid in my lungs, I was finally able to go home. I had another PICC line inserted so I could continue my IV antibiotics. Once again I left the hospital without my baby and with no hope of ever having another. My doctors had told me that if I valued my life I would seriously never try to conceive again, and my husband agreed.

While I was in the hospital recovering my mother had me fill out paperwork for adoption. I recovered and enjoyed being well again, and we pursued our "Plan B." Not long after, we adopted a little girl! The next few years flew by, and although I was always haunted by the desire to get pregnant again, teaching school kept me busy. As our new neighborhood grew in size, so did our desire to have another baby. When our daughter was eighteen months, we adopted our son. I quit teaching and was very busy with my little ones, but could not stop thinking about trying *one more time*. I honestly believed that if I could finally have a biological baby, then my demons would go away. We had also been researching HG on the Internet and knew so much more about the disease and how to treat it. I no longer felt alone and had developed some long-lasting friendships with people whose lives had also been shattered by HG. We were all talking about steroid therapy, and I was anxious to try it, although I hoped that by some miracle I wouldn't need to.

The day after our son's first birthday I tested positive. I

was thrilled and yet scared to death at the same time. We felt like we had made the right decision, but my friends and family were angry and resentful that I would put them through this again. I had a glorious three weeks where I was not sick at all and had only the "normal" symptoms such as tender nipples and extreme tiredness. I did all I could and ate all I wanted, as I knew it wouldn't last forever. I had my first doctor's appointment at six weeks. I had chosen a new, younger perinatologist in the same office as before. I'd met him only once but was impressed with his compassion. I was able to be one of the practice's few private patients and never had to deal with a regular OB again.

At seven weeks "the monster" (HG) appeared fully, and I was too sick to even lift my one-year-old out of his crib. I was immediately admitted to the hospital, and the cycle of meds and fluids began again. I went home after three days on Zofran and Reglan. For the first time the Zofran actually worked, and early on I felt well enough to actually go to the store and eat a little soup. This effect didn't last long, and although I took the Zofran the whole pregnancy and got *some* relief, it never had that first effect again.

I still vomited too many times to count, but I usually felt well enough to make it to the toilet or sink instead of my handy garbage can. I also craved cucumbers in vinegar and salt and amazingly could keep them down more than half of the time. My doctor thought this was very strange but didn't argue. I put my ice shaver to good use managing to stay hydrated through flavorless snow cones and bullion. Lemon-lime soft drinks actually stayed down most of the time as long as they were very cold.

The hardest part of the early months this time was the fact that I had two toddlers to take care of when it was hard enough taking care of myself. Unfortunately for them, Mommy was always sick, and they watched a lot of movies while Daddy was at work. Somehow I managed to keep them fed and their diapers changed. Like all good things though, this ability to stay hydrated did not last, and at eleven weeks I was again hospitalized.

Like before the combination of no work and lots of rest, along with constant IV fluids, brought me back up and kept me from the downward spiral that had plagued me in my previous pregnancies. My doctor insisted on admitting me for round-the-clock care, and it made all the difference in the world. His treatment was pro-active (unlike my former OB with his "wait and see" attitude). It worked. Within one day I felt better. Another major factor in my ability to bounce back was that I was quite overweight. In the first twelve weeks I lost forty pounds, but I had them to lose.

All of these factors though didn't keep me from returning to the hospital yet a third time at fourteen weeks. Once again I recovered quite quickly and kept my first real meal down in over three months! I'll never forget how yummy that turkey sandwich and those chips were! From fourteen to eighteen weeks I managed to keep at least one meal down a day and could move around my house enough to take care of my children. Unlike the other two pregnancies, I could watch TV and read, which helped pass the endless days. I needed no Thorazine this time and never had a PICC inserted. We did try home health rehydration once, but I was such a hard stick that I ended up coming into the doctor's office anyway. Although I was still vomiting daily and lived with constant nausea, I felt blessed that this time was so "easy." It didn't last long; I became worse and would go hours without even being able to keep my ice chips down not to mention the cucumbers or anything else.

When I reached eighteen weeks I became very depressed and nervous that I was going to lose the baby, a girl, just like I had three years before. I was once again vomiting everything up. When my doctor saw this (and when I discussed my mental state with him), he decided to use steroid therapy and put me on a tapering high to low dosage of methylprednisolone. In a short time, it made me feel well enough to eat a bowl of soup and keep it down! It was so exciting to know that steroids actually worked and that I had finally found my "miracle" drug.

The rest of the pregnancy was not as bad physically as the others, but it was more stressful emotionally. I had plenty of time to worry, as I was not doped up with Thorazine. I still felt awful enough that I was usually in bed or on a couch, but I could take care of my children and myself. The vomiting never did go away, and although most of my appetite returned, that didn't mean my stomach accepted it! I was famous for going out to eat, thoroughly enjoying it and then losing my meal before we even paid the check. I even was able to joke that I could really get my money's worth at buffet restaurants as I could come back for a second round with my empty stomach.

I made it through my dreaded thirty-two-week mark *and* the four-year anniversary of my first child's death. The fact that I was due within two days of his due date hadn't made things easy. The last eight weeks were filled with incredible anxiety that consumed me more than the physical symptoms of HG. I had expected that once my milestone passed I would be able to enjoy the rest of the pregnancy, but knowing all too well that there is never a safe date, I just stressed more.

As this pregnancy finished, I was more than ready to relinquish being sick forever and made arrangements to have my tubes tied upon delivery. I did not want to ever face HG again. I was sad knowing that it would be the last time I carried a child but anxious to finally meet the little person that had been living inside me for so long. Our new daughter was born after an emergency C-section. I had been scheduled to start induction the night before, but L&D was full so I was sent home. When I arrived the next morning it was discovered that our daughter's heart rate was going up rapidly. There went my plan of a perfect birth, and it didn't help that I was still throwing up. Just over an hour after I arrived, my wonderful doctor told us that she had to come out immediately, and I was rushed to surgery.

She was beautiful and we wept tears of relief and joy as we heard her first cry. Although she was monitored in the NICU for a while, they never found a reason for her increased heart rate, which had skyrocketed to over two hundred beats per minute. My tubes were tied on the table, and a dark chapter of my life was finally closed forever.

RARE COMPLICATIONS

SIXTEEN
Recognizing and Treating Rare Complications

No representation of HG is complete without a report on the complications that range from moderate to life-threatening. Rare complications are usually connected with severe cases of HG and/or inadequate medical treatment. Life-threatening complications are *extremely rare,* and most people receive adequate medical treatment by today's standards. By far the vast majority of hyperemetic pregnancies end very successfully, and it's helpful to remember that serious complications are much rarer than even the rarity of getting HG.

I terminated my first child due to this illness, and I personally know the unending pain and regret that this causes. The last thing I want is for anyone to read the information provided here, become frantic, and then decide to terminate. If you think that reading about rare complications will do more harm than good, you may want to skip this chapter now.

Warning Signs
Warning signs for HG complications include: bleeding, swelling in strange places, severe and localized pain, turning yellow, hallucinating, visual impairments, losing consciousness and becoming confused, or being unable to stand up or walk

without swaying or falling over. If you have any of these symptoms make your doctor aware of them.

Some complications are: gallbladder disease, Mallory-Weiss tears in the esophagus, spontaneous rupture of the esophagus, pneumomediastinum, Wernicke's encephalopathy, central pontine myelinosis, liver disease and renal failure. In extremely rare situations, a serious complication can result in the death of the baby and/or mother. These complications are extraordinarily rare. *Most HG sufferers never experience serious complications.*

Gallbladder Sludge

Sludge can be one of the more benign complications of HG. When the digestive system is slower and has even been out of commission for a significant period of time, as in TPN, the bile that is not being used to help break down food sits concentrating in the gallbladder. This concentration can become very thick and that can cause abdominal discomfort. Normally, the sludge can work itself out once the person starts eating again. In extreme cases it can lead to gallbladder disease.

Gallbladder Disease

Gallbladder disease often involves gallstones. When a stone moves out of the gallbladder and into a duct it can plug up the liver and block the flow of bile. This is called obstructive cholelithiasis and causes obstructive jaundice, which manifests itself as a yellowing of the skin. Acute cholecystitis (swollen gallbladder) can also be caused by a blockage of the bile flow in or out of the gallbladder. Gallbladder disease can cause a variety of discomforts.

Interestingly, HG can either be the cause or the result of gallbladder disease. A friend of mine who experienced severe HG and TPN had to have her gallbladder removed a few months after delivery. This left her wondering if the HG caused the gallbladder disease or if the gallbladder disease caused the HG.

For those of you who developed gallbladder problems long after an initial HG diagnosis that didn't include gallbladder evaluation, think back and determine if you had symptoms of gallbladder disease *before* pregnancy. You may have had a pre-existing gallbladder problem if you experienced any of these pre-pregnancy symptoms:

- frequent upper abdominal pain (on the right side) radiating to the back or shoulder
- pain that came on within one or two hours of eating a fatty meal
- pain that was not relieved by antacids or acid blockers
- pain that caused nausea or vomiting
- pain that subsided within one to four hours

If you didn't have any of these symptoms but experienced nausea or vomiting related to birth control pills, or if you have a history of HG in previous pregnancies, your gallbladder disease was probably more likely due to HG. If the gallbladder disease is bad you'll probably have your gallbladder removed after the baby is born although some have had the surgery during pregnancy. If the problem is causing too much pain the doctor may want to remove it during pregnancy. Even if a gallbladder is septic, draining puss and administering antibiotics can sometimes delay surgery. If you have to have your gallbladder removed, no worries. Aside from having to eat less fat, people live very normal lives without gallbladders.

Mallory-Weiss Tears

Mallory-Weiss tears are generally mild tears that take place deep in the esophagus. The tear can be disturbing as the vomiting of bright red blood usually follows. Typically, these vertical tears in the throat self-heal within ten days. *Very rarely*, they cause a significant amount of blood loss requiring transfusion. This type of severe tear can be difficult to successfully manage, as sutures are sometimes ripped open repeatedly due to prolonged vomiting. People have been known to hemorrhage from these tears, and I spoke with the mother of a woman whose tear was severe enough to be life-threatening. Mallory-Weiss tears may be treated with stitches but are usually managed with observation as they tend to be self-limiting and rarely require surgery. Initiating different antiemetic trials can also help.

Esophageal Rupture

Very rarely a "food pipe" will rupture due to HG. This is so rare that, at the writing of this book, only four cases have been reported.[165] Try not to become paranoid thinking every chest pain or tummy ache is an indication of esophageal rupture. Anyone who suffers from prolonged hyper-vomiting is going to have tummy aches and chest pains every now and again. When the esophagus ruptures, it presents with *severe* chest or upper abdominal pain. This serious complication must be treated as soon as possible. Moderate rupture usually involves an admission to the hospital, nothing by mouth, TPN, nasogastric suction, antibiotics and pain medication. In a severe case surgery may be necessary.

Pneumomediastinum

Pneumomediastinum (air in the space between the lungs) caused by HG is extremely rare. The authors of a 2001 study could find only four such cases in all the literature on HG.[166] It occurs when air leaks out of the lung and into the chest. One way this can happen is through a ruptured esophagus. Incessant high pressure vomiting can also cause the condition. A person with pneumomediastinum may not have any symptoms, but usually she will experience chest pain below the sternum that can radiate to the neck or arms. The pain may worsen upon swallowing or breathing. She may experience significant swelling of the upper chest, neck and face. Generally, medical intervention is not necessary in the context of HG-related pneumomediastinum, because it eventually disappears with the resolution of HG. Oxygen may be administered, and if a lung collapses, a chest tube is required.

Liver Dysfunction

HG can cause liver dysfunction such as jaundice. The liver can degenerate as it does in cases of starvation. Symptoms of liver dysfunction are treated, but the spontaneous resolution of liver problems correlates with the resolution of HG.

Wernicke's Encephalopathy

Liver enzyme elevation may predispose one to developing Wernicke's encephalopathy (WE). WE, which causes lesions in the brain and loss of specific brain functions, is mainly due to thiamine (vitamin B1) deficiency. IVs containing glucose can precipitate WE in a person with a compromised nutritional status. For this reason, thiamine should be given prior to such an infusion. The classic symptoms of WE are double vision and uncontrollable, jerky eye movements, difficulty maintaining balance when standing or walking, and mental confusion. Other symptoms are eyelid drooping, speech changes, loss of coordination, facial paralysis, hand tremor, profound memory loss, loss of ability to think abstractly or solve problems and coma. If not treated, WE can progress along to death. Approximately 10-20% of women who develop WE secondary to HG will die.[167] If you develop this condition, you're probably going to be acting strangely and someone will hopefully notice and get you the physical help you require. WE is uber rare. It occurs through inadequate treatment or lack of treatment altogether.

Treating WE consists of stopping the progression of the disorder by correcting thiamine levels. Some of the damage sustained may be permanent. If the loss of intellect/cognitive skills is severe, a person may need custodial care for the remainder of her life. In case reports, administering thiamine in the first twenty-four hours after the onset of neurologic symptoms was generally associated with positive fetal outcomes.[168] A woman can help prevent WE simply by making sure she is receiving thiamine supplements, particularly if she is receiving IVs with glucose or TPN. Furthermore, thiamine administration should be standard for any patient who has been vomiting for more than three weeks.[169] That applies to every case of HG. Prevention is the best medicine.

Central Pontine Myelinosis
Central pontine myelinosis causes neurologic damage and is very rare in HG. The most common cause of this complication

is rapid correction of low sodium levels in the body. Some of the symptoms are hand tremors, hallucinations, speech changes, different sized pupils, uncontrollable eye movements, double vision and the like. WE increases the risk. Treatment of Central Pontine Myelinosis requires the careful correction of low sodium levels and maintenance of normal levels. The residual effects may take years to resolve and in some cases may be permanent.

Renal Failure

In 2002 the first case of HG-induced renal failure requiring dialysis was reported, which illustrates the rarity of this condition.[170] This case was thought to be caused by intravascular volume depletion (IVD). IVD is essentially the depletion of the liquid (serum) part of the blood as opposed to the solid (cellular) part of the blood. Treatment of acute renal failure may require dialysis if severe enough.

Serious complications are almost unheard of today. Occasionally they do happen, but good medical care can prevent or treat most if not all of these complications, resulting in a favorable outcome.

Flunkey Feelings

When your body is significantly negatively affected by something most women do effortlessly, it's easy to feel defeated and defective. You may lose faith in your physical and even emotional person and assume that complications are inevitable. However, the human body is an incredible wonder that can often compensate when something goes awry, so do not lose hope. A woman's body is more complex than a man's. As one scientist put it, "Females have to be built better than males, because a woman's body carries the physical burden of sustaining another life." If you have HG, your body has thrown you a major curve, but with good health care you can work with your doctor as part of a team to reduce the risk of complications and to help your body accommodate your baby successfully. HG may be hell, but the old adage is true: anything worth having is worth fighting for. Remember your body's compensatory nature, and try not to lose faith in the miraculous process.

Kricket's Story

My husband and I had been trying for a few months to conceive, when we finally tested positive in July of 1999. The elation didn't last long when just a few days later I had the beginnings of "morning sickness."

Morning, noon and night I found myself in the bed with a bucket or running to the commode. I never ate. I couldn't. I rarely drank anything and when I did, I drank only orange juice because it didn't burn shooting out of my nose. Morning sickness is normal the first few months of pregnancy, so I thought all the nausea and vomiting I had was normal. I tried to tough it out without complaining because in a month or two it would pass.

My husband had started a new job and we were waiting for his new insurance to take effect before I saw a doctor. The very first day his insurance took affect my father and husband took me to the emergency room. I had been sick to the point of vomiting bile, so we thought that maybe I had a stomach virus in addition to the morning sickness. The ER staff said I was dehydrated, gave me an IV, and sent me home.

At nearly three months pregnant I had my first OB/GYN appointment. By now I looked pretty poor. I was pale and thin and too sick to wear makeup or even care. The doctor seemed great and truly concerned about certain pre-existing health conditions I have. You see, I also suffer from a congenital cardiac anomaly. My heart likes to act up from time to time. The doctor told my family, "Don't worry, we're going to take good care of her." But I never mentioned the continuing and constant sickness I was having. I still thought it was normal and would pass.

As time wore on the sickness didn't go away. I had to quit school. I wasn't there much anyway. Most days it was impossible for me to get out of bed. Not only was I constantly vomiting, but also I developed migraines so terrible that it seemed the walls in my bedroom were moving. School was just impossible at the time.

I'll never forget when I went to apply for WIC. The woman who interviewed me made me feel little and selfish. As she questioned my diet during this time, it was evident I had no diet. I lived on the oxygen around me and that was it. She asked me, "Don't you eat? Do you not care that you are starving your growing baby?" I said that I just hadn't realized how little I ate. I tried to explain how sick I was and how eating was a misery. The interviewer would not hear it though and had already made up her mind that I was an unfit mother.

My mother said that some women are sick their entire pregnancy. So to me, I was just going to be one of them. I was so sick that it became necessary for me to move in with my parents so they could take care of me. By then my doctor noticed that I was not gaining any weight, but he never asked why. He just said, "Go home, and for God's sake eat a candy bar!" And I would nod my head and faintly smile.

One night I awoke with severe pain right in the middle of my abdomen just under my ribs. It shot straight through to my back, between my shoulder blades. Oh what pain! It made me vomit even more. I mentioned this incident at my next doctor visit. My doctor said that it was probably acid reflux but that he wanted an ultrasound to make sure it wasn't my gallbladder. It *was* my gallbladder, but my uterus was too high up to perform the necessary surgery. If at all possible we had to try to wait till after the baby was born to remove my gallbladder. Ironically, the doctor put me on a strict diet of no fatty foods.

After that episode I developed bronchitis as well. I was really miserable never eating, always hanging over the commode, living with the daily risk of a gallbladder attack and coughing up a lung. I rarely left the house; it was too big a task for me by then. My husband had to help brush my hair some days because I was so sick.

Bronchitis became pneumonia, and antibiotics were refilled repeatedly. Fevers were not uncommon for me by then, but somehow I carried on. My mother always commented on my paleness, and my father said I looked like a third world child because I was skin and bones and had a bloated stomach.

At my next medical appointment, I was so small that the doctor began doing weekly stress tests, and my due date was moved. My pneumonia was not clearing up, and I was going downhill. The doctor said that I had to stay on bed rest for the whole week or I couldn't go to my baby shower. The shower was the only thing I had been looking forward to my entire pregnancy.

The night before my shower, my husband was at work and my mother was out of town. It was just my father and I. As I lay on the couch I said to my dad, "I don't know if I am having contractions or if I've just got the crud but it's coming every three minutes." It was scary.

When my husband got home that night, I tried to eat some toast and egg yolk to no avail. It was hopeless. It was then that both my father and my husband sat beside my bed on the floor and begged me to call the doctor. I refused. I said that at the most he would tell me to come in for an IV and then send me home. My dad almost started crying, so I finally broke down and called the doctor. Guess what he said? "Come in for an IV."

I was running a fever and had the chills. The nurses there were expecting me. They set me up for the night and even put monitors on my belly. My dad and husband went home for the rest of the night, leaving me in good care.

Later the nurse came in my room and said, "You're having contractions; can you feel them?" I said, "So that's what those are." They were contractions, not the crud. I was given medication to stop the contractions. I ran a fever all that night. Early that morning my blood was taken for a work up.

When I woke up later that morning, I was ready to go home and go to my baby shower. The doctor came into my room, said that there were some things in my blood work, and told me I couldn't leave the hospital. I begged him to let me go and told him I'd come right back if only he'd let me attend the baby shower. He said no, of course.

My family came by that morning; they were all going to go to my shower in my place. Even hubby. It's strange too. I had so looked forward to the baby shower, but as the day wore on and I drifted in and out of fever, I forgot about the shower and wondered why no one was there. I had forgotten that they were all at the party for me. I thought they had forgotten me. They all came that afternoon afterwards and tried to get me to eat the food they'd brought back from the party. Even the nurses were trying to feed it to me. Just to get them all to leave me alone about food I said I'd take a sandwich. When it came, I never ate it.

One nurse really tried to help, but I disliked her so because the smell of her perfume made me sick. I vomited twice the amount when she was there. All I wanted was for her to go away. Force-feeding was also her motto, and when that didn't work, she brought up cooks from the cafeteria to cook special meals that I might eat. Every time though, she had to hold my kidney shaped plastic bucket for me to heave those meals back up. There was always a can of Ensure in my room that the doctor and nurses urged me to drink.

At that point, my blood was taken five times a day. My liver tests were coming back showing abnormalities, and my white blood cell count was dramatically dropping. Those were the doctors' biggest concerns. All kinds of doctors, including infectious disease control doctors, were brought in to see what they could do for me, but they were never able to pinpoint a cause.

In one arm I had a special IV solution of nutrients and in the other arm I had an IV of antibiotics. After a few days, my veins were blowing and needles began coming up dry because of all the blood work and IVs. It became torturous to have my blood drawn or IV changed. I cried. I could barely see;

everything was so blurry. I'd feel so sick, and then they'd come to collect my blood, and I'd just cry. They stuck me over and over until the tiniest spot of crimson slowly inched up the needle.

IV changes were the worst. I do remember once I couldn't really see anything but blurry figures and lots of voices. I could barely make out what they were saying. The voices sounded far off and slurred. My mother later told me the nurses were trying to decide who among them was the best "stick." I do remember one of them getting it and repeatedly pushing on the spot with her thumb saying, "Does that hurt? Does that hurt?" I looked down at the blown vein in my hand and said, "It's green. What do *you* think?"

I really didn't comprehend how bad things were until the day the doctor stepped out of my room to talk to my family. Only my husband came back in minutes later. He sat on my bed, took my hand, and then his head came down and laid on me. He was crying. I started to worry that I might die. Later I learned of the sobering conversation that had taken place outside of my room. My dad had asked the doctor, "Is she going to be OK?" The doctor looked like a horse had just kicked him when he replied, "I honestly don't know."

Not only was I vomiting at that point, but I had developed diarrhea as well. Nothing was going in but everything was coming out, so my physician finally put me on TPN. Everyone said that my personality really changed during all this. They said that I became mean and nasty. I was told that I even kicked our preacher out of my hospital room. I have no memory of it, but our preacher does.

One night my fever rose above one hundred three degrees. The doctor decided that, due to all of the complications, the pregnancy was putting my survival into question and something had to be done. I either had to end the pregnancy or risk death to both the baby and I. My induction was scheduled that morning. The baby wasn't due till April eleventh and it was February twenty-third.

I have very little recollection of the events, but as soon as I realized the doctor was going to induce I kept thinking, "Where's my husband. Will he make it on time? Has anyone contacted him at work?" I learned later, that my husband had been there the whole time.

I was to have a vaginal delivery because they didn't think my body could handle the stress of a C-section. I pleaded with the doctor, "I can't; I'm too weak. *I can't.*" He firmly replied, "You *can* and you *WILL.*" I remember that clearly. He put me under a no stress policy. They wanted me to be comfortable with as little stress on my body as possible. I was to have lots of drugs and an epidural. It was all a risk, but so was staying in limbo like I had been.

When a nurse came in to check my dilation she said, "Something doesn't feel right. I'm going to get the doctor." The baby was coming out sunny side up and neck first. She'd break her neck in that position. I had to have an emergency C-section. It was a success, and I had a little girl who, at seven weeks early, weighed in at five pounds and two ounces. She was in perfect health and needed no help breathing and no incubator.

I had suffered a weight loss of thirty pounds, and after her birth I weighed in at ninety-eight pounds. When I woke up in the recovery ward, I was fine and didn't feel sick one little bit. I even announced that I wanted a cheeseburger!

Over a year later I learned of HG. I took what I learned to my doctor and discussed it with him. I had experienced all the symptoms: liver dysfunction, nausea, vomiting, weight loss, fever, gallbladder difficulties, headaches, pale skin, problems with vision, even changes in personality. None of my doctors could ever find the cause of these things. HG is a diagnosis of exclusion: you don't know what it is, but you rule out what it's not. My research convinced me that there is a high chance of HG recurrence in subsequent pregnancies, so I consulted my physician to develop a plan for the next baby. The research was right; I'm pregnant again, and I have HG.

This time I know that what is happening to me isn't normal. I have an illness and it has a name. I feel validated and have the confidence to tell my doctor when things aren't right, and he in turn listens and treats my aliments to the best of his ability. After several IVs he has given me a new drug called Zofran. It has worked miracles for me. As soon as I begin to feel nauseous I take it and am fine. In fact, I feel great! I am now five months pregnant and have *gained* ten and a half pounds. I am beginning to catch a little glimpse of what a normal pregnancy must be like... finally!

TERMINATION OF PREGNANCY

SEVENTEEN
The End of the Beginning

Even though HG is not typically fatal, its suffering can be a torture that drives many women to abort babies they desperately want. In England and Wales, between 1979 and 1992, 97% of all terminations for maternal health were due to HG.[171]

HG accounts for over fifty thousand hospitalizations annually in the U.S. In the first chapter, HG-related abortion rates were discussed. If we sort of made a semi-educated guess and pulled the rate of 2% out of the air, applying it to the entire American HG population, that would be an HG termination rate of at least one thousand pregnancies a year. A friend's doctor told her that he has seen roughly three HG-related terminations per month for the several years he has been in practice. This is one physician in one office. The number of HG-related abortions is probably staggering.

Imagine the tragic irony of being so ill that you feel physically driven to abort the child you love and want. How does this happen? It is so hard to understand or even believe that a mother could be driven to this, but the protracted duration of the intense physical debilitation, coupled with the resulting emotional suffering, can finally result in a point of absolute personal crisis. At such a point, malnutrition and dehydration may have sorely compromised a woman's cognition. Perhaps this isn't the optimal time to make life-altering decisions.

Women who are suffering from HG feel tortured and imprisoned. In nature, fettered animals have been known to gnaw off their own legs to escape a trap, so it should come as no great shock that even humans would consider making terrible sacrifices to escape an agonized confinement. Researchers in Hong Kong noted:

> "It is not uncommon that [HG] patients request termination of pregnancy because of intolerable symptoms and psychological stress."[172]

How many women feel physically forced to terminate a pregnancy for the sole purpose of relieving the devastating symptoms of HG?

At-Risk Moms

Women most at risk have other children and lack the necessary physical health and support to care for them properly. The care of young children (especially toddlers and children with special needs) is a challenge for any mother. Mothers who cannot physically take care of themselves may find it impossible to meet the needs of other children. Eileen experienced this:

> "In addition to my physical suffering I felt like a failure as a mother. I felt totally unable to care for my boys. One day one of my sons came to the side of my bed and begged me for an egg. It was noon and neither of my children had been given breakfast. I could not get out of bed to feed them. My little boy

just stood there at my bedside begging for food. He and his brother ended up eating peanut butter out of the jar all day. I'll never forget that; it was a very low moment in my life."

Eileen did not have enough help. Without adequate support some hyperemetic mothers invariably turn to abortion as the only way of ensuring the care of other children.

HG is a dramatic illness for a child to witness. Often she will be quite fearful that Mother is going to die. She may cry often, pitch angry fits, cling to Mother, abandon and fear Mother, emulate Mother by pretending to vomit, stop eating, over-eat, lose sleep, have nightmares, have trouble at school, suffer from tummy aches, and worry excessively about personal health or the health of other family members. Susan experienced this with her son:

"My four-year-old son went through a miserable phase, where he was convinced I was dying and could not cope. He is normally a really good kid and pretty fearless, but he became a mess. He had complete meltdowns over things that never bothered him in the past, obsessed about my health, and was hurting his friends daily at school. Since I started doing better and can play with him every day, he is doing much better. "

The realization that a mother's illness is hurting her children can be more than she can bear. Support for the family is essential.

Importance of Support

Canadian researchers were interested in learning more about abortion and HG, and for two months they collected data from one thousand, one hundred women.[173] In the study, forty-two hyperemetic women thought about terminating, and an additional seventeen actually did. Interestingly, the major difference between these two groups seemed to be support.

That a woman would abort a child she loves and wants is the most compelling evidence for the severity of this illness, and it bears glaring witness to the low-grade social and medical support that some women receive. No matter how temporary the situation, it is paramount that those with seriously impaired health are given every available medical option that is positive to their overall well being, and it certainly wouldn't hurt to add the support that family and friends have a moral obligation to provide. Without social and medical support, HG can end with a broken heart.

The Vanishing

People are often shocked to feel abandoned by those on whom they believed they could rely. Unfortunately, the myriad acquaintances that make up the brunt of our day-to-day social lives can often be counted on as fair weather friends. HG is so severe and misunderstood that, outside of one's own family, there is not much social support.

Supports may find the condition overly ominous, while others may have read a poor description of HG, its symptoms and treatments, and they may get the errant idea that HG is little more than a minor inconvenience, easily managed by medications. This type of support may be annoyed by the way you are "carrying on." Some may compare their pregnancies to yours, and they may share the sentiment that you are only pregnant, not sick. One friend told me, "Well, I had terrible morning sickness too, but I just ate two crackers when I got up in the morning and didn't make such a big deal out of it." Every time I see this dear lady, she tells me that it's time for me to have another baby. (If two crackers would do it I'd have enough children to start my own football team.) Your pregnancy can also bother those with fertility problems or child loss. They may be hurt by *anyone* who becomes pregnant and resent especially pregnant women who complain. It's true that peoples' personal issues can sometimes make them unsupportive, and while it's regrettable, it's a common phenomenon.

Do not be surprised if someone regards you as whiney, stubborn, or unpleasant. You may hear that you are overreacting, seeking attention or others may believe you to be weak. One friend, who is aware of my situation, "diagnosed" her daughter as having HG and proudly proclaimed that the daughter continued to work fifty-five hours a week in a merchandising position. When I expressed surprise that someone with HG could maintain such a schedule, she replied, "Yes, well my daughter is a *strong* girl."

Her commentary was unintentional, though a little of me couldn't help but take it personally. I wanted to tell her that I have a fairly high level of endurance and pain tolerance and that I didn't wince once while undergoing a two-hour tattoo. I wanted to tell her about the time I gave myself nine stitches or about the time a nurse said I *couldn't* have broken my broken bone, because I was laughing too hard. I wanted to tell my friend that at eighteen-years-old I went to funeral college, embalmed human remains for four hours straight in lab every Monday, and that I was able to make plans for lunch while elbow-deep in autopsied viscera. I wanted to ask her if any of that made *me* "strong enough." Instead I smiled and said, "That's really something."

I recall the time a friend compared her mastitis to my HG and then negatively judged my character because I didn't handle four months of starvation and severe vomiting as well as she handled a few days of fever and sore breasts. (I've had mastitis, and it's cake in comparison.) Another time co-workers at a meeting described my feminine constitution as deficient due to my inability to work around what they called "normal" morning sickness. I could fill up a separate book with the cruelty of others and the pain they have caused. The only point would be to illustrate ad nauseum that it happens to others and you are not alone. I got through it, and so can you. We have to accept the fact that, intentional or not, some people make personal judgments regarding the character of women who suffer from HG. The best I can offer is that they know not what they do.

Family Support

At a funeral I attended, the deceased man's son stood up and shared a very powerful moment in his life:

> "When I was a kid I once asked my dad, a veteran, if a nuclear bomb was the most powerful thing in the world, and he said, 'No, Son. The most powerful thing in the world is a family's love.'"

When a person is in a crisis, she seeks out those she can rely on to help her. Who better to assist her than the members of her own family? Generally, pregnant women can have a tendency to cling to their mothers because they are assuming the same type of role and want someone who can relate. It can be an especially difficult time for the hyperemetic woman who has no maternal support.

Abandonment isn't always personal or preventable. Occasionally a main support will die. My social support disappeared when I lost my most avid fan and caretaker, my grandmother. She was my mother figure in life, and I lost her to cancer ten months before I experienced my first bout of severe HG. I often wonder how different my life would be had she been alive and healthy enough to physically care for me during my initial HG. She was my mom and my best friend, and she died just when I needed her the most.

My mother figure was "unsupportive" through no fault of her own. It must be particularly painful when a mother is alive and well and yet fails to offer loving support. Mary had problems with hers:

> "My mother constantly needled me to get off the couch and go for a walk. She did not understand at all what I was going through and made me feel worse for being unable to accomplish something as small as a short walk outside. I got the feeling she thought I was just being uncooperative and that I didn't want to get well. She also told me to 'get a hobby.' Instead of acknowledging how bad I was feeling, my mom seemed to say, 'You're not really sick; you're just

uninterested.' I was shocked and felt abandoned by her attitude."

Conversely, a mom's functional support can make all the difference. In the beginning, many members of Pam's family didn't understand her illness. Because of this, negative attitudes formed and contributed to Pam's feelings of defeat. Eventually, she considered termination, but her mother, Jenny, was a fierce advocate who sprang into action. She got on the Internet and dug up as much information as she could find. Because of her initiative, Jenny was able to offer information that not only comforted Pam but educated the rest of the family. In a letter she wrote:

"I believe that an act of God helped me find the information I got. And I do believe it made a big difference in how we reacted to everything. Before, family members thought I was crazy for believing that Pam's nausea and vomiting were abnormal and serious, but because of the information I was able to give them, even they were able to realize that HG involves a real illness and does not mean Pam is 'just a wimpy little girl.' I also believe that the change in their attitude made a big difference in how Pam was able to look at her situation. Things are much better now."

Jenny's efforts paid off. She did not leave Pam to her own devices. Offering nothing in the way of suggestion or assistance, becoming physically and emotionally distant, or, more overtly, literally leaving the person are all forms of abandonment. After my first pregnancy, a family member told me, "Well, you're so independent that we just assumed you'd take care of yourself." That attitude did not pay off. Support is crucial.

Every now and again I get a letter from a woman whose husband is not fulfilling his wedding vows. Instead of actively showing her the love she needs most in sickness, he accuses her of trying to get attention or being lazy and gets mad when she can't clean the house, prepare meals, care for children, and go to work. It is cruel to suggest that a woman's HG symptoms are somehow a controllable behavior. The idea that HG is morning sickness normalizes something that is most certainly *not* normal. When a woman with HG is expected to act like a woman with morning sickness, the results can be harmful. A husband's unsupportive attitude is probably due more to ignorance than anything else. If the wife had a recognized illness like cancer and was going through chemotherapy the husband probably wouldn't act this way. However, pregnancy is supposed to be little more than a mild inconvenience. The idea that it can cause massive complications is something altogether foreign to many husbands, especially if they have had prior pregnancy experience in a former marriage.

People who invalidate the sufferer's sickness can exacerbate HG by browbeating or inflicting guilt on the woman as "motivation" to perform tasks that should not be undertaken by a sick person. The sick mom may try to maintain her former superwoman pace in order to please a disgruntled family member or to prove to herself that she is strong. The exertion can cause a relapse that necessitates a hospital stay or other type of intervention. Conversely, if she doesn't attempt to maintain her former activity level, she may begin to resent the fact that a person for whom she cares deeply is attacking her character and neglecting her physical needs.

Some husbands or main supports are sensitive and want to be helpful but are terrified at what they are witnessing. One man said, "I don't want to sound overly dramatic, but it was like she was possessed." HG often results in multiple hospital stays and occasionally involves complications. This can be very exhausting and scary for both the mother and her supports. However, when a support constantly worries aloud if the baby and the sufferer are going to be OK, it can cause the sufferer considerable stress. Also, when a main support is already worn out from assuming the same role in prior HG pregnancies, there can be great fear of the prospect of going through it again. This dread can exert significant pressure on the sufferer. Beth's husband was so anguished about having to go through HG again that he implored her to terminate:

> "I had HG in the first pregnancy and it brought me to the point of kidney failure. During my second pregnancy I made it through without going to the hospital. In my third HG pregnancy I was admitted to the hospital nine times in eight weeks and I lost thirteen kilograms. I was just pregnant for a fourth time, but unfortunately at six weeks the vomiting started so bad that I dehydrated very quickly. My doctor gave me a Maxalon (Reglan) injection, a pat on the head, and sent me home. My husband was so distressed that he begged me to terminate. I did. Now I suffer from terrible depression and fail to understand a medical profession that can sew hands back onto people but couldn't help me get through vomiting."

OBstacles

Medical support is so important. There are many options available for women with HG. The problem is that these options are being withheld from women. Due to cost, some physicians and HMOs may delay or avoid some options such as Zofran or TPN. Options may also be limited if the physician's view of HG is unrealistic. One OB resident shared her and her peers' perception: "Most of us view [HG patients] as whiners." She added, "HG cases are not technically exciting."[174]

Whether due to the astronomical expense of optimally treating HG or the physician's lack of concern, some women are robbed of life-saving treatments that would otherwise prevent the abortion of their children.

Armchair Psychology

Some doctors, who don't understand HG, think the condition is mentally precipitated in the easily-flustered woman. Anyone who complains of being terribly sick during her pregnancy is mentally suspect. If you are dealing with an unplanned pregnancy and HG, the armchair psychologist may make an effortless leap from "unplanned" to "unwanted," and this attitude has the potential to negatively affect medical treatment.

If the doctor thinks you do not want your baby, your pseudo-shrink may feel that your HG is primarily a psychosomatic problem to be dealt with on a psychiatrist's sofa. No matter how you try to reassure this type that your baby is a welcome surprise, she will ever harbor lingering doubts. To her, you have emotional issues that you need to identify and resolve before you can recover from HG. She is not familiar with the study that shows no difference in the incidence of nausea and vomiting in planned and unplanned pregnancies.[175] Neither has she considered the report in which a woman's first HG pregnancy was unplanned and brought to term while her second HG pregnancy was planned and terminated.[176] The latter scenario is more common than people think. I have personally heard from many women who aborted the second, planned child because they woefully discovered that HG prevented them from caring for their first. If your doctor inquires whether the pregnancy was planned or not, makes an issue of an unplanned pregnancy, or suggests that you see a psychotherapist in lieu of the medical treatment you feel you need, she may be an armchair psychologist, and you may need a new doctor.

If you are single, have HG and the pregnancy was unplanned, you may encounter double discrimination. Incredibly, some still assume that single women, in particular, can not experience the unplanned joy of an unplanned pregnancy. Additionally, if you are single, have HG, an unplanned pregnancy *and* unrelated emotional issues, may God help you, because the armchair psychologist won't. And for the sake of all that is good and pure in the world, never ever tell the armchair psychologist that at fourteen you couldn't eat for a month after your boyfriend broke up with you. If you do, you will be under suspicion for somehow giving yourself HG to avoid becoming fat. It's unbelievable how low some professionals will stoop. If the doctor who is treating you for HG constantly refers to the circumstances under which your child was conceived or any other irrelevant personal issues, *you don't have to put up with it.* Consider finding a better obstetrician.

Rotation Policy

One major problem in multiple partner practices is the rotation policy. The general philosophy is that if you see every doctor, assistant and midwife in the practice, you will be familiar with the on-call professional when the time comes to deliver your baby. This is silly. When a woman is in active labor, any individual with a catcher's mitt will do. Some practices will suspend the rotation rule in a complicated pregnancy, but that requires acknowledgement that HG goes beyond normal morning sickness. If this does not happen, consider consulting another doctor, because the rotation policy may be grossly inappropriate for women with HG. Physical deterioration is a process; it is extremely important that this process is monitored as closely and continuously as possible. Limiting HG examinations to one or two doctors could be helpful for a variety of reasons.

It bears repeating: if an HG patient sees a different professional every time she goes for an appointment, by the time she gets around to the third or fourth person, she may have lost a significant amount of weight. If the medical staff doesn't carefully examine and compare her previous weights they may not realize that she is uncharacteristically thin and therefore has been very sick and suffering as greatly as she conveys. In addition, a patient who, prior to HG, paid meticulous attention to personal appearance may come into the doctor's office unbathed, with no makeup, stringy hair, unshaven grizzly bear legs and shrubbery growing where armpits once were. An unfamiliar health care professional may glance at her and assume she has always been a slob, whereas the doctor who has seen her from day one will know that "Miss Priss" wouldn't dare let herself look like a junkie unless something was horribly wrong. If the process is followed closely, the sufferer will have a better chance of avoiding the delays that have caused unnecessary agony for many sick moms.

I am particularly thankful that my Matria home health care nurse, who called and spoke with me *every single day* in my fourth pregnancy, could tell that something was wrong with me one day just by listening to my voice. I told her I was just as sick as any other day and not to bother my doctor who I would see the following week, but she insisted. She got me an appointment right away. He took one look at me and admitted me for tube feedings and a five-week hospital stay. Because of her familiarity with me, the Matria nurse was able to get me the care I needed, which spared me an entire week of agonizing debilitation. *That* is support.

Re-Dehydration

Doctors are pretty good about rehydrating the dehydrated but, as previously discussed, the way they go about it can cause additional suffering. For instance, HG is not something that magically goes away after a single IV. HG involves ongoing dehydration and therefore, hydration should be fairly constant. Dehydration takes its toll, even affecting cognition. In the context of therapeutic abortion for HG, how can a sick mother be expected to make rational, life-altering choices if her cognitive process is on the fritz? If someone has had two or three IVs within a short period of time, it may be time to consider in-home IVs. I'm a firm believer in uninterrupted fluids for an uninterrupted pregnancy.

The Slow Fast

Because of persistent, prolonged vomiting, HG usually involves an extended period of involuntary fasting which results in a rapid and unhealthy weight loss. When a pregnant person has fluid and electrolyte imbalances and has lost 5% or more of her total body weight, it's appropriate to consider supplemental nutrition to diminish suffering and improve the physical condition.[177]

Too many doctors are slow in prescribing alternative nutrition, the simultaneous administration of nutrients and fluids. There are many available formulas and several methods of administering this nutrition, but a doctor must prescribe it first. If a doctor will not feed you when your inability to feed yourself has resulted in significant weight loss and malnutrition, you are being neglected, and that is abuse. It little matters if effective treatment is expensive or tedious. What is important is appropriate care for you and your child.

Drug Dragging

Some women reach the point where none of the conventional antiemetics are effective. This, combined with poor medical support, can cost a woman her child. No one should lose a child because her doctor will not prescribe drugs that literature shows to be helpful in her situation.

Corticosteroids are systemic, and some doctors, who aren't familiar with the studies, drag their feet in using them. Even faced with the abortion of a child, some doctors will not prescribe corticosteroids. Ask them why. Birth defects? Although corticosteroids have not generally been linked to birth defects in humans,[178-179] doctors in a sue-crazy society may think twice before being "unconventional," If you want to try corticosteroids but your doctor refuses due to anxiety over birth defects, ask her to supply you with studies that support her fears. If she still persists, ask her to compare and contrast the risk of birth defects caused by corticosteroids and the risk of "birth defects" caused by abortion.

Corticosteroids can be an incredible, magic bullet if used correctly and administered by a physician. Just the other day, I witnessed an ultra-healthy "corticosteroid baby" playing and laughing her head off at the park, her mother smiling in adoration beside her. At thirteen weeks, that child had a time and day set to be terminated in a therapeutic abortion, but a different doctor and a corticosteroid prescription combated HG and saved her life. Within a year after her uncomplicated birth the mother underwent a total hysterectomy for an unrelated health problem. Imagine if those first few doctors had succeeded in preventing this mother from receiving corticosteroid therapy! I too received gobs of steroids in pregnancy four, and my baby is perfect in every way.

HMO Shuffle

When HG has not been taken seriously and not been treated adequately, women and children have died. Sufficient technology is available to treat HG, so why aren't women given the treatment options they need? In an HMO's fervent attempt to keep costs down, they may refuse to pay for necessary treatment. If the patient cannot pay for that treatment, she will not receive it.

HMOs may also pressure a doctor to keep treatment costs to a minimum. So the physician may not even make her patient aware of treatment options, which she knows the HMO will not pay for. Insurance companies can be vile in their fervent observation of the bottom line: money. Watch them like a hawk. In my most horrible HG pregnancy, my insurance caseworker frequently attempted to thwart my health care in order to limit costs, all under the guise of being *my advocate*. She directly contradicted orders from the IV therapy team who inserted four of my PICC lines. From the very first PICC line they said I needed a pump, but my HMO caseworker said I only needed a gravity drip. When I questioned her logic I was told that the hospital was only trying to get more money. "It will cost..." she said before catching herself and reasoning, "I mean, you just don't need it."

I pressed, "IVT says I need it, they should know, and excuse me, but did you just say something about how much it costs?" My HMO caseworker giggled nervously, told me that as a nurse she knew more about HG than I did, and quickly changed the subject. I did not get the pump that day, and it caused me, a person on a PICC line for constant fluids, to become dehydrated. I had to have that PICC line replaced, which took multiple attempts due to my state of dehydration. My livid husband called from the procedure room and got into an argument with the caseworker who again did not want to pay for a pump. The IV team wanted to talk to her, and my husband mentioned our attorney, when lo and behold, she finally miraculously understood that what I needed was the appropriate medical treatment.

Prior to my long hospitalization this same woman went out of her way to repeatedly explain to me that hospitalization was out of the question. She went into great, comically frightening detail of how nasty and germ-filled hospitals are. "They are dangerous," she warned constantly. "Bacteria pour in through the air ducts. You do not *need* to be there; you do not *want* to be there." It turns out that although I did not *want* to be there, I *needed* to be there for five weeks. In spite of knowing how loathsome my HMO caseworker's motives were, I must admit that every now and again I caught myself looking at the mid-century A/C unit wondering about the "germs." Health care was *always* a battle with my insurance company caseworker, and her motive was never more obvious than the day I got the call.

I was in the hospital fighting for my baby's life and feeling like the living dead, but I was stable and hanging in there. When I reached what I suppose would normally be around the sixty-five thousand-dollar treatment mark, with miles still to go, the insurance caseworker had the nerve to call me and make sure I "understood" that I had the right to terminate my pregnancy. I was shocked, offended, and infuriated, and my doctor agreed that the call had been inappropriate.

Beware, beware. Watch out for HMOs who want to dictate the course of your health care. That is not their job. They are there to pay for the health care your doctor orders and *that is it*. Do not allow them to rob you of your physical and emotional health by contradicting your doctor's orders or by subtly (or not-so-subtly) making inappropriate suggestions that could negatively affect you for the rest of your life.

Variations in Medical Support

The level of medical support is as varied as the level of symptom severity. Some who suffer terribly are offered little to nothing by way of medical support. Others, who seemingly didn't have HG at all, receive the royal treatment. Occasionally, people with large financial resources, high profiles or prestigious occupations develop HG, and they seem to receive a curiously high level of medical care.

If you're the President of the United States or a ditch digger, your doctor has a duty to provide the best care available. It is her responsibility to offer you cutting-edge medical treatment, which consists of appropriate monitoring, rehydration when you can't drink, nutritional support when you can't eat and available, effective medications. Your responsibility is to yourself and to your child. You are not legally or ethically bound to a doctor or her practice. Your doctor works for *you*. If she refuses to give you the help you need, find someone else. Chances of having a positive pregnancy outcome are optimized by social and medical reinforcement.

When Enough Isn't Enough

Even when all supports are in place, the best therapy may be unable to relieve intense suffering. Severe HG that is unresponsive to treatment is a rare, miserable and disabling condition associated with several hospital stays, months of bed rest, loss of employment, etc. Life-preserving treatments can be invasive and scary and can carry significant risks (though the probability of these risks is low). Furthermore, if HG is inadequately or inappropriately treated, it can eventually lead to maternal death, although this is nearly non-existent. The point is that HG goes beyond morning sickness. It can be severe and excruciating, and a minority of women surrenders in the form of a request to terminate. Unwanted terminations can also result due to *very rare* occasions when medical treatment is insufficient to preserve maternal life otherwise.

The mother of a woman who developed life-threatening Mallory-Weiss tears shared that when doctors sutured the tears, vomiting continued reopening the wounds. One night the daughter was found lying in crimson-stained snow just outside the hospital door. They rushed her into the ER, placed her in a drug-induced coma, and contacted her mother explaining that they could not keep the young woman in a drug-induced coma for the remainder of the pregnancy. Doctors expressed their opinion that the situation was clearly life-threatening, and when they allowed the patient to come out of the coma vomiting resumed as predicted. The patient, who was single and had other children, reluctantly agreed to an unwanted termination.

Therapeutic termination is a particularly dreadful subject because it deals with mothers who abort children they want, and I think there is no greater conflict. A significant amount of moms terminate for HG, and so I have included a chapter of relevant information on abortion procedures. It is a good idea to be informed regarding the benefits and risks of any procedure used to treat HG, particularly one as permanent as abortion.

See Chapter 13 for tips on how you can help someone suffering from HG.

India's Story

Some things in life are simply taken for granted. Like children. I never imagined a life without children. Having a family of my own was something that I always knew would happen. Unfortunately, many people do not realize the miracle that takes place each time a child comes into being. Children are a great and wondrous gift from God, a gift that, because of an illness, I chose not to accept.

I regret the decision that I made every day of my life. This is my story, written in the hopes that it will shed light on an epidemic that is ruining the lives of women and children all over the world. HG is a horrific medical condition that has forever changed my life.

I found out I was pregnant when my husband and I had been married almost a year. We were both excited and nervous about the news. Right away I told everyone I knew. I wanted everyone to share in my joy, and I never once gave thought to the notion that something might go wrong.

I remember feeling tired, ravenously hungry and quite emotional during the first few weeks after I found out about the baby. I bought pregnancy books and read them from front to back trying to learn everything I could. I was relieved to find out that all of my symptoms appeared to be normal. I did what all of the books told me. I stayed away from fatty foods, waited an hour before lying down after a meal, etc. I was doing pretty well.

While at work one day, I noticed some light brown spotting. I called the doctor immediately and he told me to come in right away. I cried all the way to the doctor's office, and I remember sitting in the waiting room praying to God to let my baby be all right. My doctor performed an ultrasound and found a heartbeat right away. I was so relieved. The ultrasound showed the baby at seven weeks. He then told me that I was not out of the woods yet and that while the chance of having a miscarriage after seeing a heartbeat is very low, it does happen about five to ten percent of the time.

At around eight weeks I began to get sick. I remember the very first day I threw up. I had eaten some canned ravioli and lay down for a nap. When I awoke I immediately became sick, but then the nausea went away. According to all the books I was reading I had just completed my first bout with "morning sickness." No big deal. If that's what morning sickness consisted of, I could manage it. I was in for a rude awakening.

By nine weeks I was a bloodhound. I could smell meat cooking a mile away. My gag reflex was in full force. I was perpetually nauseous. Within days the nausea gave way to vomiting, sometimes as often as twenty times a day. I couldn't keep any food or liquid down.

Things came to a head one Sunday when I awoke in the middle of the night vomiting. I threw up until there was nothing left in my stomach and then I moved on to dry heaves. Needless to say, I didn't go to work the next day. By Monday night things had not improved. At around two in the morning I called my doctor to let him know that I had not been able to keep food or liquids down for over twenty-four hours. I was told to go to the emergency room if I felt I could not make it until morning. I drove myself to the hospital, was immediately hooked up to an IV drip, and fell asleep. The doctor admitted me to a private room the next morning to monitor my ketones and electrolytes. I remember being absolutely miserable, unable to eat, and getting up every ten minutes to drag my pole to the bathroom to shed all that IV fluid. I was released from the hospital the next day with myriad drugs that were supposed to help me deal with the "morning sickness." Even though I still felt horrible, I had hope that if I could get these prescriptions filled and take them like a "good girl," I would be OK. I was so incredibly naïve.

For the next few days, I took the Reglan and the Phenergan as directed. I was still not able to eat, still vomiting, and now I was sleepy to boot! I was getting scared, and my husband was running out of patience with me. It's sad to think that I was just trying to survive from day to day, and then I was worried that I was not being a good enough wife, a good enough daughter, a good enough employee. I was trying to keep myself afloat, and I was worried that my husband would be mad or disappointed because I could not cook dinner for him. The emotional stress that came from worrying only exacerbated the sickness.

After a week and a half of taking the medications I continued to be violently ill. Everything I ate came back up, and all smells made me vomit. I lost five pounds in just a couple weeks. All the books tell you to get "plenty of rest" to avoid morning sickness. I would lie down to go to sleep around ten at night, and I would wake up every ten to fifteen minutes throughout the night to dry heave. I never slept more than a few minutes at a time. My husband started getting scared that I wasn't going to be all right. Even though he wanted the baby and was concerned about his child's health, he was frightened that he might lose me. That made me even more nervous, because I started to worry that my illness was becoming a heavy burden to him.

Over the next few weeks, the doctor put me on a couple of different medications that did absolutely nothing for me. I would go to the doctor, get a shot of Phenergan, fall asleep for a couple of hours, and then wake up vomiting again within an hour. At eleven weeks the doctor noticed some blood during an internal exam. The ultrasound showed the strong beating heart of my perfectly healthy baby. Yet I was miserable. I was frail, sick, pale, couldn't work, and couldn't do anything except lay on my couch.

I *begged* my doctor to do something, but he just said, "What's happening here is a beautiful thing. Many women get sick when they are pregnant. We've done everything that we can do to help you without risking the baby's wellbeing. It's time to tough it out." My hope disappeared.

At twelve weeks I was sicker than ever. I had lost nearly ten pounds in a month, was severely depressed, and could think of nothing but getting better. I was so sick for so long with no real help or understanding from anyone, and my natural survival instincts started kicking in. I no longer focused on what was best for my baby but what I could do to be well again. I remember lying on my couch one afternoon, tortured by stale cigarette smoke from my husband's addiction and thinking of my doctor's opinion that there was nothing else anyone could do, when a thought occurred to me: "*I* can do something."

I realized I could terminate my pregnancy and not be so terribly ill anymore. No more throwing up and no more trips to the doctor only to have him tell me I was making a big deal out of nothing. I could have my life back. I wouldn't have to rely on anyone else for the simple tasks of life. I could cook for my husband, I could clean my house, I could visit with friends, I could work. It wouldn't be so bad. Maybe later they would even find the cure for HG and I could get pregnant again then. But right then and right there I felt I had to reclaim my health, myself, my life. That was it. The decision was made. Hope dawned on me for the first time in over a month. I was finally going to get well.

I called the next morning and made the appointment. All I could think of was "Four hundred dollars, and I'll be me again." What a dreadful memory to have now, four years later, desperately wanting a child and regretting every day the decision that I made. But I was desperate then, obsessed with getting the pregnancy over with and feeling normal again. It seemed the only logical solution at the time.

The memories I have of that morning are absolutely horrific. Oh my God! What did I do! How could I have walked into that clinic and let those people take my child from me? I suffered so that my baby could live, and then I let some stranger undo my little child whom, only weeks before, I was terrified of losing to miscarriage! My gift from God…returned to Sender.

In one brief instant my child was no longer with me. As I awoke from sedation I realized that I was no longer deathly ill. I didn't feel great, but I didn't feel as if I was going to die. I told myself that I could deal with what I'd done. I told myself that things would be OK. I left the clinic, went home, and fell asleep on the couch. When I awoke some hours later, the reality of what I had done sank in and I have never experienced such pain, such unbearable LOSS. The thought of how I felt when I awoke that day still brings tears to my eyes. I have never known such grief over anything else in my life. It was at that moment that I began to realize how precious, how fragile, how miraculous life is. If I could have gone back and changed what had just been done, I would have done it in an instant. If I could have traded my life for my child's life I would have. But I knew that my child was gone forever and that I had sealed that fate.

Then I became angry. How could this have happened? We bring people back from death, but we cannot find a cure for HG? I was furious that so many in the medical community do not even recognize HG as a serious or even real illness. Children are dying every day because women are not getting the care they need. Moms are driven to the brink of insanity by a physical condition that leads them to terminate their pregnancies, yet the doctors still call it "morning sickness." "Eat crackers, drink soda, take antiemetics, and everything will be better." Nothing made it better, yet doctors weren't interested. I was supposed to go on as if it was normal while women all around me were coasting through their pregnancies saying they wouldn't know they were pregnant if it weren't for their big bellies. HG is obviously a life-threatening illness; my child died because of it.

Over the past four years I have succeeded in becoming pregnant four times but have never carried past eight weeks. I have not seen a heartbeat in any of the ultrasounds that have been performed since my first, terminated pregnancy. I know in my heart that our first child would have survived if I had given her the chance. I wish I had been given better medical care.

I understand a woman's decision to terminate a pregnancy due to HG, but I also understand the hell that comes with that decision. HG eventually goes away, but I am living proof that the agony of losing a child never does.

EIGHTEEN
Abortion Procedures & Complications

Warning

This section on abortion procedures is for those HG sufferers who are considering termination and want information on surgical options. Abortion is not pretty and can be upsetting. *If you do not want to read detailed descriptions of different abortion procedures, skip this chapter now.*

Abortion Methods

In America abortion is legal throughout all nine months of pregnancy. Roughly three percent of all abortions are for maternal health reasons.[180] There are several types of abortion methods, the most common being the vacuum suction method, dilatation and curettage (D&C), dilatation and evacuation (D&E) and dilatation and extraction (D&X) also known as "partial birth abortion." By no means are these the only methods of abortion in use. However, these are the methods most commonly offered. Most HG sufferers who terminate do so in the first trimester, although some fatigue of the HG battle later in pregnancy and request termination then.

Since HG-related therapeutic terminations are performed solely to end maternal illness, I do not include a description of the D&X abortion method. The HG mother wants her child, and a child that far along could be delivered prematurely with a chance of survival.

Vacuum Suction Method

This method is used very early in pregnancy. In the early first trimester of pregnancy the baby's bones are flexible and muscle tissue is very fragile, coming apart with very minimal effort. At around seven weeks of pregnancy the baby is about the size of the nail on your index finger. Due to the combination of these factors, a cannula alone can abort the baby. A cannula is a straw-like instrument. One end is attached to a hose, which is attached to a suction machine. The other end, the end that goes into the uterus, has a scooped opening. First, the abortion performer quickly dilates the cervix using solid tubes that gradually get bigger. She pokes one small tube in, pulls it out, pokes a bigger tube in, pulls it out, and so on and so forth until she creates a big enough cervical opening. Next, she inserts the cannula into the cervix and up through the uterus. When the cannula comes into contact with the baby it sucks her down the tube and into a little container. The cannula is moved in all directions to make sure the baby, umbilical cord, placenta and amniotic sac have all been removed.

D&C

Near the end part of the first trimester the D&C is the usual method of abortion. At this point of growth, the baby's bones are just barely beginning to calcify. Muscle tissue is getting stronger. At twelve weeks of pregnancy, the baby is about two and a half inches from head to bottom and she weighs as much as fourteen paperclips (fourteen grams).

In the D&C procedure, the dilating tubes are used, but now they get bigger to open the cervix wider. A cannula is still used along with the addition of a curette. A curette is a sharp spoon-shaped instrument with no basin. That is to say, the edges are curved out and upward like a spoon, but there is nothing in the middle. The abortion performer inserts the spoon shaped end into the cervix and up through the uterus where she blindly scrapes away at the uterus. The sharp oval of the curette cuts through the baby's harder bone and tougher muscle tissue. The curved lip of the curette scrapes the baby and placenta away from the walls of the uterus like a spoon removes seeds from a cantaloupe. Once the baby and gestational structures have been reduced to biological goo, everything is sucked out through a cannula. The abortion performer will alternate between the curette and the cannula until she feels she has removed all traces of the baby's body and pregnancy structures.

D&E

When the second trimester is under way, the baby is even more developed. At fifteen weeks she weighs in at almost two ounces, and is five inches long from her head to her tiny little bottom. Her bones are harder to break and her muscles are tougher to tear apart.

Because the baby's spine and skull are much stronger in the second trimester, removal of the body requires more force. In order to abort a baby in the second trimester, the cervix has to be forced open fairly wide. Because quick cervical dilation with graduated tubes can easily damage the cervix, laminaria is typically used. Laminaria is made of seaweed. It is long and thin and resembles matchsticks. When moist, it expands. To open a cervix, several of these laminaria sticks are wedged into it. Over the course of a day or two, the laminaria absorb the mother's bodily fluid. They slowly expand, which may reduce the risk of damage to the cervix. After the abortion performer inserts a suction cannula, breaks the bag of waters, and then introduces forceps into the womb, she tears the limbs off of the living child. Next, the spine is snapped into pieces. Lastly, the baby's skull is crushed. While the person performing the abortion is working, her assistant will often press on the mother's abdomen to feel for pieces of the baby left inside. By doing this, the assistant can help the abortion performer in the important task of removing all of the body parts. Pieces of the baby's body are pulled out of the woman's womb, through her vagina, and placed on a tray. As with any abortion, someone must rifle through the remains and piece them together like a rough jigsaw puzzle. This ensures that all of the parts have been removed. If parts of the baby are retained in the womb, they can cause infection or an unpleasant surprise when a mother later passes recognizable pieces of her child such as a hand or, as one woman lamented, her child's dismembered head. I am very familiar with this particular procedure. It is how my first pregnancy ended.

Maternal Complications

Most children are aborted without serious physical harm to the mother. However, abortion is an invasive procedure and carries with it the risk of maternal complication ranging from mild to serious. Risks increase along with a child's development and in settings with minimum standards. Hospitals are expected to adhere to stringent health regulations put in place to protect a patient's safety, but due to advocacy for unrestricted abortion, abortion clinics are less regulated than veterinary clinics in some states. Therefore, aborting a child at an abortion facility may increase the risk of maternal complication. Some complications are laceration and perforation, infection, hemorrhage, infertility, recurrent miscarriages and death of the mother. Abortion is also linked to breast cancer.

Laceration and Perforation

Maternal lacerations are cuts or tears that the abortion performer accidentally exacts on parts of the mother's anatomy such as the cervix and the uterus. Lacerations can cause heavy bleeding and scarring. Maternal perforation is much more than a laceration and happens when the abortion provider accidentally pokes a hole in a mother's organ. If the instrument is attached to a suction machine, the instrument can suck up part of the bowel. Older women who have had several deliveries are at a higher risk than the general population. Risks also increase if the person performing the abortion is inexperienced. General anesthesia can also increase risk as it relaxes the uterine muscles causing them to be more easily perforated.

Lacerations may be minor and heal on their own or they may be significant requiring surgery. Similarly, perforations may self-heal or require surgery such as a hysterectomy. When bowel is sucked out, a colostomy may be required. In a colostomy, a doctor makes an artificial anus by attaching the colon to an opening in the abdominal wall. A colostomy bag is attached to the opening in the abdomen to collect fecal matter until it needs to be discarded and a clean bag attached. Depending on the severity of injury the colostomy may be temporary or may last for the remainder of one's life. One woman, who had to have a permanent colostomy following an abortion procedure, described how personally humiliating having a colostomy is. She said she constantly worries about the smell and about the noises it makes. Because of this, she doesn't like to leave her house; the colostomy has severely limited her social life.

Infection

Unless the person performing the abortion is using an ultrasound machine, abortion is a blind procedure. The abortion performer, no matter how skilled, cannot see what she is doing inside a woman's body. She is merely relying on her prior knowledge of human female anatomy and the anatomy of pregnancy. This is sufficient most of the time. However, on rare occasions a part of the baby's body is left her mother's womb. For example, the older baby's bones begin to calcify. Once they do, they can splinter when broken apart. One little bone splinter can cause a woman to get a dangerous infection. Among other things, infections can lead to scarring and infertility.

Treatment for infection may include a second abortion procedure to remove any leftover parts, drugs to cause contractions in an effort to empty the uterus or drugs to treat the infection.

Hemorrhage

Retained fetal parts, perforation, and a failure of the uterus to contract can cause excessive blood loss. Generally, treatment is successful, but in one case an abortion provider tore a two-inch by three-quarters-inch hole in a woman's uterus.[181] The thirty-three-year-old mother did not survive and left two children behind.

Medication to stimulate uterine contractions may be used to effectively control hemorrhaging. Another abortion to remove retained parts may also stop the hemorrhage. If the hemorrhage is due to a large perforation, a surgical hysterectomy is often the only life-saving option. Blood transfusions are sometimes required.

Infertility

Infertility can occur if a woman's uterus has been perforated requiring a hysterectomy. Infection can also cause infertility if it causes scarring in the fallopian tubes. This can prevent the egg from traveling to meet with sperm. Bone fragments from the aborted child can also lodge into the uterine lining where they can cause infertility and remain undetected for years.[182]

Removing bone fragments can correct some cases of abortion-related infertility. Infertility can also be treated with in vitro fertilization (IVF) or gestational surrogacy where another woman carries and delivers the baby created via IVF. Occasionally, abortion-related infertility is untreatable. In the case where a woman undergoes a complete hysterectomy, adoption or childlessness are options.

Recurrent miscarriages and Premature Birth

Scarring from injury to the uterus can prevent the embryo from implanting properly in the uterine wall. Intrauterine scarring can also obstruct blood flow to the placenta and cause bleeding which can be life-threatening for both mother and child. Both of these situations can cause miscarriage. Any surgery that involves the uterus can cause uterine scarring. Abortion has also been linked to placenta previa (low-lying placenta), which can result in death to the mother and child.[183] Additionally, abortion has been linked to premature birth (which can cause serious disabilities) and low birth weight in at least forty-nine studies.[184]

Scarring can sometimes be treated with surgery. If this isn't effective, other infertility treatments can be considered.

Placenta previa usually means strict bed rest. If the bleeding cannot be controlled, abortion via C-section is the life-saving treatment in cases of severely low placentas. Sometimes the baby is mature enough to survive, sometimes not. If the previa is marginal, children may be born vaginally, otherwise birth requires a C-section.

Incompetent Cervix

Abortion can also weaken the cervix. The risk rises with repeated or second and third trimester abortion procedures. The cervix is not designed to open at will. It is a muscular ring that is strong enough to hold a heavy baby in a woman's womb 24-hours a day, seven days a week. If this ring is damaged and loses its awesome strength and durability, a baby can literally drop from a woman like an apple from a tree. I sustained an incompetent cervix (IC) due to the HG-related abortion of my first child in the second trimester. Later, my other pregnancies required months of tedious and even painful bed rest. HG and an IC, by the way, are incompatible, as the force of vomiting can put pressure on the cervix. Theoretically you could vomit your baby right out of your body. IC pregnancies are rife with perpetual anxiety and feelings of helplessness. The condition is permanent and will affect every pregnancy you ever have.

Cervical incompetence has no cure, but there are treatment options. Staying in bed on strict bed rest until the baby is born is one way to try and prevent premature birth, and putting something like a book or a brick under the legs of the bed can tilt a woman in a position that supposedly helps to hold the baby in. This is called the Trendelenberg position. If cerclage is indicated and chosen, the cervix will be sewn shut. Cerclage stitches sometimes rip, and the result can be the expulsion of a tiny little passenger who is too young to survive. Cerclage is usually recommended at around fourteen weeks, but the vomiting of HG has not ordinarily resolved by this time. Those with particularly forceful vomiting may find that pressure is exerted on the stitches, endangering the pregnancy. The sutures also pose a risk for infection, which can cause pregnancy loss. Though indicated, I opted out of cerclage, stayed strictly in bed, and that worked for me.

Some women think they don't have to consider sustaining an IC or any other future pregnancy risk from abortion, because they don't intend to get pregnant again. However, many HG moms who terminate are shocked to discover a compulsion to get pregnant again. Mothers who have lost a child often experience a strong desire to have a "replacement child." This has been a relatively common phenomenon throughout history.[185]

Death
Some sources say aborting a child is safer than bearing a child, but it is impossible to make such a claim. National abortion reporting is not mandatory in the United States. No one really knows how many abortions take place nationally or how many women die due to legal abortion procedures per year, so no one can accurately compare the number of abortion-related maternal deaths with the number of birth-related maternal deaths. Problems with reporting are the reason for this lack of information.

How Safe Is Abortion For Women?
In America, a significant number of women die in legal

abortion-related events each year. However, the reporting of these deaths has always been low. For example, one year Dr. Jack Willke, of Cincinnati, Ohio, reported that the official statistics in his state showed no legal abortion-related deaths, yet he personally knew of two. In another example, a reporter for the Chicago Sun-Times uncovered twelve legal abortion-related deaths in one city alone while government statistics listed only sixteen such deaths for the entire nation that year.[186] Because those who perform legal abortions do not accurately report related maternal deaths, our government simply stopped collecting these statistics in 1987, as they saw no point in gathering invalid data.

Even researching death certificates will not help determine the number of women who die in legal abortions each year, because legal abortion-related death is not always listed as such. If a certificate lists the cause of death as "hemorrhaging due to uterine perforation," we do not know if the woman was impaled in a car accident or if the woman was involved in an abortion. We have no way of knowing how many abortion-related maternal deaths occur in America. However, approximately one and a half million abortion procedures are performed each year, and the vast majority of women survive. We can hope that the risk of a woman dying in an abortion procedure is lower than her risk of getting HG, but no one can honestly claim that abortion is safer than childbirth.

Clues from Abroad
Unlike the U.S., Finland has socialized medical care, so its death certificate records are very accurate and complete. In 1997, a study of pregnancy-associated deaths was undertaken, and the results showed that the risk of dying within a year after an abortion was almost four times higher than the risk of

dying after a miscarriage or successful birth.[187] Some of these abortion-related deaths were immediate in nature while others were delayed.

Immediate Vs. Delayed Risks

Hemorrhage, infection, and allergic reaction to anesthesia or other medications are a few abortion-related complications that have the potential to cause maternal death. These complications can occur within minutes, hours or over a period of days following an abortion. However, abortion-related complications can also present months or even several years later. These complications range from physical (such as breast cancer) to emotional (as with Post-Traumatic Stress Disorder) and are potentially fatal.

Breast Cancer

Scientific evidence on the abortion/breast cancer (ABC) link is thusfar recognized by eight medical organizations.* Sixteen out of seventeen statistically significant epidemiological studies and biological evidence support a cause and effect relationship between abortion and breast cancer.[188] Women have a right to know.

Abortion is only one of several risk factors for breast cancer, so it cannot be said that all women who have breast cancer have had abortions. In the medical literature twenty-nine out of thirty-eight epidemiological studies worldwide support the ABC link.[189] Fifteen of these studies were done in the United States, and thirteen of those support the finding that abortion is an independent risk factor for breast cancer. Epidemiological studies explore a statistical relationship between an exposure to a possible risk and a disease.

A 1994 study by Dr. Janet Daling and her colleagues found that abortion caused a 50% increase in a woman's chances of getting breast cancer.[190] Teenagers under the age of eighteen, women aged thirty and older, and women with a family history of breast cancer were found to be in high-risk groups for the disease if they had abortions. Teenagers under the age of eighteen and women aged thirty and older who had abortions more than doubled their risk for the disease. Women with a family history of the disease were found to increase their risk by 80%. Twelve of the study's subjects belonged to two of these high-risk groups; they had abortions before age eighteen and also had a family history of the disease. All twelve women developed breast cancer by age forty-five. Daling, who supports abortion, says:

> "I would love to have found no association between breast cancer and abortion, but our research is rock solid and our data is accurate. It is not a matter of believing it, it is a matter of what is."

The lifetime risk of breast cancer for the average American woman is 12.5%. If a woman boosts that risk by 50%, then her lifetime risk climbs to nearly 19%. If the abortion occurred in her first pregnancy, then her risk climbs even more. Around eight hundred thousand women abort their first child annually. Statistically, forty-four thousand of them would have avoided breast cancer if they had given birth to their children instead. Of these forty-four thousand women, eleven thousand will die from breast cancer, and although they will not be listed as such, these are abortion-related deaths.[191]

A cause and effect relationship between abortion and the disease is also supported by biological evidence. This includes a 1980 study on rats, which demonstrated that 77.7% of post-abortive rats could be reliably caused to develop breast cancer if they were exposed to a carcinogen.[192] In contrast, 66% of virgin rats and 0% of rats with full term pregnancies developed the disease when exposed to a carcinogen.

Scientists know that overexposure to estrogen is related to most of the risk factors for breast cancer. They know that this female hormone promotes the growth of tumors. In fact, estrogen replacement therapy (ERT) was added to the nation's list of known carcinogens in 2001. ERT is largely the same chemical form of estrogen as that made by a pregnant woman's ovaries.

Scientists know that women are overexposed to estrogen starting early in their pregnancies. By the end of the first trimester, estrogen climbs 2000% in a woman's bloodstream if she is carrying a normal pregnancy (one not destined to miscarry).[193] Estrogen causes normal and pre-cancerous cells to multiply. This is why many women experience breast tenderness and swelling before they have even found out that they are pregnant. If the woman has never had a full term pregnancy before, then her breast cells are predominantly primitive and immature. In this state, they are known as "undifferentiated" cells. Undifferentiated cells are known to be cancer-vulnerable.

Scientists hypothesize that it is only in the third trimester that a woman's overexposure to estrogen is neutralized. Starting at thirty-two weeks gestation, another process called "differentiation" kicks in to shut off cell multiplication and to shape the breast cells into milk-producing tissue. Scientists know that differentiated cells are mature and therefore cancer-resistant. Hence, the woman who has a full-term pregnancy is left with more cancer-resistant cells than she had before she ever became pregnant. This is why women who bear more children are known to have a significantly reduced breast cancer risk.

In contrast, the woman who has an abortion does not experience the differentiation process. Therefore, she is left with more immature and cancer-vulnerable cells than she had before she became pregnant. Scientists have never challenged this hypothesis because too much of it is already widely accepted by medical experts, and it is consistent with what is already known about human biology. Consequently, the hypothesis has never been disproved.

If you have experienced child loss through abortion, there is health care information that can help you minimize the risk of dying from breast cancer. At the writing of this book, you can find this information at this Web site: http://www.abortionbreastcancer.com/have_had_an_abortion. htm

Abortion-Related Post-Traumatic Stress Disorder

Many women who have undergone an abortion procedure find it difficult to cope with the fact that they have ended the life of their child. Directly after losing the child or even years later, they may suddenly develop a serious negative emotional response known as Post-Traumatic Stress Disorder (PTSD).

In general, PTSD results from having experienced something so traumatic that it goes beyond the realm of usual human experience. It is a response to an extreme, out of the ordinary occurrence such as war, rape, witnessing a violent crime or sustaining serious injury or illness. Causing the death of a living human child is a traumatic event. It's a monumental occurrence, and that is why it is often described as "the most difficult decision a woman will ever make." Abortion-related PTSD is so common that it has received the nickname "Post Abortion Syndrome." Termination for maternal health reasons puts the mother at particular risk of PTSD, because it is contrary to her desire to protect her child and is therefore outside the scope of usual human experience.

Expectant mothers who terminate for maternal health reasons experience many of the same feelings of deep loss and despair that other expectant mothers feel upon losing a gestating child "naturally." However, due to the nature of the self-imposed experience, there exist certain differences. For instance, it may be harder, at least initially, for religion to comfort the mother of a terminated child. She may feel that her actions have displeased God; she may feel unworthy of comfort. Fetal pain is often a frightening issue for those who suffer from abortion-related loss. Whereas I am easily convinced that the child I miscarried slipped away from life peacefully, it's impossible for me to believe that my first child, who died in a D&E, experienced a peaceful death. Though many mothers of miscarried children wonder if they might somehow be guilty of accidentally causing their child's death, the mother of the terminated child knows for certain the part she has played.

ASHLI FOSHEE MCCALL

A parent's worst nightmare is a child's life cut short. The mother who miscarries and feels that her doctor or someone else is to blame may become angry at that individual. The mother of a child killed by a drunk driver may focus her rage on the drunk behind the wheel. Grief becomes complicated, however, if *she* was that drunk. So it is with the expectant mother who aborts. Who does she ultimately blame? Where does her rage go? Although others may have contributed, she knows her name was on the dotted line. Enter the symptoms of abortion-related PTSD.

Risk Factors for Emotional Trauma Post-Abortion

Are you at risk of suffering from seriously negative psychological effects after an HG-related abortion? Run down the checklist of risk factors. If one or more apply to you, you are at risk for suffering from abortion-related emotional trauma. In general, the more that apply, the more risk and trauma there can be.

Characteristics that raise the risk of emotional trauma after abortion:[194]

- Difficulty making decisions
- Personal moral belief against abortion
- Religious beliefs
- Strong concerns about keeping abortion secret
- Originally wanted pregnancy
- Abortion due to maternal health issue
- Strong maternal orientation
- Being married
- Prior children
- Feeling pressured or forced
- Feeling decision is her only option

- Feeling pressured to choose quickly
- Decision is made with inadequate info
- Being an adolescent
- Prior emotional or psychiatric issues
- Poorly functioning coping mechanisms
- Prior low self esteem
- Poor work pattern
- History of sexual abuse/assault
- Lack of social support
- Few friends
- Made decision alone without help from partner
- Lack of support from family
- Partner accompaniment to abortion event
- Prior abortions
- Thinks often of the baby; wonders the sex and knows the due date
- Second or third trimester abortion (indicates woman is strongly conflicted)

Symptoms of Abortion-related PTSD:

- *Despair* - over the loss of one's child and one's future with that child
- *Guilt* - for destroying the child and violating one's own ethical code and inclination to protect
- *Anxiety* - irritability, hyperactivity, upset stomach, worry, etc.
- *Emotional numbness* - unconsciously avoiding feeling
- *Sudden and uncontrollable crying spells* - unpredictable and intense
- *Deterioration of self-image* - a feeling of unnaturalness, unworthiness, "loss of soul"

- *Interruption of sleep patterns* - too much or too little sleep
- *Sexual dysfunction* - associating sex with the child's death and the "surgical rape" of the abortion procedure itself
- *Appetite disturbances* - eating too much or too little
- *Loss of motivation* - inability to muster genuine interest in much of anything
- *Flashbacks* - occasionally occurring at inopportune times; triggered by gynecological exams, sound, scent, motion, sight or seemingly nothing at all
- *Dreams or nightmares* - can involve the child and be graphic and highly disturbing
- *Remorse/regret* - wanting one's child back to no avail; endlessly formulating solutions that would have saved the aborted child
- *Rage* - may lurk palpably beneath a thin veneer and manifest as a newly-short temper
- *Frustration* - at being misunderstood, misrepresented, abandoned, powerless to reverse the situation
- *Survival guilt* - inability to enjoy the beautiful and happy things in life, experiences that were "stolen" from the child
- *Preoccupation with becoming pregnant* - in an attempt to atone and/or replace; to ground one's self, to find a reason to live
- *Substance abuse* - to escape the hopelessness of the situation, anything to relieve the impossible pain
- *Self-punishing or self-degrading behaviors* - Self-harm,[195] burning or cutting, intentionally starving, failing to take care of one's self medically or otherwise
- *Anniversary reactions* - an increase of any of these or

other negative experiences on the due date or death date

- *Suicidal thoughts* - mulling over, in desperation, a solution for some lasting form of pain relief

Any of these symptoms has the potential to affect not only us but also those with whom we share our lives. None of the emotional side effects are easy or pleasant, and any combination can cause us to make choices that are not compatible with a healthy life.

Emotional State, Physical Risk

In the previously mentioned Finland study, seven years worth of death certificates were examined.[196] Two hundred eighty-one women died within a year of a pregnancy event (whether pregnancy ended in abortion, miscarriage or birth). Results of the study concluded that the women who had aborted a child were seven times more likely to commit suicide, four times more likely to exhibit risk-taking behavior that resulted in accidental death, four times as likely to die in homicide and had a 60% higher chance of dying of natural causes.

Suicide

Most sick mothers don't feel good about aborting a child they wanted. Later on when we're dealing with all the fallout, we may inadvertently stumble across developmental facts or images of babies who were the same age as our baby at the time of abortion-related death. Facing such a reality can be devastating, but what's done is done. This is hard to live with, and some decide that they can't go on. For them, moments that formerly made life worth living undergo a strange metamorphosis and evoke instead confusion and intense emotional pain. Day after day, the pain can chip away at a person. At times, I myself still experience this pathology, not because I was a psychopath to begin with but because such an extremely negative experience has made me very sad in some respects.

The abortion of my first child has been a terrible blow to my overall self-esteem. Just the other day, when my toddler asked me if monsters were real, and I told him "No," I secretly felt that I was lying. He was looking for a big, pointy-fanged, child-killing beast when the real "child-killer" has soft hair, a pretty face, and tucks him into bed every night. What will he think when he finds out I killed his sibling? What will I say? For me there are moments... like watching children in a park and trying to pick out the one who is the age that my dead child would be. Often I wonder who she was, how she was going to look, act, sound, smell, be... I miss her. I want her.

I have talked to a number of women who terminated for HG, and I hear over and over that it was like jumping out of the frying pan into the fire. As I wrote this chapter, I was in touch with a woman who was in the dreadful process of ticking down the days until the first due date of the aborted child she had deeply wanted. While she is able to "hold it together" all day, she cries at night when her son is sleeping. It's no wonder that abortion-related suicide has been documented in the United States.[197] In one examination approximately 30-55% of women polled reported having suicidal thoughts post-abortion, and 7-30% actually attempted suicide.[198] Of the attempts and completed suicides, a significant number coincide with the anniversaries of due dates or abortion dates.[199]

Risky Behavior

Some women who have lost a child in an abortion procedure don't care whether they live or die. Others may engage in risky behaviors as a way to divert their attention away from the pain. The rush of adrenalin felt in dangerous situations may momentarily alleviate depression. Sometimes risk-taking is so dangerous that it leads to accidental death.

Homicide

At least one survey of two hundred fifty-six women who aborted a child showed that roughly 60% became short tempered afterwards.[200] Forty-eight percent said they became more violent when angered. Anger and violence were linked to substance abuse, suicidal tendencies and fatal confrontations with others.

"Natural" Death

In the Finland study, only one woman who aborted did so for a health reason.[201] In other words, she was already sick, and she died within a year of that event. Everyone else was apparently relatively healthy at the time of pregnancy. Women who aborted had a 60% increased risk of dying within a year. This suggests that abortion produces an unnatural physical and psychological stress that can negatively impact a woman's general, overall health. A doctor offered a few insights. First, depression may suppress immune responses.[202] Next, emotional conflict consumes energy that would be better spent doing healthier things. Last, prolonged, unresolved mourning may distract a woman from taking care of herself. She may not monitor an existing health issue as closely and may not notice changes in condition. She may neglect check ups. She may not eat or sleep well; she may begin drinking more heavily than usual; and so forth. The disturbing emotions that accompany the trauma of losing a child to abortion can wear down the strongest personality. If a mother cannot find the help she needs to live with this type of child loss, the situation has serious potential.

Prevention

As always, prevention is the best medicine. Very rarely is therapeutic termination necessary for the treatment of HG. I have talked to scads of women who aborted due to this illness, and *not one of them* was satisfied with that choice. All of them had some type of resulting complication whether it was physical, emotional or both. The *only* way to ensure that abortion-related complications will not negatively affect you and your family is to avoid abortion. Each of us has a right to carry our children to term. We have a right to excellent health care, and we must never falter in the demand for it.

This publication is intended to help sick moms obtain appropriate and supportive treatment from medical professionals, family, friends, employers and others so that hopefully, none are left with the regrets that too many of us must live with.

Though HG is a horrible disease *it will end* within a nine-month period. Buy the outfit you plan to take your baby home in, tape pictures of children to your bedroom wall, and surround yourself with symbols, anything that reminds you of the person you are fighting for. Demand excellent health care, accept the illness, be patient in your suffering, and search for the beauty of the sacrifice you're making for your child. It is there. Dig deep in your heart, find your strength, and *do not be afraid.*

You can beat HG!

❧

*Medical Organizations that recognize the ABC link:

- National Physicians Center for Family Resources
- Breast Cancer Prevention Institute
- The Polycarp Research Institute
- Ehtics and Medics
- MaterCare International
- Breast Care Center-EAMC
- Catholic Medical Association
- American Association of Pro-Life Obstetricians and Gynecologists

Dr. Lana's Story

I'm a physician, and I've been married for eight years. After a year of trying to get pregnant I was thirty-six and still childless. We consulted a fertility specialist, and IVF was indicated.

We went out of state for the best IVF doctor we could find. We spent our life savings on five cycles, with no success. Our sixth try was going to be the last. If it was not successful we were going to adopt. The sixth time was the charm; our daughter was conceived.

Thirty days into the pregnancy, before the first prenatal visit, bang, HG. I was sick 24-hours a day and even woke up in the night vomiting. I ran a private practice and felt forced to work which exacerbated my symptoms. Because this was an IVF situation, I was never really accused of not wanting my daughter although I sensed that a psychological component was suspected.

At the ER I was given Compazine, and I had a reaction. It made me really anxious and agitated, and I ended up signing release forms and leaving against medical advice. No one told me the feelings were related to the Compazine. Medical staff didn't recognize the reaction, and didn't give me Benadryl to counteract the effects. The next time I went back, I expressed my feeling that the anxiety and agitation could have been caused by the Compazine and they said, "Yeah, we see that all the time." I tried Phenergan but had a dystonic reaction to it.

Once again, I was not given Benadryl. My legs were literally twitching off the hospital bed. Reglan and Kytril were also administered, but they just didn't work. At eight weeks they gave me Zofran. It really seemed to help for about a week and then mysteriously, the beneficial effects just stopped. I was H. pylori negative and so was not given antibiotics. The HG peaked between nine and sixteen weeks. After losing 15% of my total body weight I got a PICC and TPN was started.

We consulted a high-risk perinatologist for a second opinion. Bizarrely, she told me if I still had HG after the sixteenth week then it wasn't HG. She told me that at that point we needed to suspect a GI problem with the main therapy being behavioral therapy. No one said I didn't want my daughter, but they did suspect that I had "issues" with eating. It was ridiculous.

By eighteen weeks I was only puking once a day but I still needed nutritional support. Finally, at eight months, the PICC line clogged and they removed the TPN. I was forty-one at my daughter's birth. After she was born I still experienced abdominal pain and vomiting. The TPN had caused gallbladder disease, and I had to have my gallbladder removed.

We had frozen tots left over from IVF, so when I was forty-three we tried again and were successful. I had the same physicians as in the first pregnancy, and the HG returned on cue. This time I had an NG tube. I was not given a naso-numbing agent and placement was horrible. I had to actively participate by swallowing a tube that was gagging me. I puked it out the day after placement. They put it in again and two days later I puked it out again. Puking it up is an unpleasant experience. I vomited, and all of a sudden the thing was just hanging out of my mouth. I was hooked like a fish from my nose through my mouth. The second time I just cut off the tip and pulled it out myself. That was enough.

After losing 15% of my total body weight, my doctor, who had a new gadget, convinced me that central TPN was less risky than peripheral TPN and more comfortable. This line was inserted in my neck where it stayed for two weeks. As a doctor, I felt very anxious about the centrally inserted TPN. These are things I prescribe for in-patients in the intensive care unit. They are managed in the hospital; I don't expect patients to go home with central TPN. They are *sick* folks. We're talking critically ill people who have had massive heart attacks or strokes.

My mother and husband introduced and somewhat encouraged the idea of termination. This made me feel really deflated and unsupported in my arduous endeavor; everyone else had apparently given up on the pregnancy. It seemed more important that I regain my health rather than continue to inconvenience family and doctors. Truth be told, not suffering was a very appealing concept. The broad support of termination as the solution made it easy to ignore the emotional impact that the loss of the baby might have.

I mentioned termination to my doctor along with my reluctance to do it. I asked for more options. I was told that termination was the only option left that we had not tried. The doctor encouraged termination but said he was not comfortable with carrying out the act. Instead he referred out. I believe doctors don't like to feel like failures, and not knowing the etiology or effective treatment for something puts us at a disorienting disadvantage. Termination is a sure "cure" for HG, places the physician back in control, and carries the advantage of getting rid of pesky patients for whom "nothing" can be done. I needed more options and my doctor wasn't willing to put forth the extra effort to give them to my child and me.

I was referred to a physician and scheduled the termination for a Friday. I showed up for the procedure but couldn't do it and left. What followed was a horrible weekend at home with central TPN and Zofran that was not working. I vomited fifty times in forty-eight hours. You do the math. It was absolutely miserable. In my desperation I called the referred doctor and asked for the termination. It was scheduled for later that day. When I arrived, the physician wanted to perform the termination in his office without anesthesia. I demanded anesthesia and was told that the abortion would have to be performed in the OR (operating room). I agreed.

In the OR, the anesthesiologist refused to administer anesthesia due to the HG-related physical deterioration. He told me the risks outweighed the benefits. I told them there was no way I would do it without anesthesia, so the anesthesiologist consented. When everything was a go, I started crying and saying I didn't really want to do it. I wished aloud that there were some other option that would keep this from happening. Everyone heard me. In my medical records I was described as being "mournful, depressed and tearful." My pleas were ignored. No one dared to offer anything in the way of alternatives. I suppose they didn't want to question "my choice."

The HG totally resolved after the termination. Initially, I was relieved. I was out of the physical crisis and back in control of my life. It was the kind of relief that comes after being under water for too long; just before you think you're lungs are going to burst, you finally break the surface and take the most comforting breath of your life. Physically it's great to have that kind of resolution. Emotionally it's quite a different story.

Within days it became apparent that termination had been the wrong answer. Major grieving for the baby initiated along with anguish over the way the baby died. I cried every day. I was extremely depressed at the loss of our child. I needed to find help so I contacted a hospital, familiar with women's issues, in search of a professional. I was referred to a grief counselor. When I related events to the counselor, she was appalled at the poor quality of treatment I had received. She said the hospital social worker or clergy or *someone* other than people who were ready to perform a termination should have been called upon when I clearly expressed that I had major reservations and did not want to terminate but didn't know what else to do. My seriously conflicted feelings were evident not only in my words but also in the fact that I canceled my first termination appointment.

I saw a therapist on a weekly basis and was diagnosed with Post-Traumatic Stress Disorder (PTSD). I found it somewhat helpful to talk. Once I called a Catholic-run post-abortion "healing" program, and I was very hurt by the judgmental attitude of the person running it. I immediately abandoned the idea, and my self-esteem plummeted.

My marriage (including my sex life) was negatively affected by the termination. There is a lot of hostility and resentment after something like that. Other family relationships were also negatively affected. Parenting my living child became difficult. I felt unworthy of her, and being faced with her value and preciousness forced me to acknowledge the value and preciousness of my dead child. I became overprotective and clingy.

I am angry with doctors who did not do their jobs to the best of their abilities. They were unsupportive and their concern was false and limited to getting rid of my case.

I have identified four main areas that explain why the second pregnancy ended in termination:

1. *The second pregnancy was worse.* I vomited twenty to twenty-five times a day compared to the ten to fifteen times a day of my first pregnancy.

2. *There was a lack of medical support.* At one point my doctor said, "Go sit in the sun; you'll feel better." There was far too much rotation and no continuity between doctors. No one sufficiently monitored my health decline. Once a doctor told me: "You look great!" I couldn't believe it. I asked outright, "Do you need glasses?" I feel I was possibly discriminated against for being a doctor. I felt there was an overall "Physician, heal thyself!" attitude. I was expected to take care of myself. I was also told I had to leave the hospital with the central line because my insurance

refused to pay for in-patient stay, so there was definitely a managed care component.

3. *There was a lack of social support.* My husband took care of himself and our daughter, but he wasn't very supportive of me. I felt isolated and somewhat abandoned. I would have liked daily periods of concerned conversation, and physical comforting such as hugs or handholding would have been nice. The support I received was limited to termination, and I feel a fair amount of resentment over that. I needed strength and positive messages at a time when I couldn't be strong or positive for the baby or myself. Occasionally my husband made accusatory comments like, "I don't see any other pregnant women like this. Why are YOU like this?" I felt blamed and guilty. My mom was in the house with my husband and sometimes I felt "double-teamed" by these attitudes. The rest of my family did not realize how desperate the situation was, and no one was actively brainstorming aggressive interventions for a positive outcome.

I really would have liked supportive intervention such as finding childcare for my daughter and taking care of life outside my bedroom door so I could just be sick and focus wholly on getting through the debilitation of severe HG. At that point it was time to drop out of life and have everyone pick up the slack in the face of the extreme task that was before me. People did not respond like it was an emergency, like it was a life or death situation. No one had much to say regarding the termination. It was easier to have no opinion. It was simpler to support abortion in the face of a health crisis as the "easy" way out for everyone. We all totally lacked understanding of what termination fully entailed. No one came to the rescue; I just couldn't handle HG by myself.

4. *I kept working.* I was in a private practice and was afraid to lose my job like I had in the first pregnancy. I dragged myself into work half-dead and tried to perform a job when I couldn't even perform the simple tasks of daily living. I didn't know when to quit. I tried to be Superwoman.

The termination left a massive wound that is difficult to work through. I experienced an unexpected yet strong drive to get pregnant, to complete a pregnancy after not completing a pregnancy. I couldn't bear the thought of signing off with defeat. We had some frozen tots left, but because of the combination of my age and the fact that the kids were on ice, my chances of becoming pregnant again were next to nil. However, five months later, I became pregnant with *twins*.

For the third pregnancy I had a wonderful new doctor whom the grief counselor recommended. When I lost 15% of my total body weight I was put on TPN via PICC again. I actually had a PEG/J done, but it turned out to be ineffective because my peers wanted to run 70ccs an hour and I couldn't do twenty without getting sick. This wasn't adequate nutrition for the three of us.

This last time I was given more pharmaceutical options: Halidol (slightly beneficial), Kytril (again nothing), Marinol (nothing). I could have tried marijuana, but I felt weird about that and didn't want to do it. I also had hydrocortisone and Decadron but both steroids did nothing and caused me to be very irritable and paranoid, and I suffered from bouts of sleeplessness. On the occasions that I did sleep, I had strange, disturbing dreams.

Incredibly, termination did cross my mind in the midst of extreme suffering and debilitation. But this time my sister was very proactive and exhausted herself trying to support me through the pregnancy. It helped to know that I had someone in my corner cheering me on and giving me the pep talk when I needed it most.

The HG didn't improve until twenty weeks. I had sporadic vomiting afterwards. Some days I threw up and some days I didn't. I averaged about once a day after twenty weeks. Severity and duration in the first and third pregnancy were comparable. It's interesting, because you'd think the twin pregnancy would have been the worst, but I was twice as sick in my second pregnancy. My third pregnancy involved carrying a boy and a girl, so I don't think the sex of the second baby had much to do with it.

At the time of delivery I was too weak (physically and emotionally) to give birth, so I had a C-section. My healthy, precious twins were delivered after a third arduous pregnancy, and while they do not take the place of the child I lost, they add such joy to my life. I have had three pregnancies, and I have three children to love and nurture. I can't help feeling that somewhere, somehow this all makes sense.

I lost a child because of HG, and I have a great desire for something good to come out of something so terrible and tragic. I hope that sharing my story is a start.

NINETEEN
Abortion: Thinking It Through

Dehydration and clinical starvation affect the brain and can impair judgment. The lack of sufficient medical and social support may exacerbate symptoms and add further stress and pressure on a woman who is battling a monster illness. This is a bad time to make a life or death decision, but too many mothers feel they have run out of positive options. If you are considering abortion, identify the reasons why and explore the possible outcomes. Do any of the following apply to you?

I am leaning towards abortion because:
- I want my health back.
- I don't want to lose my job.
- I want to get rid of the depression and fear.
- I want to put an end to the chaos of HG!
- I can be well again *and* accept the terms, as this is a health issue.
- I want to return to my former self.
- I want to restore my relationships with others.
- I want to restore my confidence in the idea that medicine is able to give me control over my life.

If you share any of these reasons, consider what abortion can ensure and what it cannot ensure. Compare your list with mine to get a broader perspective.

What abortion can ensure:
- *Abortion will permanently solve the temporary health problem of HG in the pregnancy being terminated.*

Once the child is gone the HG will end.

What abortion cannot ensure:
- *It will not absolutely ensure your physical health.*

As with any invasive procedure there are risks associated with abortion. (See Chapter 18.)

- *It will not ensure your job*

Often, by the time an HG mom really begins to consider abortion, she has already missed a considerable amount of work. Though an employer is sorry that an employee has been ill, a lot of missed work can threaten job security. If the sufferer has tried to go to work but could never stay long, vomited enough to disturb others, and could not do her job as well as she did before, her employer may be ready to let her go. If she terminates and people find out about it at work, she may have problems with social attitudes, and "other" reasons may be found for firing her. By that time, it might be very difficult to fight legally, because an employer might already have enough justification (through missed work and decreased job performance) to terminate her job.

If, after all this, a woman's job has not been terminated, it is still not guaranteed. All mothers experience depression after losing a child they want. Some become so deeply depressed that they lose interest in their jobs. Hyperemetics are no different. Those who have lost a child due to HG-related abortion may lack the motivation for many things including their career.

If the occupation was one of the pressures that even remotely factored into the loss of the child through abortion, it can become a source of pain and anger. Often a mother will need time off to deal with the issues surrounding the death of her child. Having missed so much work already, she may not be allowed to take more time off. Nonetheless, she may absolutely have to have it. In addition, emotional repercussions that accompany the loss of a child may affect job performance. I am not suggesting that all women who terminate lose their jobs. Some do and some don't. What I *am* suggesting is that terminating a child you want is not a simple bump in the road of life. It's more like a mountain, and often time is the only thing that helps.

- *Abortion will not ensure emotional health.*

The woman who wants her child does not normally feel emotionally better after abortion. An expectant mother's heart is shattered when her child dies. Abortion is not a natural death. It is purposeful with a set time and date and a fee paid for procurement. Abortion is also not pretty. Losing one's child is bad enough, but the circumstances surrounding abortion-related child loss serve to complicate the experience.

- *Abortion will not ensure that you are finished with HG.*

Many women who lose a child to abortion feel a compulsion to conceive another child. This commonly happens with women whose children were miscarried or stillborn. An abnormal pregnancy condition does not end a woman's normal propensity for childbearing. Neither does abortion. In fact, hard as it may be to believe, abortion can actually increase the drive. Some women feel compelled to conquer the disease that robbed them of their child, and some find that they just don't want death to be their last experience with childbearing. Some may even be unconsciously trying to get the aborted child back. Because of the compulsion to have another child, abortion may actually mean *starting HG all over again.*

- *Abortion due to a "health issue" will not ensure peace.*

Death can't touch love. Often the rationalization that the HG is unbearable does not survive after the illness and baby are gone. And even devout religious belief, with all its comforting beauty is sometimes not enough to fill arms that ache to hold a child.

- *Abortion will not ensure a return to your former self.*

Abortion will not turn back the hands of time. Once pregnant, you are ever after the mother of the child conceived. Abortion will not bring you back to your old, pre-pregnant self, for then you were not the mother of your child. It may be unrealistic to think that you can go on living as though the child you loved and wanted never existed. Abortion will not divorce you from your child; it will simply remove her from life, leaving you to deal with the aftermath.

- *Abortion will not ensure a restoration of relationships with others.*

Some folks have earned special places in our hearts. HG is a very traumatic experience that is difficult to handle alone. Initially, most of us begin looking for those closest to us to support us with kind and encouraging words and helpful acts. How common it is to feel completely shocked and deeply abandoned by those from whom we expected the most but got the least! Many HG sufferers say that, when they got HG, they really found out who their friends were, and it turns out they didn't have many. Even when an HG pregnancy ends *successfully*, these negative feelings of abandonment and resentment can linger. Along with the development of penetrating chasms within the family, even the best friendships may be permanently over.

Abortion does very little to restore relationships and may actually make them much worse. Some family members may secretly or openly resent a person for taking from them a unique and precious family member whom they already loved and looked forward to sharing their lives with. Their grief at losing a family member is valid even if they did nothing to prevent it. Conversely, if individuals feel that the child was just a nascent blob of biological minutia and not a child at all, it can be devastating to a deeply grieved mother and can cause an irreparable rift.

Those who abort may also come to the conclusion that they lost the support they needed to manage the illness and culminate the pregnancy successfully with the birth of their living child. It can be nearly impossible to feel anything positive towards those who, through their negative, nonexistent, or otherwise unsupportive attitude, contributed to the death of one's child.

Relationships with children can be negatively affected by termination. If a pregnancy is terminated to restore a standard of childcare, unfortunately, consciously or subconsciously, resentment can be directed towards children. When one child is sacrificed for another, uncomfortable, confusing emotions can surface. Women may also experience the agonizing conflict that comes with the inconsistent nature of loving both the unborn and born child but having destroyed one while fiercely protecting the other. Many HG moms who abort tend to come away with a new and pointed appreciation for life and children. However, all abortion-related perspectives are not positive, and the personal emotional damage can have a lasting negative impact on relationships with children.

You may have seen the horrific pictures of aborted children. These images only portray the reality of what occurred. Besides the personal loss of the child, the graphic and terrible nature of the death is one of the most difficult aspects to deal with. In dark moments, a mother may succumb, not only to the fact that she caused her child to die, but also to the possibility that her child was subjected to unspeakable agony. Because of this, a mother may develop a heightened emotional sensitivity towards people in pain. This can cause a parent to recoil from anything that might cause a surviving child any type of pain, physical or emotional, which can result in abandoning the person during their period of suffering. In an extreme form, this coping mechanism can be dangerous. If a child sustains illness or injury and a mother can't deal with it, she may flee the accident scene or deny an illness exists. Also, in light of possible pain inflicted on the aborted child, a parent may feel that she has no right to cause the other child any pain at all. Discipline may suffer due to hypersensitivity and/or overcompensation.

Finances can be affected if a parent feels compelled to overcompensate. This may be unconscious self-reassurance that, despite aborting one child, one still has the ability to be a good parent who is capable of caring for and protecting another child. Financial or other types of overcompensation may also be an unintentional attempt at emotional, physical or spiritual restitution. The compulsion to *do something* to remedy a painful situation sometimes prevails over reason.

Aborting a child you want can be so hard to deal with that you are simply unable to do so. Some women develop the coping mechanism of "shutting off." It's a sort of psychic numbing. If a woman has learned to "shut off" in stressful situations she may become unsupportive to her living children. Conversely, if a woman cannot shut off her emotions but is brimming with endless anger and sorrow, her forbearance may be at a minimum. A formerly longsuffering mother may develop a very short fuse. Tending a child's somewhat extreme emotional ups and downs can be very challenging when a parent is having a hard time coping with her own.

Emotional and physical closeness can be affected by abortion. A mother must emotionally distance herself from her child before aborting her. Afterwards, for some mothers, the subconscious inner workings may dictate emotional proportion between children. This "consistency" may be a dysfunctional way to restore some semblance of order or control. To be fair to the lost child, Mom may feel compelled to emotionally distance herself from her surviving children. She cannot repair her relationship with the aborted child, but she can stunt or even ruin her relationships with living children. This is more likely an unconscious compulsion rather than a conscious decision. It adds inner conflict, as the "consistency" of distancing one's self can be internally comforting while at the same time very unhealthy and disturbing.

The majority of moms I've interviewed go to the other extreme after losing a child in an abortion. Rather than distancing themselves from their surviving children, they cling to them for dear life, not letting them out of their sight for fear that something will happen to them. Excessive worry over children and reliance upon them can be oppressive.

Maybe a mother doesn't experience any of the overtly negative effects mentioned above. Maybe it's merely an issue of a few depressive episodes a year. Perhaps, the surviving children will come out unscathed. Maybe once or twice the two-year-old who sees his mother's unintentional expression will ask, "Mommy, are you sad?" and Mom will lie her way out of it without further incident. In any case, children can and do suffer from the abortion of siblings whether they are ever aware of the baby's existence or not. I saw a T-shirt that read: "When Mama's not happy, NOBODY'S happy." It was a perfect illustration of how abortion can affect relationships with children (and everyone else).

- *Abortion will not ensure restoration of confidence in the idea that medicine is able to give you control over your life.*

When a patient feels that she has run out of medical options and this leads to the abortion-related death of her child, she may arrive at the opinion that her doctor betrayed her by not offering her existing, positive options. Doctors may hastily suggest abortion to solve the temporary yet difficult problem of HG, and I have heard from many women who feel this was the case in their experience. Abortion as a medical option may cure HG, but its fee is the life of a child who can not be replaced. It may be difficult to have faith in medicine if its answer to a temporary illness is so costly, and this may cause a sense of distrust in medical professionals, which may in turn result in feelings of helplessness.

Because of repeated exposure to hospitals and medical staff, HG sufferers are already susceptible to developing phobias or negative feelings in connection with all things medical. When a medical procedure results in the death of a child, health care aversion can certainly be compounded, and a woman may develop a long-term avoidance of routine medical procedures such as annual gynecological exams. These exams, which were never really pleasant to begin with, may remind her of the loss of her child and her distrust in physicians, and she may be unwilling to submit herself to such an emotional assault. Avoiding exams can put her at risk for certain gynecological ailments and life-threatening conditions. Due to the loss of my child through abortion, I have to fight against the tendency to avoid annual exams.

And again, abortion has its own risks. When a patient ends up with a permanent colostomy bag, or worse, due to an abortion gone awry, it typically does not evoke feelings of control.

All Things Considered

If you are contemplating termination for HG, you may be inclined to discuss it with trusted friends and family members who are physically healthy and may have a better cognitive ability. However, understand that their thought processes may be negatively affected by the crisis of watching you suffer or by their own ignorance. Someone who is witnessing your illness and thinks you are going to die may advise you differently than someone who understands HG. You might also consult your physician, but even then if you are not viewed as a whole person with a real relationship to your child, you may be perceived as a number and thusly advised. If ending the HG is the only aspect considered, then perhaps the advice will be inappropriate for your particular situation. You might contact a grief counselor to inquire about information on losing a child before birth, which could give you a fuller representation of what you might deal with should you choose abortion.

If you are weighing the decision to abort or continue a health-related crisis pregnancy, you might try talking to other HG moms who survived HG and also those who have terminated due to HG. If you go to http://www.yahoo.com and type "hyperemesis gravidarum message board" (without quotes) in the search box, it will pull up many online message boards for HG. Currently, you can contact moms who terminated, at http://www.hyperemesis.org and at The Shadowlands online.[203]

Helen's Story

I had HG with three of my pregnancies. My husband and I weren't married the first time, and my doctor questioned whether the baby was planned and wanted. He did not diagnose HG, but sent me home to eat crackers and drink flat soda even after I wasn't able to keep food or liquid down. He told me I would be OK as long as I kept it down for fifteen minutes. I started the pregnancy at one hundred ten pounds, and by the time I lost fourteen pounds I changed to another doctor in the same office. She sent me to the ER and wrote "hyperemesis gravidarum" on my hospital slip. She never told me what it was or gave me any information. I had an IV in the ER and was sent home where I immediately threw up. Nothing changed, and I went back for another IV in the ER. Finally, they hospitalized me for two days with an IV. Phenergan made me sleepy but otherwise wasn't working by pill or suppository and Reglan did nothing for me. They sent me home, but I was back a few days later, hospitalized for another two days. When I went home again, I was still very nauseous but the vomiting was starting to let up. By twenty weeks the sickness was about gone, but I still had some nausea. I was relieved to be able to go back to work, because management gave me a really hard time when I requested my leave of absence in the first place. I had bad heartburn, but other than that the rest of the pregnancy went well, and I had a beautiful boy weighing in at nearly eight pounds.

Two years later I was pregnant again. The same exact thing happened. It started at four weeks and lasted until twenty weeks. This time I had a new doctor. I was still sent to the ER for IVs but was hospitalized only once. I received Reglan again, and again it didn't help. In this pregnancy, I had IV therapy at home with a visiting nurse. I was unable to care for myself much less my son, and he went to my mother all day while my husband was at work. Somehow I managed to get through that pregnancy, and I had another lovely boy who weighed six pounds.

My third pregnancy was a surprise like the others but wanted just the same. We were happy at the thought of a new little life. At the time, I had not been educated on my medical condition; no one ever really talked about it. I hoped I could finally have a normal pregnancy, but I became sick at four weeks again. This time it seemed worse than the others. I couldn't get my oldest son to school, my four-year-old was sitting in front of the TV all day, and I couldn't move. I remember asking him to get me a piece of bread, because I had been told: "Eat before you get out of bed and wait about fifteen to thirty minutes before you get up." It doesn't help when you have HG. It can even make you throw up. My husband could only take so much time off of work, so my son and I were on our own. I had another new doctor in the same office as the others. You think they would know my history and just go ahead and hospitalize me when it started up, but no. I had to go through the whole ordeal of being sent to the ER, being sent home and then being admitted to the hospital as usual. They waited until I got down to some really heavy suffering to admit me to the hospital to pull me back up only to send me back home where it would all start over. It's infuriating to suffer when people can help you but refuse to do so until you are reduced to a whimpering, begging dog. This time I felt weaker than before and had a low fever and sometimes chills. When I finally got admitted again,

I had my worst night ever. They tried IV Reglan again because it had worked so well before-NOT! Of course it didn't work, and I was throwing up every hour on the hour. When they put the Reglan in I started to feel like the hospital walls were closing in. I was panicky and very depressed. It was unusual, and I felt like I was losing it. All I wanted to do at this point was sleep and be unconscious of the pain of constant nausea and vomiting. And then finally it occurred to me that I simply couldn't stand to be sick another minute.

My husband came to visit me and I begged him to tell me it was OK to terminate. They started Zofran but it didn't seem to work. The only thing that helped a little was when they gave me an injection to help me sleep. Sleep was what I wanted to get me OUT of this situation. Why couldn't I sleep until twenty weeks when the HG went away? After about a day or two the Zofran started kicking in, but by this time I had made up my mind to get out of this misery. I was six weeks along when my doctor set up the appointment.

Once the baby was out, the sickness went away immediately. I was able to eat again and feel physical comfort and get back to my normal routine, and it was initially excellent. However, after a couple of days I began to feel a terrible guilt and sadness. I wanted my baby; I just couldn't stand the sickness anymore. Of course I wonder how things might have been if I continued with the Zofran and had the IV therapy at home with a visiting nurse. Maybe I could have gotten through it. I try to tell myself that abortion was the right decision at the time, but I don't really believe it. In fact, I'm going to try again in a few months, because I have this strong feeling that I just have to complete a new pregnancy. I also wonder and hope that if I have another child it will somehow replace the one I lost. I dealt with the suffering of HG and now I'm dealing with the suffering of abortion. Abortion is worse than HG.

I wish I had had a better support system in place because I just felt like I couldn't get through the HG. I wish that my doctor had suggested other treatments or offered the IV therapy at home or *something*. When I told her that I decided to abort the baby, she didn't bat an eye. You think she would have taken some time to talk more openly with me about the whole thing. She could have offered me some hope and some other options, because I had been fighting up until that point, and that's what I really wanted and needed.

Things could have been different.

TWENTY
Living in the Shadow

As a mother who aborted due to HG, it's important for me to give a personal account of what it is like to live in the shadow of such a decision. To begin, abuse, physical and emotional, was a painful part of early childhood and something I will always have to live with. Abortion is not like that. I have suffered the loss of friends who died young and tragically. Those were bewildering times. Abortion is not like that. My dear parents died after lingering, dehumanizing periods of illness. I was in my mid-twenties; it was stunning and left me feeling a bit like a lost orphan. Abortion is not like that. In fact, no sad experience I've ever had compares. Abortion is absolutely the most terrible thing I have ever known.

The death of a child is a perpetual cardiac pang. Underneath the surface, the weight of a gaping void is always somehow there. Formerly beautiful aspects of life can become bittersweet as joy is tinged with sadness. Finding help can be a slow and aggravating process.

Because abortion is a complicated, controversial type of loss, it cannot be as easily, openly shared as other types of losses. Society allows abortion but generally negatively considers a mother who makes such a choice. The woman who aborts her child due to vomiting and starvation is hard pressed to find sensitivity and compassion from others who do not understand and who think "morning sickness" is a stupid reason to end a child's life. Because of this, a mother may not have many opportunities to seek support and share pain with others. Indeed, the social options are to lie, tell the truth about the pregnancy's end, suffer in silence, or seek asylum in professional, religious or other venues.

Living a Lie

Women who seek abortions for health reasons rarely report them, thus creating a false impression that abortion is not a likely consequence of severe/inadequately treated HG. Lying about the demise will evoke the sympathy and sensitivity that any mother who loses a child deserves, but the concern of others may seem hollow and even painful when it is a response to a half-truth. Some have informed others of their "miscarriage" and had to endure explanations like, "It's really a blessing in disguise; you wouldn't want to be saddled with a 'messed up' kid for the rest of your life." An insensitive comment like this is disturbing enough when a woman actually does miscarry, but the last thing anyone wants to hear after the loss of a child through abortion is that the death was somehow the child's own doing or God's doing or any number of the crazy things people say when a child dies. Of course, none of these can compare to the hate-filled comments a woman gets if she *doesn't* lie about the loss.

The Painful Truth

Those who tell the truth about the abortion are most likely in for it. Some people who do not support abortion may have a hard time sympathizing with such grief. They may feel that the mother deserves whatever misery she has coming to her and are happy to tell her this to her face. They don't want to be bothered with explanations of what it is like to have HG. They don't care. They are convinced that the mother is horrible, and, if they can add to the pain, so much the better. Thankfully, only a small number of abortion opponents are like this. In fact, a large number of abortion opponents used to be abortion advocates until they were hurt by abortion, so generally their crowd is very compassionate.

If you are outspoken and many people learn of the abortion, you may be surprised to discover that friends and family begin pouring out of the woodwork to confess their abortion-related losses. The number of people in your life who have been negatively touched by abortion can be astounding. In a way, it helps to know you're not alone, but in another way, it hurts to wonder why no one ever warned you.

Many abortion supporters are somewhat contradictory in believing in the sacredness of abortion for others, while acknowledging how horrible and wrong they think it is personally. It may be difficult to get any sympathy from these folks if they perceive a mother's pain as self-inflicted, somewhat deserved, or "just a choice; get over it already." Also, some abortion advocates are more concerned with protecting abortion than protecting women hurt by abortion. Such a person offers little compassion for a hurting mother. In fact, hurting moms may get fury and disgust if they are seen as some sort of threat to Roe v. Wade. These people don't allow discussion that involves negative, abortion-related feelings. Other abortion supporters are very sensitive to a mother's pain, but they may tend to invalidate any guilt or shame experienced by an individual, opting instead to try and convince a mother that there is no real moral implication. While this may be a kind attempt, the hurting mother may not find that it connects honestly with her sense of the experience, and so she may feel cared for but unheard.

Talking It Over (And Over And Over)

Many times women express their grief by talking it out with family members who witnessed the debilitating toll the illness took. Problems can arise when family members, who also lost a relationship with the child, find their own pain difficult to manage. Many of them may want to avoid and "forget" it, and they steep themselves in denial. They may resent being reminded of the event in repeated one-way conversations. They may feel assaulted and become angry, and this may threaten the relationship. Even so, it may not be easy for a grieving mother to refrain from immersing her partner in her anguish.

When the physical health crisis is over, aborting a child due to maternal illness can be difficult even for the mother to understand. If she finds someone she can talk to, she may naturally want to discuss the same aspects time and again in an attempt to make sense of what happened. Most friends and family members will reach a breaking point where they just can't listen to it anymore, either because they are sick of it or just find it too painful. When friends and family couldn't be paid to listen to the details one more time, a professional therapist could.

Professional Help

Seeking professional counsel is nearly always the first suggestion others make. Some moms take this advice because they feel it will help, while others take the advice merely to please the people who keep pressuring them to do so. Either way, there is potential. The key is finding sufficient counsel. Interestingly, outside of sectarian groups, there aren't many counselors who are specifically trained to deal with the subject of abortion, and I don't know of anyone specifically trained to address the relatively rare circumstance of abortion for maternal illness. Women are caught between the options of consulting those who went to school to learn psychology (but not the effects of abortion on women) and consulting those who have learned about the effects of abortion on women (but know little of psychology). One group of counselors is mainly secular and mostly professional while the other group is sectarian and mainly lay.

Secular Help

Secular help is non-religious help. While I don't know of any secular groups that offer any type of program for women who have lost a child through abortion for maternal health reasons, there are grief counselors who lead groups, some of which deal specifically with pregnancy-related child loss. This may or may not be appropriate for those who have experienced illness-related abortion. Other counselors deal specifically with Post-Traumatic Stress Disorder (PTSD). However, knowing how to deal with PTSD doesn't make one an authority on child loss.

On the positive side, professional grief and PTSD counselors are more educated on the subject of grief and its processes and are qualified to dabble in the psyche. Unfortunately, all their education still may not tell them what to do for the mom who has aborted a child due to a maternal illness such as

HG. Treatment models deal mainly with parents who have lost children through no choice of their own. Unwanted as it is, therapeutic abortion is still intentional child loss. It creates problems that don't necessarily exist within the frame of non-consensual child loss. Those who specialize in prenatal child loss may be able to adapt a treatment model, but inclusive group therapy settings may not ever be appropriate. A group of miscarrying moms may find it difficult and even offensive to be asked to support a mom who, for whatever reason, aborted her child. It may also be disturbing for an HG mom to hear other mothers, with normal pregnancies, lament that they would have suffered through "*anything*" to have saved their own children.

Some private, secular counselors who support abortion may be perplexed at grief over "choosing to end a terrible illness." This type may find it difficult if not down right impossible to validate the individual experience. Tell her you've lost a breast and she will commiserate unto eternity, but tell her you've lost a child in an abortion and the response may be "What child?" Being encouraged to see the lost child as an insignificant nothing or merely a choice can be a slap in the face. It implies that the patient is grieving over minutia that merely *seems* significant. One "feminist" counselor, who advertised that dealing with abortion was her specialty, told my husband and me that the spirit of a child does not enter until the ninth month and so our "fetus" was only worthless biological putty and nothing to concern ourselves with. I tried other secular counselors who refused to attribute grief to abortion; they chose instead to delve deeper into my childhood and relationship with my mother. Sigh.

Good therapists do exist, but it can be tough to find one. It may take several attempts with various personalities, and this is possibly not the type of personal story one wants to share habitually, with stranger after stranger. Finding a suitable therapist can be expensive even with insurance that covers part of the payment. For those who do not have such financial resources or for those who find comfort in Christianity, turning to faith-based counsel may be a viable option.

Sectarian Help

Sectarian help is faith-based, that is, based on religion. There are plenty of organizations and crisis pregnancy centers that offer what they call "post-abortion counseling." Over 95% of all abortions are classified as elective, so it should come as no surprise that this type of counseling is mainly geared towards those who aborted electively. On the positive side, this group will validate the reality of the lost child. They believe and acknowledge that you are a parent, will always be a parent, and that you lost a child before birth. They are also Christians, and so automatically have something deeply in common with other Christians.

Unfortunately, this type of group may be more prepared to deal with guilt, forgiveness, and social rehabilitation than they are to deal with actual child loss. They may be at a complete disadvantage to help a husband and wife deal with the agony of losing their child and the dream of the life they wanted to share with that child. Some of the usual counseling focus may not apply and may even add insult to injury. For example, I went through a program that discussed the perils of premarital sex. The implication was that monogamy and marriage prevent abortion. While partly true, it was somehow insulting to me, a married woman who remained faithful and yet aborted a child I wanted due solely to illness.

Generally these "counselors" expect, and some even insist, that you be "healed" from the death of your child by the end of their "post-abortion" program. If you are not, some of these folks are offended. They can make hurtful accusations. For example, after a sectarian program I still felt devastated and unhealed and was told that I was rejecting Christ's death on the cross. Genuine Christianity is more compassionate than that. Truth be told, the majority of these sectarian helpers are "pro-life" volunteers who do not hold any type of professional counseling certification.

Some organizations claim to be sectarian and also support abortion. Since they believe abortion is Biblical, they will probably approach the grieving mother at that angle. I don't know how this could possibly validate the parents' feelings that their child was, as the Bible says, a precious and unique "gift from God," but I imagine they find a way. As of the writing of this book, I know of no sectarian post-abortion programs other than Christian and no real counseling programs, sectarian or otherwise, specifically for mothers who have aborted a child due to maternal health issues. If you can find one, write and let me know.

As with HG, expecting to find a "cure" or a professional who truly understands may be unrealistic, but there *are* good counselors even if you have to go through a million of them to find one. There are also ways to manage life after expecting a child and then losing her in an illness-related abortion. As previously mentioned, online forums address the issue specifically and offer an opportunity for others in similar situations to communicate. Helping others cope with HG in positive ways is something that helps me tremendously. For believers God can work wonders, and for everyone time *will* hang its faithful cobwebs on the crisis of fresh mourning. If you are suffering because you lost a child in an abortion due to HG, hang in there. Do not lose hope. Keep breathing. You are not alone.

Ophelia's Story

I just terminated a planned first pregnancy because of severe HG. I vomited twelve times a day with eventual vomiting of blood. Unbelievable. I lost twelve pounds in two weeks and mentally could not cope. NOTHING helped. All the things they tell you... things like: "Don't drink and eat at the same time. Don't drink liquids that are too hot or too cold..." well, it just doesn't work! I was so sick that I did not take a shower for six days.

The decision to terminate was heartbreaking. My husband actually thinks that maybe I really did not want to be pregnant because admittedly, I had some ambiguous feelings, but doesn't everyone? Being a parent is a HUGE responsibility. I thought a little anxiety was normal. However, I was not prepared for my life to change so completely and drastically and scarily within just one week of finding out I was pregnant. For something that was supposed to be the best experience of my life, it was the worst. I was supposed to be so happy but was only sick beyond belief, depressed and scared. What my doctor does not understand is that within one day of the termination I felt 95% better.

I want to get pregnant again and will definitely handle things differently. Next time I will get into the hospital immediately after those symptoms start (and you know it when they do) and I'll try hypnotherapy.

I regret not insisting to be admitted to the hospital, although I kept informing my doctor that I had not eaten in six days and could not even bear swallowing my own saliva, which was being excessively produced.

I would not wish this on anyone.

EPILOGUE

It feels like it has taken multiple lifetimes to write this book. I could work on it for the rest of my days and it would still seem unfinished. HG is plainly more than a book ever can say. I wish the answer to the problem of our illness had been hidden in these pages. I wish I could have identified the cause and shared a simple cure. I so want to demystify what, for centuries, has been a conundrum and to ensure positive pregnancy outcomes for all. But I can't. The truth of the matter is that HG is likely going to be a terrible plague on families for ages to come.

While I can not supply a solution, I believe the information in this book can help you fight for your baby and yourself. I believe, because I've shared what I've learned and have seen the beautiful difference it has made. Knowledge is power, and you should have it. I also want to recognize, validate, and encourage you in your valiant battle against HG. The message I'm sending is clear: hyperemesis gravidarum is a real physical illness that is terribly debilitating, but *you can beat it!*

In the limited space that a book allows, I strove to be realistic and accurate, to provide information on plenty of positive options, and I have tried my best to represent a broad spectrum of the HG experience. I know that some of the risks can be scary, but <u>Beyond Morning Sickness</u> is an effort to replace anxiety with the hope that information and personal stories offer. I want you to feel educated and released from fear. I want you to be confident in knowing what you need, when you need it and how to get it.

The main goal of this book is your overall health and happiness. I hope that reading it helped you as much as writing it helped me. May you conquer HG so that you and your child can enjoy one another for the rest of your truly precious lives.

Ashli Foshee McCall
November 4, 2006

RORI'S NOTE

Hello, Great News! This past Saturday Jenine, my daughter, woke up...and *didn't feel sick!* YEA!!!!!!!!!!!!!!! She is now nineteen weeks and has started eating. First a bowl of soup and now she's trying other foods! So of course her spirits are up. It looks like we have turned the corner. I'm still not quite ready to let my guard down, but I'm enjoying watching her go back to her old self. What a great Mother's Day gift! I am wondering if this nightmare has finally turned into a wonderful dream come true. I should just sit back and enjoy it. (Boy, God sure works in mysterious ways.)

I talked to Jenine tonight. The advice you gave us really worked. She said it helped when everyone finally backed down and let her go at her own pace. Looking back, in my opinion, I think she would have had a rough time with the HG by itself, but the gallbladder problems stirred things up worse. After all the confusion with trying to force-feed her after the surgery, I think she was starting to feel better but was still afraid to eat. With the help of your letter everyone agreed to give up suggesting food to her, and she was able to try something when she *could*. Before she knew it she was starting to enjoy food, and the fear of having a relapse went away. Right now she has a 24-hour PICC but will probably go to twelve hours later this week. I'm unsure when she will be off of it, but she is planning a PICC party. Wish you could be here!

Looking at her now, smiling, I could almost forget what a nightmare this was.

I got your pamphlet today. It is wonderful! I'm going to take one to my daughter's doctor and start spreading the word. I do know that for the rest of my life I will have one ear open listening to anyone who talks about someone who is abnormally sick in her pregnancy. I'll be there to try and steer her in a good direction.

I want to thank you from the bottom of my heart for all the support you have offered me. Whether I needed a hug or a kick in the rear, there have been times when you have saved my sanity with what you have said.

I have a beautiful daughter with the biggest smile you have ever seen, and I missed it so much. I'm glad to have it back. I can't even imagine what it would be like for someone without enough support. I just want to let you know that all the suffering you have endured and all the research you have done has made a BIG difference in the lives of everyone in my entire family.

Have you ever heard the country song about the hundred-dollar bill? Someone gives it to someone in need, and that person helps someone else, and it becomes a never-ending chain of compassion. Well, you have passed me a 'hundred-dollar bill,' and I won't break the chain. I will be there to pass it along to the next person who needs a friend."

APPENDIX A
Drug Information

I am not a medical professional. I did not complete a recognized course of study culminating in a pharmacological degree. This list concerns drugs for use in the United States and is not a complete list. Drugs are constantly being developed and studied. Their forms and usage are in perpetual flux, which is why authoritative works like the Physician's Desk Reference are reissued annually. By the time you read a copy of this book, some drugs may have new forms or new uses or may not be in use at all. I am not recommending any particular drug but only offering information about drugs you may be taking.

Where possible I have listed the drug class so that you can understand how the medication works. This knowledge may help to reassure you, and it may help you to communicate with your doctor. Most people do not know the difference between antihistamines and phenothiazines. Your unusual knowledge may comfort you. The uniqueness of it may also pique your doctor's interest, and you may be able to reclaim a little of the respect that is sometimes automatically lost just by suffering from HG.

While knowledge is power, many times the exact anti-vomiting mechanism of a medication is unknown. Even the ones that are known may fall under more than one type. For instance, Phenergan is an antihistamine and a phenothiazine. To keep it simple though, I only list at least one category where I can. Also, where I only list a few side effects, there are oftentimes more. Actual drug references carry the most extensive information on this subject. My objective is to provide a well-rounded information resource consisting of a good many options.

If you have concerns about the medications you are taking, discuss it with your doctor. If she seems annoyed that you are questioning her, instead of encouraged by your interest in being part of your own healing team, then you may want to consider getting a second opinion or switching doctors altogether. No one should make you feel guilty for your concern; it is healthy and good to be interested in what is happening to you and your baby.

Antihistamines

Antihistamines block histamine, a chemical in the body that can manifest as allergic reaction when released. Simply put, antihistamines relieve the symptoms of allergies. If HG involves allergy, this may explain one way antihistamines can be an effective treatment. Another way antihistamines may help relieve nausea and vomiting is by sedating the vomiting center of the brain and making it less sensitive to the nausea and vomiting messages it receives.

Common side effects are dry mouth, blurred vision and difficulty urinating.

Phenothiazines

Phenothiazines block dopamine, a neurotransmitter

responsible for sending messages in the brain. By blocking this "messenger" from delivering vomit-inducing information to the chemoreceptor area in the brain, nausea and vomiting can sometimes be relieved.

Common side effects are expressionless face, shaky hands, lowered blood pressure, shakiness, and uncontrolled movement of the face and tongue.

Serotonin Receptor Antagonists

An overabundance of serotonin can cause nausea and vomiting. Serotonin receptor antagonists block the body's ability to detect such an overabundance of serotonin.

Common side effects are headache, sedation, diarrhea and constipation.

Corticosteroids

Corticosteroids occur naturally in the body. They reduce inflammation by blocking prostaglandins and are commonly used to prevent organ transplant rejection because they suppress allergic reaction and immune system activity. One drawback to a reduction in immune system activity is a susceptibility to infection.

Common side effects are an elevated sense of well-being and a sense of euphoria (psychotropic effects).

FDA Ratings and List of Drugs

The Food and Drug Administration (FDA) has rated drugs for use in pregnancy. What follows is an explanation of these ratings. Additionally, a list of drugs and related information is provided.

Category	Interpretation
A	Controlled studies fail to show a risk to the fetus, and the possibility of fetal harm appears remote.
B	Either animal studies showed no fetal risk but there are no controlled studies in pregnant women -or- animal studies showed a risk that was not confirmed in controlled studies.
C	Either animal studies showed a risk to the fetus and there are no controlled studies in women -or- studies in animals and women are not available. It is reasonable to take these drugs if the potential benefit justifies the potential fetal risk.
D	There is positive evidence of human fetal risk, but the benefits from use in pregnant women may be acceptable despite the risk (as in a life-threatening situation).
X	Animal or human studies showed fetal abnormalities -or- there is evidence of fetal risk based on the human experience -or- both, and the risk of the use of the drug in pregnant women clearly outweighs any possible benefit. The drug is contraindicated in women who are or may become pregnant.

Antihistamines:
All antihistamines cause drowsiness.

Generic:	**cyclizine**
Pronunciation:	*SYE kli zeen*
Brand:	**Marezine**
Class:	antihistamine
FDA Category:	B
Forms:	pill
Common Side Effects:	dizziness, drowsiness, blurred vision

Generic:	**dimenhydrinate**
Pronunciation:	*dye men HYE dri nate*
Brand:	**Dramamine, Driminate**
Class:	antihistamine
FDA Category:	B
Forms:	pill, injection, oral liquid
Common Side Effects:	dizziness, drowsiness, blurred vision

Generic:	**diphenhydramine**
Pronunciation:	*dye fen HYE dra meen*
Brand:	**Benadryl, Unisom, Nytol caplet, Sominex, etc.**
Class:	antihistamine
FDA Category:	B
Forms:	pill, injection, oral liquid
Common Side Effects:	dizziness, drowsiness

Generic:	**Doxylamine & pyridoxine**
Pronunciation:	*dox ILL a meen & peer i DOX een*
Brand:	**Bendectin, Diclectin SR**
Class:	sedative antihistamine and vitamin combination
FDA Category:	C
Forms:	pill
Common Side Effects:	drowsiness, dizziness, restlessness, constipation, headache, dryness of mouth and eyes or stomachache

Generic:	**meclizine**
Pronunciation:	*MEK li zeen*
Brand:	**Antivert, Bonine, Dramamine 2, Driminate 2**
Class:	antihistamine
FDA Category:	B
Forms:	pill
Common Side Effects:	dizziness, drowsiness, blurred vision

Corticosteroids:

Generic:	**dexamethasone**
Pronunciation:	*dex a METH a sone*
Brand:	**Decadron, Dexone, Hexadrol**
Action:	decreases immune response
FDA Category:	C
Forms:	pill, injection, oral liquid
Common Side Effects:	insomnia, stomach upset, dizziness, muscle weakness, diabetes control issues, increased hunger/thirst

Generic:	**hydrocortisone**
Pronunciation:	*hye droe KOR ti sone*
Brand:	**Cortef, Hydrocortone**
Action:	decreases immune response
FDA Category:	C
Forms:	pill, injection
Common Side Effects:	insomnia, stomach upset, fatigue, dizziness, muscle weakness, joint pain, diabetes control issues, increased hunger/thirst or nausea

Generic:	**methylprednisolone sodium succinate**
Pronunciation:	*meth ill pred NISS oh lone SEW dee um SUCK sin ate*
Brand:	**Solumedrol**
Action:	decreases immune response
FDA Category:	C
Forms:	injection
Common Side Effects:	same as with prednisolone

Generic:	**prednisolone**
Pronunciation:	*pred NISS oh lone*
Brand:	**Prelone**
Action:	decreases immune response
FDA Category:	C
Forms:	pill, injection, oral liquid
Common Side Effects:	insomnia, stomach upset, fatigue, dizziness, muscle weakness, joint pain, diabetes control issues, increased hunger/thirst or nausea

Generic:	**prednisone**
Pronunciation:	*PRED ni sone*
Brand:	**Deltasone, Liquid Pred, Meticorten, Orasone, Prednicen-M, Sterapred, Sterapred DS**
Action:	decreases immune response
FDA Category:	C
Forms:	pill, oral liquid
Common Side Effects:	same as with prednisolone

Phenothiazines:
These are used in combination with antihistamines, to reduce side effects.

Generic:	**chlorpromazine**
Pronunciation:	*klor PROE ma zeen*
Brand:	**Thorazine**
Action:	changes the actions of chemicals in the brain; should be used with an antihistamine to reduce side effects
FDA Category:	C
Forms:	pill, suppositories, oral liquid
Common Side Effects:	dizziness, drowsiness

Generic:	**prochlorperazine**
Pronunciation:	*pro klor PER a zeen*
Brand:	**Compazine**
Tip:	use with an antihistamine to reduce side effects
FDA Category:	C
Forms:	pill, injection, suppositories, oral liquid
Common Side Effects:	decreased sweating, restlessness, tremor, difficulty urinating jaw clenching

Generic:	**promethazine**
Pronunciation:	*pro METH a zeen*
Brand:	**Phenergan**
Class:	antihistamine
FDA Category:	C
Form:	pill, injection, suppositories, oral liquid
Common Side Effects:	dizziness, drowsiness, increased sensitivity to sunlight, nausea/vomiting; call your doctor if any of these occur: uncontrollable movements of eyes/lips/face/tongue/legs, dizziness, headache

Generic:	**thiethylperazine**
Pronunciation:	*thye eth ill PEAR a zeen*
Brand:	**Torecan**
Class:	phenothiazine
FDA Category:	C
Form:	pill, injection, suppositories
Common Side Effects:	headache, dizziness, drowsiness, agitation, tremor, increased heart rate; if anything starts to move involuntarily, call your doctor.

Miscellaneous Drugs:

Generic:	**dronabinol**
Pronunciation:	*droe NAB i no*l
Brand:	**Marinol**
Class:	cannabinoid
FDA Category:	C
Forms:	pill
Common Side Effects:	anxiety, euphoria, dizziness, paranoia, sedation

Generic:	**droperidol**
Pronunciation:	*dro PAIR id all*
Brand:	**Inapsine**
Class:	butyrophenone; tranquilizer
FDA Category:	C
Forms:	injection
Common Side Effects:	drowsiness, dizziness, floating feeling, anxiety, restlessness, change trouble breathing, EKG changes, rapid heart rate, muscle stiffness

Generic:	**haloperidol**
Pronunciation:	*hal o PAIR id all*
Brand:	**Haldol**
Class:	butyrophenone; tranquilizer
FDA Category:	C
Forms:	pill, liquid, injection
Common Side Effects:	drowsiness, dizziness, fainting

Generic:	**metoclopramide**
Pronunciation:	*met oh KLOE pra mide*
Brand:	**Reglan**
Class:	substituted benzamide; speeds up gastric emptying (the rate at which the stomach and intestine move during digestion) and strengthens the lower esophageal sphincter
FDA Category:	B
Forms:	pill, injection, oral liquid
Common Side Effects:	uncontrollable spasms of arms/legs/lips/tongue/face or other body part, unexplained anxiety, aggitation, jitteriness, insomnia; these could be early warning signs of a serious side effect to come so contact your doctor.

Generic:	**ondansetron**
Pronunciation:	*on DAN se tron*
Brand:	**Zofran**
Class:	serotonin receptor antagonist; reduces nausea and vomiting in chemotherapy, radiation treatments and surgery
FDA Category:	B
Forms:	pills, injection, oral liquid
Common Side Effects:	anxiety, drowsiness, dizziness, headache, fewer side effects than any other antiemetic

Generic:	**pyridoxine (B6)**
Pronunciation:	*peer ih DOCK seen*
Brand:	**Nestrex**
Class:	vitamin that helps to break down protein, fat and carbohydrates in food
FDA Category:	A
Forms:	pill, injection
Common Side Effects:	none if taken as prescribed; overdose can be dangerous

Generic:	**trimethobenzamide**
Pronunciation:	*try meth oh BEN za mide*
Brand:	**Tigan**
Class:	anticholinerginic
Forms:	pill, injection, suppositories
FDA Category:	C
Common Side Effects:	drowsiness

Antacids:
Many women have heartburn/acid issues from repeated vomiting. These problems can actually cause more vomiting, so I have included a small list of helpful drugs that your doctor might prescribe.

Generic:	**cimetidine**
Pronunciation:	*sye MET I deen*
Brand:	**Tagamet, Tagamet HB**
Action:	antacid
FDA Category:	B
Forms:	pill, injection, oral liquid
Common Side Effects:	dizziness, headache, diarrhea, constipation, nausea

Generic:	**famotidine**
Pronunciation:	*fa MOE ti deen*
Brand:	**Pepcid AC**
Class:	antacid
FDA Category:	B
Forms:	IV, pill, powder
Common Side Effects:	headache, diarrhea, constipation, elevated liver enzyme levels

Generic:	**nizatidine**
Pronunciation:	*ni ZA ti deen*
Brand:	**Axid AR, Axid Pulvules**
Class:	antacid
FDA Category:	C
Forms:	pill
Common Side Effects:	swollen lips/tongue/face/throat, hives, unusual bruising

Generic:	**omeprazole**
Pronunciation:	*oh MEH pra zol*
Brand:	**Prilosec**
Class:	antacid
FDA Category:	C
Forms:	pill
Common Side Effects:	drowsiness, dizziness, headache, diarrhea, gas, bloating, itching

Generic:	**pantoprazole sodium**
Pronunciation:	*pan TOE pra zole SEW dee um*
Brand:	**Protonix**
Class:	acid blocker
FDA Category:	B
Forms:	pill, IV
Common Side Effects:	gas, constipation, headache, cough, abnormal liver function test results

Generic:	**ranitidine**
Pronunciation:	*ra NYE te deen*
Brand:	**Zantac**
Class:	antacid
FDA Category:	B
Forms:	pill, injection, oral liquid
Common Side Effects:	dizziness, headache, diarrhea, constipation, nausea

APPENDIX B
Basic Needs & Resources

If you can't meet any of you or your family's needs, do not hesitate to call on extended family, friends, churches or even crisis pregnancy centers (listed under "Abortion Alternatives" in the Yellow Pages). If these are not an option, it is good to know there are still positive alternatives! The following is a list of very basic needs and some helpful resources:[204]

Child Care:

- _Child Care Aware_ - This organization offers information on general options, local resources and referrals. By dialing 1-800-424-2246, you can get information about subsidized child care programs in your area. Emergency child care due to maternal health issues is a reality! In addition to child care information, Child Care Aware can help you address other necessities. Tell the agency what you need and when you need it, and they'll work on helping you find someone in your area who can provide it.

Clothing:

- _Thrift Stores_ - A volunteer can take the kids' measurements and then go to a thrift store such as Goodwill or Salvation Army and purchase low-cost, name brand clothing that is stylish and will last.

- *Auctions* - Online auctions such as www.ebay.com can be a wonderful resource for inexpensive clothing purchased in large lots. A volunteer can go to a library and use a computer to bid on items of clothing for your children.
- *Garage Sales* - Inexpensive clothing by the barrel-full. Volunteers can scout garage sales for clothing or any other item the family might need.

Food:

- *Various Food Assistance Programs* - Wonderful food assistance programs, such as WIC, Food Stamps, School Meals and many more, can be found at http://www.usda.gov by clicking on "Food and Nutrition" on the homepage and clicking on "Food Assistance" after that.
- *Local Charities* - Sometimes these entities offer food banks/pantries. Call the county welfare office for more info.

Housing:

- *Local Human Services or Social Services Dept.* - This listing is found under the name of your town and then "Administrative Offices" in the government section of your phone book. They can provide information on emergency housing in the event of an eviction.
- *Town Clerk's Office* - If your town is small, and you can not find a local Human or Social Services organization, the town clerk's office may be able to offer you a referral to someone who can help.
- *Emergency Services Organizations* - The American Red Cross, Salvation Army, Catholic Charities, and the

United Way are all emergency services organizations that can help find low-cost housing. They can be found in the yellow pages under "Social Services."

Medical Care for Children:

- *State Health Insurance Plan* - www.insurekidsnow.gov says every state offers an insurance plan for children from babies to teens. Contact 1-877-KIDSNOW for more info.
- *Medicaid* - Call your local Medicaid office to see if you meet the guidelines and can apply for emergency Medicaid.
- *Free/low-cost clinics* - Some counties provide such health programs. Call your local health dept for more info.

Transportation:

- *Bus Pass* - In the event that the loss of income causes a loss of transportation, family, friends or other volunteers can usually provide transportation to and from the doctor's office/hospital. For the spouse who could not keep up the car payments alone, a bus pass can be purchased if available in your area. The bus will get the spouse to and from work, to the grocery store, and most other places. The local transit usually does a good job of locating bus stops within walking distance of important destinations.
- *Car Pooling* - If taking the bus is not an option, car pooling might be. If you live far out in the country but work in town, chances are that someone else in your area also commutes. Check with local friends and churches. If you explain your situation and your

finances to a compassionate and able person, she should be happy to car pool with you and will likely donate the service for free.

Resources
Helplines:

- *Hygeia Foundation, Inc.*
  Hygeia maintains a Web site where grieving moms can go and talk about their losses. HG and termination for HG are mentioned within the site. In addition, they have a message board for moms on bed rest, and advocates can call a toll-free number to try and locate excellent and dignified health care.
  Web site: http://www.hygeia.org
  Toll free information: 1-800-893-9198

- *Matria Healthcare, Inc.*
  Matria is a U.S. provider of home health care services that specializes in obstetric home care for women with HG.
  Web site: http://www.matria.com/ob/services/faq/nvp_faq.html
  Toll free information: 1-800-456-4060

- *Motherisk*
  The Motherisk program was established in 1995 for nausea and vomiting of pregnancy (NVP) and features a book on NVP with twelve sections on HG.
  Web site: http://www.motherisk.org/sickness/index.php
  Toll free helpline: 1-800-436-8477

- *Sidelines*
  Sidelines addresses pregnancy complications with a focus on prematurity. They are a source of good support for those on bed rest.
  Web site: http://www.sidelines.org (A printable coloring book called Mommy and the Hospital can be found by clicking on "Resources" on the site's home page.)
  Toll free helpline: 1-888-447-4754

Supportive Web sites:
- http://www.hyperemesis.org
- http://www.angelfire.com/nt/hugs/
- http://www.hyperemesisgravidarum.com
- http://www.extrememorningsickness.com

Books with good references to HG:
- Nausea and Vomiting of Pregnancy: State of the Art 2000
  by various contributors; edited by Gideon Koren and Raafat Bishal
  Ordering Information: Amazon.com

- No More Morning Sickness
  by Miriam Erick
  Ordering Information: Amazon.com

- Managing Morning Sickness: A Survival Guide for Pregnant Women
  by Miriam Erick
  Ordering Information: Amazon.com

- The Proving Grounds
  by Barbara Mangini
  Ordering Information: Amazon.com

- <u>Body Mutiny: Surviving Nine Months of Extreme Morning Sickness</u>
  by Jenna C. Schmitt
  Ordering Information: Acacia Publishing (866) 265-4553

Patient Advocacy Pamphlets:
- "Speak Up: Help prevent errors in your care"
  Ask for the general Speak Up pamphlet and the home health care pamphlet if applicable.
  Ordering Information: (630) 792-5800
  (All pamphlets are provided as free downloads at their Web site: http://www.jointcommission.org/PatientSafety/SpeakUp/)

Products:
- ReliefBand (electrical acustimulation device):
  Ordering Information: 1-888-297-9728
  Web site: http://www.reliefband.com

- Ketone Test Strips (for testing urine for ketones):
  Ordering Information: 1-800-Drugstore (378-4786)
  Website: http://www.drugstore.com/qxp37671_333181_sespider/ketostix/reagent_strips_for_urinalysis.htm
  (Test strips can also be purchased from local drug stores and medical supply companies.)

- Hypnosis Audios for Nausea:
  Harwell Hypnosis & Healing Arts
  Sam Bass Professional Center
  1315 Sam Bass Circle, Suite B-6

Round Rock, Texas 78681.
Ordering Information: (877) 341-2567
Email: harwellhypnosis@msn.com
Web site: http://www.harwellhypnosis.com/selfhyp.
asp

- Amazing Changes Hypnosis
  1001 Boulders Parkway Suite 140
  Richmond, VA 23225
  Ordering Information: (804) 272-3330
  Email: Info@Hypnosis.ac
  Web site: http://www.hypnosis.ac/Morning_
  Sickness.html

Services:
- To find a hypnotherapist:
  The American Society of Clinical Hypnosis
  140 N. Bloomingdale Rd.
  Bloomingdale, IL 60108-1017
  Voice: (630) 980-4740
  Fax: (630) 351-8490
  Email: info@asch.net
  Web site: http://www.asch.net/

- To find a homeopath:
  Council for Homeopathic Certification
  PMB 187
  16915 SE 272nd Street, Suite 100
  Covington, WA 98042
  Phone: (866) 242-3399
  Fax: (815) 366-7622
  Email: chcinfo@homeopathicdirectory.com

Web site: http://www.homeopathicdirectory.com/

Helping Children Cope

Children need many fun opportunities to spend time away from Mother's scary illness. If you are helping with the children here are some ideas for you.

You might take the children to:

Parks, parades, playgrounds, hiking and biking trails, nature centers, zoos, the beach, outdoor recreational areas, arcades, skating rinks, swimming pools, museums, galleries, gardens and botanical sites, springs, movies, school sporting events, free concerts and plays at colleges, an airport observation tower (for plane watching), libraries (for books, audio-visuals, computers and free programs), classes (some large hardware stores offer free kids' classes), parades, theme parks, craft shows, an exciting place for a fun vacation, scouting, 4-H Club, local events, YMCA/YWCA, historical reenactments, church, youth groups, fairs, concerts, festivals, campgrounds, letterboxing, geocaching, etc.

Use good judgment when deciding on experiences for children. All activities should be fun, age appropriate, and most importantly, safe.

In addition, here are some books that may be helpful to adults who care for children:

- <u>How to Help Children Through a Parent's Serious Illness</u> by Kathleen McCue and Ron Bonn

- <u>Parenting Through Crisis: Helping Kids in Times of Loss, Grief and Change</u> by Barbara Coloroso

- <u>Helping Children Cope with Separation and Loss</u> by Claudia Jew Jarratt (This one might be good for helping children deal with time away from Mother due to hospitalizations.)

These books may be beneficial to young children:

- <u>When Mommy is Sick</u> by Ferne Sherkin-Langer

- <u>Mommy's in the Hospital Again</u> by Carolyn Stearns Parkinson

- <u>Raymond's Perfect Present</u> by Therese On Louie

I'd love to hear from you!
ashli@beyondmorningsickness.com

APPENDIX C
The World Wide Web: Misinformation Highway

If you look up HG on the Internet, you can find great information and advice. However, you'll find misinformation too, some of it from honored sources. Just because a source is respected doesn't mean it is right about everything. However, some people who read these pages will accept misinformation as fact, and this can be damaging. Once I had an argument with a person who knew nothing about HG. She didn't believe me when I told her how bad this disease is, so she looked it up on the Internet to find out more about it. She returned from her research thoroughly disgusted and asking, "What's the big deal? You puke a little too much and they give you drugs to stop it. Whoop-dee-doo." Whoop-de-doo, indeed. Here is a sample of eleven pieces of misinformation/misrepresentation gleaned from a brief examination of only 19 web sites that shall remain nameless:

- Site claims the expected length of work-related disability for a woman with HG and metabolic disturbance is 3 weeks maximum for a job that requires "very heavy work."

- Often even one small meal is impossible yet a Web site suggests 6 small meals a day as part of the treatment for HG.

- Site suggests seventeen small meals and sixteen liquid drinks (including several doses of ½ cup of ice chips) per day.

- Physician's site says that not wanting the baby has been linked to HG. Also says that young single women whose parents accuse them of "sinning" get HG and that remarkable improvement is seen once they are placed in the hospital. It goes on to say that once these personalities go back to the hostile home environment they experience relapses. It also says, and this is my favorite part, that being hysterical and immature are risk factors for the disease.

- Site says HG does not persist after the twentieth week.

- Medical site suggests that eating crackers before rising in the morning helps HG.

- Medical site says getting involved in work or other activities helps many women with HG.

- Major respected medical site says nausea and vomiting normally stop (for good) within a few days of being placed in the hospital but sometimes a person needs to be readmitted "once or twice."

- Site advises small, frequent meals and suggests an avoidance of spicy foods. (Like people who can't keep down water are going to have to be told to cut down on the jalapenos.)

- Site says nuts, cheese and milk should be eaten several times a day for the mildly hyperemetic but that fatty foods should be avoided. Also says antiemetics are only given to severe cases. Says emotional problems can contribute to the *cause* of HG.

APPENDIX D
Bed Rest, Pregnancy and Blood Clots

Many times HG is so debilitating that women find themselves bed ridden. Pregnant women have an increased chance of developing blood clots (thrombi) as do those on bed rest. Pregnant women who are on bed rest or lying on the couch all day long may reduce the risk of developing potentially dangerous blood clots by walking up and down the hall at least three times a day. If you can't walk without vomiting or have some other issue that prevents walking, alternatives exist.

Most hospitals employ physical therapists who have a set of exercises specifically intended to reduce blood clot risks for those on bed rest. Your doctor may refer you to a physical therapist or may be able to write for the bed rest exercise protocol. Sources for clot-preventing exercises can be found at the end of this appendix. Talk to your doctor before attempting any type of exercise.

If movement causes vomiting or you have some other issue that prevents bed rest exercises, graduated compression or anti-embolism stockings can be worn. These are long stockings that begin at the feet and end with a built-in elastic garter around the thigh. They are fairly consistently tight and this constricts blood vessels enough to increase blood pressure in the legs.

The elevated pressure helps to prevent slow-moving blood that can cause clotting. Pneumatic compression cuffs can also help. These are worn up to the thigh and are automatically inflated and deflated every few minutes to stimulate and compress leg veins.

It is important to try and prevent blood clots because, though rare, blood clots can embolize or break off and travel through the body, ending up in places like the lungs. This is known as a pulmonary embolism and is potentially fatal. Blood thinning drugs can also be used to help prevent or disperse blood clots. Heparin (pregnancy category C) is one such drug. Ask your doctor if she has written guidelines for preventing blood clots.

Blood Clot Symptoms:
- Pain or tenderness in the area
- Swelling of the area
- Warmth of the area
- Redness of the area
- Unusually pronounced veins

Embolism Symptoms:
- Difficulty breathing
- Tachycardia (increased pulse rate)
- Coughing up blood
- Malaise
- Chest pain
- Excessive sweating
- Fainting

Sources for Clot-Preventing Exercises

- Bedrest exercises can be found in the book: <u>Days In Waiting: A Guide to Surviving Pregnancy Bedrest</u> by Mary Ann McCann.

- A 64-page book called <u>Preterm Birth Prevention</u> can be downloaded at: http://www.permanente.net/homepage/kaiser/pdf/23671.pdf
  (Pages 18-21 feature information on bedrest exercises specifically.)

- Various exercises are explained by accessing: http://www.medicalcenter.osu.edu/patientcare/
  Once there, follow this pathway:
  "Health Information"
  "Patient Education Materials"
  "Exercise/Rehabilitation"
  "Lower Body"

APPENDIX E
Companion Pamphlet

I hope you have found <u>Beyond Morning Sickness</u> helpful. I have also developed a companion pamphlet for your convenience. Are there others who don't seem to understand HG, what you are going through or how to help? You can share this pamphlet with them. The companion pamphlet is an easy way for you to explain your illness without actually having to explain your illness! It is free and in PDF form. If you would like one click on "Companion Pamphlet" at:

http://www.beyondmorningsickness.com

Please feel free to copy these pamphlets for your own, non-profit distribution.

CONSULTED WORKS

Abortion and HG

Erick, M More on NVP (Letter)
Midwifery Today (Summer 1997)n42pMT-7

Erick, M *No More Morning Sickness*
New York, NY: Penguin Group, 1993

Gawande, A A Queasy Feeling: Why Can't We Cure Nausea?
The New Yorker (July 5, 1999)p34-41

Johnson N *A Doctor Explains The Abortion Procedure*
Cleveland, OH: American Portrait Films

Mazzota P, et al. Factors associated with elective termination of
pregnancy among Canadian and American women with nausea
and vomiting of pregnancy
J Psychosom Obstet Gynecol (Mar 2001)v22n1p7-12

Mazzota P, et al. Therapeutic abortions due to severe morning
sickness: unacceptable combination
Can Fam Phys (Jun 1997)v43p1055-7

Nugent, MP *Having Your Baby When Others Say No*
Garden City Park, NY: Avery Publishing Group,1991

Willke JC, et al. Abortion: Questions and Answers
Cincinnati, OH: Hayes Publishing Company, 1988

Breast Cancer and Other Abortion Risks
Brind J, et al. What every woman in the world has a right to know!
(Brochure) Endeavour Forum, Inc. (Toorak, Victoria, Australia) and the Abortion-Breast Cancer Quarterly Update (Poughkeepsie, NY)

Daling JR, et al. Risk of breast cancer among white women following induced abortion
Am J Epidemiol (Aug 15 1996)v144n4p373-80

Daling JR, et al. Risk of breast cancer among young women: relationship to induced abortion
J Natl Cancer Inst (Nov 2 1994)v86n21p1569-70

Elford K, et al. Novel treatment of a patient with secondary infertility due to retained fetal bone
Fertility and Sterility (Apr 2003)v79n4p1028-1030

Ewertz M, et al. Risk of breast cancer in relation to reproductive factors in Denmark
Br J Cancer (Jul 1988)v58n1p99-104

Gissler M, et al. Pregnancy-associated deaths in Finland 1987-1994 -- definition problems and benefits of record linkage
Acta Obset Gynecol Scand (1997)v76p 651-657

Howe HL, et al. Early abortion and breast cancer risk among women under age 40
Int J Epidemiol (Jun 1989)v18n2p300-4

Laing AE, et al. Breast cancer risk factors in African-American women: the Howard University Tumor Registry experience

J Natl Med Assoc (Dec 1993)v85n12p931-9

Lasovich D, et al. Induced abortion and breast cancer risk
Epidemiology (Jan 2000)v11n1p76-80

Malec K The abortion-breast cancer link: How politics trumped
science and informed consent
J Am Phys Surgeons (Summer 2003)v8n2p41-45

Malec K Homepage
Coalition on Abortion/Breast Cancer; Rev 6/03
http://www.abortionbreastcancer.com

McFadden A The link between abortion and child abuse
Family Resources Center News (January 1998) 20

Ney PG, et al. The effects of pregnancy loss on women's
health
Soc Sci Med (1994)v48n9p1193

Pike MC, et al. Oral contraceptive use and early abortion as
risk factors for breast cancer in young women
Br J Cancer (Jan 1981)v43n1p72-6

Reardon D Psychological Reactions Reported After Abortion
The Post-Abortion Review (Fall 1994)v2n3p4-8

Reardon D Women at risk: abortion and the high-risk patient
(Brochure) Retrieved on August 22, 2004 from
http://www.afterabortion.org/women_a.html

Rohan TE, et al. A population-based case-control study of diet and breast cancer in Australia
Am J Epidemiol (Sept 1998)v128n3p478-89

Rookus MA, et al. Induced abortion and risk for breast cancer: reporting (recall) bias in a Dutch case-control study
J Natl Cancer Inst (Dec 4 1996)v88n23p1759-64

Rooney B, et al. Induced abortion and risk of later premature births
J Am Phys Surgeons (Summer 2003)v8n2p46-9

Russo J, et al. Susceptibility of the mammary gland to carcinogenesis.ll. Pregnancy interruption as a risk factor in tumor incidence
Am J Pathol (Aug 1980)v100n2p497-512

Tischler C Adolescent suicide attempts following elective abortion
Pediatrics (1981)v68n5p670

Willke JC The deadly after-effect of abortion: breast cancer (Brochure) Hayes Publishing Company, Cincinnati, 2000

Woman begged for help before her abortion killed her
Arizona Republic (Jan 30, 2001)

Replacement Child
Ansfeld L, et al. The replacement child. Variations on a theme in history and psychoanalysis.
Psychoanal Study Child (2000)v55p301-18

Statistics
Torres A, et al. Why do women have abortions?
Fam Plan Perspect (Jul/Aug 1988)v20n4p170

Alternative Treatments
General Information
Aikins M Alternative therapies for nausea and vomiting of pregnancy
Obstet Gynecol (Jan 1998)v91n1p149-55

Ernst E, et al. Health risks over the Internet: advice offered by "medical herbalists" to a pregnant woman.
Wien Med Wochenschr (2002)v152n7-8p190-2

Thorp, et al. Long-term physical and psychological health consequences of induced abortion: review of the evidence
Obstet Gynecol Survey (2003)v58n1p67-79

Acupressure
Ernst E Hyperemesis gravidarum (Correspondence)
Postgrad Med J (Jul 2002)v78n921p443

Kuscu NK, et al. Hyperemesis gravidarum (Correspondence)
Postgrad Med J (Jul 2002)v78n921p443-4

Roscoe JA, et al. Acupressure and acustimulation bands for control of nausea: A brief review
Am J Obstet Gynecol (May 2002)v186n5pS244-7

Strong TH Alternative therapies of morning sickness
Clin Obstet Gynecol (Dec 2001)v44n4p653-60

Werntoft E, et al. Effect of Acupressure on Nausea and Vomiting During Pregnancy. A randomized, placebo-controlled, pilot study
J Reprod Med (Sep 2001)v46n9p835-9

Acupuncture
Carlsson C, et al. Manual Acupuncture Reduces Hyperemesis Gravidarum: A Placebo-Controlled, Randomized, Single-Blind, Crossover Study
J Pain Symptom Manage (Oct 2000)v20n4p273-9

Habek D, et al. Success of acupuncture and acupressure of the Pc 6 acupoint in the treatment of hyperemesis gravidarum
Forsch Komplementarmed Klass Naturheilkd (Feb 2004)v11n1p20-3

Knight B, et al. Effect of Acupuncture on Nausea of Pregnancy: A Randomized, Controlled Trial
Obstet Gynecol (Feb 2001)v97n2p184-188

Electric Stimulation
Golaszewski T, et al. Treatment of hyperemesis gravidarum by electrical stimulation of the vestibular system
Am J Obstet Gynecol (Aug 1994)v171n2p577

Golaszewski TM Treatment of hyperemesis gravidarum by electrical stimulation of the vestibular system
J Psychosom Obstet Gynecol (Sep 1997)v18n3p244-6

Slotnick RN Safe, successful nausea suppression in early pregnancy with P-6 acustimulation
J Reprod Med (Sep 2001)v46n9p811-4

Ginger (Powdered)
Erick M Maternity—Morning Sickness
The Boston Parents' Paper (June 1995)

Niebyl JR, et al. Overview of nausea and vomiting of pregnancy
with an emphasis on vitamins and ginger
Am J Obstet Gynecol (May 2002)v186n5pS253-5

Dental Erosion
Scheutzel P Etiology of dental erosion—intrinsic factors
Eur J Oral Sci (Apr 1996)v104n2(Pt 2)p178-90

Drugs (Teratogenicity, Side Effects, Fear of Taking Meds)
Ditto A, et al. Evaluation of treatment of hyperemesis
gravidarum using parenteral fluid with or without diazepam:
A randomized study
Gynecol Obstet Invest (1999)v48n4p232-6

Gardner DK, et al. Hyperemesis Gravidarum
Pharmacist (Aug 1997)p47-66

Heikkilla AM, et al. Use of medication during pregnancy—a
prospective cohort study on use and policy of prescribing
Ann Chir Gynae Suppl (1994)v208p80-3

Jewell D, et al. Interventions for nausea and vomiting in early
pregnancy.
Cochrane Database Syst Rev (2002)n1:CD000145

Koch KL et al. Nausea and vomiting during pregnancy
Gastroenterol Clin North Am (Mar 2003)v32n1p201-34, vi

Koren G, et al. The teratogenicity of drugs for nausea and vomiting of pregnancy: Perceived versus true risk
Am J Obstet Gynecol (May 2002)v186n5pS248-52

Magee LA, et al. Evidence-based view of safety and effectiveness of pharmacologic therapy for nausea and vomiting of pregnancy (NVP)
Am J Obstet Gynecol (May 2002)v186n5pS256-61

Mazzota P, et al. Pharmacologic treatment of nausea and vomiting during pregnancy
Can Fam Phys (Jul 1998)v44p1455-7

Nageotte MP, et al. Droperidol and diphenhydramine in the management of HG
Am J Obstet Gynecol (June 1996)v174n6p1801-6

Peleg D, et al. Prescribing antiemetic therapy during pregnancy
Contemp OB/GYN (Jun 1997)p164-71

Prevost R Treatment of Pregnancy-Related Illnesses
Am Pharm (Oct 1995) vNS35n10p25-32

Rohde A, et al. Mirtazapine (Remergil) for treatment resistant hyperemesis gravidarum: rescue of a twin pregnancy
Arch Gynecol Obstet (Aug 2003)v268n3p219-21

Seto A, et al. Pregnancy outcome following first trimester exposure to antihistamines: meta-analysis
Am J Perinatol (Mar 1997)v14n3p119-24

Diclectin (aka Bendectin)
Brent R Medical, social, and legal implications of treating nausea and vomiting of pregnancy
Am J Obstet Gynecol (May 2002)v186n5pS262-66

Diclectin info packet from Motherisk at the Hospital for Sick Children in Canada
555 University Ave, Toronto, Ont. M5G 1X8
www.duchesnay.com/prodcenter.html
(Web site for the Canadian manufacturer of the drug)

Reglan
Buttino L, et al. Home Subcutaneous Metoclopramide Therapy for Hyperemesis Gravidarum
J Perinatol (Sep 2000)v20n6p359-62

Steroids
Chan GC, et al. Complications of the use of corticosteroids for the treatment of hyperemesis gravidarum
Br J Obstet Gynaecol (Jun 1995)v102n6p507-8

Chan LY, et al. Successful treatment of recurrent, intractable hyperemesis gravidarum with methylprednisolone. A case report.
J Reprod Med (Apr 2003)v48n4p293-5

la Marca A, et al. Hyperemesis gravidarum is not associated with hypofunction of the pituitary-adrenal axis (Correspondence)
Am J Obstet Gynecol (Nov 1998)v179n5p1381-2

Moran P, et al. Management of hyperemesis gravidarum: the importance of weight loss as a criterion for steroid therapy. QJM (Mar 2002)v95n3p153-8

Nelson-Piercy, et al. Complications of the use of corticosteroids for the treatment of hyperemesis gravidarum (Response) Br J Obstet Gynaecol (Jun 1995)v102n6p508-9

Nelson-Piercy C, et al. Corticosteroids for the treatment of hyperemesis gravidarum Brit J Obstet Gynaecol (Nov 1994)v101n11p1013-5

Nelson-Piercy C, et al. Randomised, double-blind, placebo-controlled trial of corticosteroids for the treatment of hyperemesis gravidarum BJOG (Jan 2001)v108n1p9-15

Ozdemir I, et al. A case of primary Addison's disease with hyperemesis gravidarum and successful pregnancy Eur J Obstet Gynecol Reprod Biol (Mar 2004)v113n1p100-2

Safari H, et al. The efficacy of methylprednisolone in the treatment of hyperemesis gravidarum: A randomized, double-blind, controlled study Am J Obstet Gynecol (Oct 1998)v179n4p921-4

Safari H, et al. Experience with oral methylprednisolone in the treatment of refractory hyperemesis gravidarum Am J Obstet Gynecol (May 1998)v178n5p1054-8

Subramaniam R, et al. Total Parenteral Nutrition (TPN) and Steroid Usage in the Management of Hyperemesis Gravidarum

Aust. NZ J Obstet Gynaecol (Aug 1998)v38n3p339-41

Taylor R Successful management of hyperemesis gravidarum using steroid therapy

Q J Med(Feb 1996)v89n2p103-7

Whittaker R Randomized, double-blind, placebo-controlled trial of corticosteroids for the treatment of hyperemesis gravidarum. (Correspondence)

BJOG (Jan 2003)v110n1p88

Wong CY, et al. Complications of the use of corticosteroids for the treatment of hyperemesis gravidarum

Br J Obstet Gynaecol (Jun 1995)v102n6p508

Yost NP, et al. A randomized, placebo-controlled trial of corticosteroids for hyperemesis due to pregnancy

Obstet Gynecol (Dec 2003)v102n6p1250-4

Ziaei S, et al. The efficacy of low dose prednisolone in the treatment of hyperemesis gravidarum

Acta Obstet Gynecol Scand (Mar 2004)v83n3p272-5

Zofran

Siu SS, et al. Treatment of intractable hyperemesis gravidarum by ondansetron

Eur J Obstet Gynecol Reprod Biol (Oct 2002)v105n1p73-4

Sullivan CA, et al. A pilot study of intravenous ondansetron for hyperemesis gravidarum
Am J Obstet Gynecol (1996)v174n5p1565-8

Tincello DG, et al. Treatment of hyperemesis gravidarum with the 5-HT3 antagonist ondansetron (Zofran)
Postgrad Med J (Nov 1996)v71n853p688-9

Drug Ratings
Briggs GG, et al. Drugs In Pregnancy and Lactation
Fourth Edition. Williams & Wilkins 1994; xix:xx

Eating (Hindered Ability)
Erick M Battling morning (noon and night) sickness
J Am Diet Ass (Feb 1994)v94n2p147-8

Linehan S Drug therapies for hyperemesis gravidarum (Correspondence)
Can Fam Phys (Sep 1997)v43p1499

Enteral Feeding
American Gastroenterological Association Medical Position Statement: Guidelines for the use of enteral nutrition

Enteral Nutrition
Harrison's Principles of Internal Medicine 11th Edition
Chapter 74: Diet Therapy: Alteration of the feeding route
p400-1, 403-4

Erick M, et al. Nutrition via jejunostomy in refractory hyperemesis gravidarum: A case report
J Am Diet Ass (Oct 1997)v97n10p1154-6

Garcia-Luna, et al./Godil, et al. PEG and PEG-J for nutrition support in pregnancy (correspondence)
JPEN J Parenter Enteral Nutr (Nov-Dec)v23n6p367-8

Godil A, et al. Percutaneous endoscopic gastrostomy for nutrition support in pregnancy associated with hyperemesis gravidarum and anorexia nervosa
J Parenter Enteral Nutr (Jul-Aug 1998)v22n4p238-41

Hsu JJ, et al. Nasogastric Enteral Feeding in the Management of Hyperemesis Gravidarum
Obstetrics and Gynecology (Sept 1996)v88n3p343-6

Irving PM, et al. Percutaneous endoscopic gastrostomy with a jejunal port for severe hyperemesis gravidarum
Eur J Gastroenterol Heptatol (Sep 2003)v16n9p937-9

Pearce CB, et al. Enteral nutrition by nasojejunal tube in hyperemesis gravidarum
Clin Nutr (Oct 2001)v20n5p461-4

Pereira JL, et al. Percutaneous endocscopic gastrostomy and gastrojejunostomy. Experience and its role in domiciliary enteral nutrition
Nutr Host (Jan-Feb 1998)v13n1p50-6

Sanders S, et al. New Protocol To Manage Hyperemesis Gravidarum
J AM Diet Ass (Dec 1994)v94n12p1367-8

Sanders S, et al. Doctor's script for nasogastric feeding
Personal correspondence; copy of script obtained by writing S. Sanders, MS, RD at:
Cedars-Sinai Medical Center, 8700 Beverly Blvd, Los Angeles, CA 90048-1869, Attn: Department of Medicine, GI 7511

Serrano P, et al. Enteral nutrition by percutaneous endoscopic gastrojejunostomy in severe hyperemesis gravidarum: a report of two cases
Clin Nutr (Jun 1998)v17n3p135-9

Tapia J, et al. Jejunostomy: techniques, indications and complications.
World J Surg (Jun 1999);v23n6p596-602

Trovik J, et al. Nasoenteral tube feeding in hyperemesis gravidarum. An alternative to parenteral nutrition
Tidsskr Nor Laegeforen (Aug 1996)v116n20p2442-4

van de Ven CJ Nasogastric enteral feeding in hyperemesis gravidarum (Commentary)
Lancet (Feb 1997)v349n9050p445(2)

Etiology (Causal Theories) & Risk Factors
Al-Yatama M, et al. Hormone profile of Kuwaiti women with hyperemesis gravidarum.
Arch Gynecol Obstet (Aug 2002)v266n4p218-22

Bailit JL Hyperemesis gravidarum: epidemiologic findings from a large cohort
Am J Obstet Gynecol (Sept 2005)v193n3(part 1)p811-4

Black FO Maternal susceptibility to nausea and vomiting of pregnancy: Is the vestibular system involved?
Am J Obstet Gynecol (May 2002)v186n5pS204-9

Broussard CN, et al. Nausea and vomiting of pregnancy
Gastroenterol Clin North Am (Mar 1998)v27n1p123-51

Crotti M, et al. Evaluation and treatment of hyperemesis gravidarum
Minerva Ginecol (Dec 2001)v53n6p413-9

Demir B, et al. Adjusted leptin level (ALL) is a predictor for hyperemesis gravidarum
Eur J Obstet Gynecol Reprod Biol (Feb 2006)v124n2p193-6

Dokmeci F, et al. Trace element status in plasma and erythrocytes in hyperemesis gravidarum
J Reprod Med (Mar 2004)v49n3p200-4

Eliakim R, et al. Hyperemesis Gravidarum: A Current Review
Am J Perinatol (2000)v17n4p207-18

Fait V, et al. Hyperemesis gravidarum is associated with oxidative stress.
Am J Perinatol (Feb 2002)v19n2p93-8

Fatum M, et al. Hyperemesis gravidarum: an updated review
Harefuah (Jan 2003)v142n1p61-5, 77

Furneaux EC, et al. Nausea and vomiting of pregnancy: endocrine basis and contribution to pregnancy outcome.
Obstet Gynecol Surv (Dec 2001)v56n12p775-82

Galanakis E Sickness and sex of child (Correspondence)
Lancet (Feb 2000)v355p756

Gherman RB, et al. Intractable hyperemesis gravidarum, transient hyperthyroidism and intrauterine growth restriction associated with hyperractio luteinalis. A case report.
J Reprod Med (Jul 2003)v48n7p553-6

Glick MM, et al. Molar pregnancy presenting with hyperemesis gravidarum
J Am Osteopath Assoc (Mar 1999)v00n3p162-4

Goodwin TM Hyperemesis Gravidarum
Clin Obstet Gynecol (Sept 1998)v41n3p597-605

Goodwin TM, et al. Increased concentration of the free beta-subunit of human chorionic gonadotropin in hyperemesis gravidarum
Acta Obstet Gynecol Scand (Nov 1994)v71n10p770-2

Goodwin TM Nausea and vomiting of pregnancy: An obstetric syndrome
Am J Obstet Gynecol (May 2002)v186n5pS184-9

Hasler WL Serotonin receptor physiology: relation to emesis
Dig dis Sci (Aug 1999)v44supplement8p108S-113S

Hershman JM Human chorionic gonadotropin and the thyroid: hyperemesis gravidarum and trophoblastic tumors
Thyroid; (Jul 1999)v9n7p653-7

Hod M, et al. Hyperemesis gravidarum. A review
J Reprod Med (Aug 1994)v39n8p605-12

Hummel T, et al. Olfactory modulation of nausea during early pregnancy?
BJOG (Dec 2002)v109n12p1394-7

Imperato F, et al. Hyperemesis gravidarum: etiology and treatment
Clin Ter (Sep-Oct 2003) v154n5p337-40

James WH A potential cause of hyperemesis gravidarum: evidence from the sex ratio of associated infants (Correspondence)
Acta Obstet Gynecol Scand (Apr 2001)v80n4p337

James WH Hyperemesis gravidarum and sex of child (Correspondence)
Lancet (Jan 29 2000)v355n9201p407

James WH The associated offspring sex ratios and cause(s) of hyperemesis gravidarum (Correspondence)
Acta Obstet Gynecol Scand (Apr 2001)v80n4p378-9

Jordan V, et al. Acidic isoforms of chorionic gonadotrophin in European and Samoan women are associated with hyperemesis gravidarum and may be thyrotrophic
Clin Endorin (May 1999)v50n5p619-27

Jordan V, et al. The incidence of hyperemesis gravidarum is increased among Pacific Islanders living in Wellington
N Z Med J (Aug 25, 1995)v108n1006p342-4

Kallen B, et al. Relationship between vitamin use, smoking, and nausea and vomiting of pregnancy.
Acta Obstet Gynecol Scand (Oct 2003)v82n10p916-20

Kaplan PB, et al. Maternal serum cytokine levels in women with hyperemesis gravidarum in the first trimester of pregnancy
Fertil Steril (Mar 2003)v79n3p498-502

Koch KL Gastrointestinal factors in nausea and vomiting of pregnancy
Am J Obstet Gynecol (May 2002)v186n5pS198-203

Kuscu NK Interleukin-6 levels in hyperemesis gravidarum
Arch Gynecol Obstet (Nov 2003)v269n1p13-5

Leylek OA, et al. Immunollogic and biochemical factors in hyperemesis gravidarum with or without hyperthyroxinemia
Gynecol Obstet Invest (1999)v47n4p229-34

Loh KY Understanding hyperemesis gravidarum
Med J Malaysia (Aug 2005)v60n3p394-9

Maes BD, et al. Gastric emptying in hyperemesis gravidarum and non-dyspeptic pregnancy
Aliment Pharmacol Ther (Feb 1999)v13n2p237-43

Melero-Montes M, et al. Hyperemesis Gravidarum and the Sex of the Offspring
Epidemiology (Jan 2000)v12n1p123-4

Miller F Nausea and vomiting in pregnancy: The problem of perception-Is it really a disease?
Am J Obstet Gynecol (May 2002)v186n5pS182-3

Minagawa M, et al. Mechanisms underlying immunologic states during pregnancy: possible association of the sympathetic nervous system
Cell Immunol (Aug 1999)v196n1p1-13

Murata T, et al. Relation between plasma adenosine and serum TSH levels in women with hyperemesis gravidarum
Arch Gynecol Obstet (Mar 2006)v273n6p331-6

Nesheim BI A potential cause of hyperemesis gravidarum: evidence from the sex ration of associated infants (Correspondence)
Acta Obstet Gynecol Scand (Apr 2001)v80n4p337

Nwobodo EI, et al. Twin births at University of Maiduguri Teaching Hospital: incidence, pregnancy complications and outcome.
Niger J Med (Apr-Jun 2002)v11n2p67-9

Outlaw WM Impaired fatty acid oxidation as a cause of liver disease associated with hyperemesis gravidarum
Med Hypotheses (Jan 2005)v65n6p1150-3

Panesar N, et al. Are thyroid hormones or hCG responsible for hyperemesis gravidarum? A matched paired study in pregnant Chinese women
Acta Obstet Gynecol Scand (2001)v80n6p519-24

Panesar NS, et al. hCG: its pancreatic and duodenal receptors and in vivo electrolyte secretion in female rats
Am J Physiol (Cec 1998)v275n6part1pG1430-6

Panesar NS Human chorionic gonadotropin: a secretory hormone
Med Hypotheses (Aug 1999)v53n2p136-40

Philip B Hyperemesis gravidarum: literature review.
WMJ (2003)v102n3p46-51

Rakheja D, et al. Long-chain L-3-hydroxyacyl-coenzyme a dehydrogenase deficiency: a molecular and biochemical review
Lab Invest (Jul 2002)v82n7p815-24

Rochelson B, et al. Low prepregnancy ideal weight: height ratio in women with hyperemesis graviarum.
J Reprod Med (Jun 2003)v48n6p422-4

Sahakian V, et al. Vitamin B6 is effective therapy for nausea and vomiting of pregnancy: A randomized, double-blind placebo-controlled study
Obstet Gynecol (Jul 1991)v78n1p33-6

Samisoe G, et al. Does position and size of corpus luteum have any effect on nausea of pregnancy?
Acta Obstet Gynecol Scand (1986)v65p427-9

Sekizawa A, et al. Cell-free Fetal DNA Is Increased in Plasma of Women with Hyperemesis Gravidarum
Clin Chem (Dec 2001)v47n12p2164-5

Sherman PW, et al. Nausea and vomiting of pregnancy in an evolutionary perspective
Am J Obstet Gynecol (May 2002)v186n5pS190-7

Signorello LB, et al. Saturated Fat Intake and the Risk of Severe Hyperemesis Gravidarum
Epidemiology (Nov 1998)v9n6p636-40

Sipiora ML, et al. Bitter taste perception and severe vomiting in pregnancy
Phys Behav (May 2000)v69n3p259-67

Slager J, et al. Midwifery Co-Management of Hyperemesis Gravidarum
J Midwif Wom Health (Nov/Dec 2000)v45n6p457-64

Snell LH, et al. Metabolic Crisis: Hyperemesis Gravidarum
J Perinat Neonat Nurs (Sept 1998)v12n2p26-37

Sorensen HT, et al. Hyperemesis gravidarum and sex of child (Correspondence)
Lancet (Jan 29 2000)v355n9201p407

Teksen F, et al. Copper, zinc and magnesium status in hyperemesis gravidarum
J Obstet Gynaecol (2001)v21n1p46-8

Trogstad L, et al. Recurrence risk in hyperemesis gravidarum
BJOG (Dec 2005)v112n12p1641-5

Verkuyl D Sickness and sex of child (Correspondence)
Lancet (Feb 26 2000)v355n9205p756

Vilming B, et al. Hyperemesis gravidarum in a contemporary population in Oslo
Acta Obstet Gynecol Scand (Aug 2000)v79n8p640-3

Yoneyama Y, et al. Plasma 5'-nucleotidase activities increase in women with hyperemesis gravidarum
Clin Biochem (Oct 2002)v35n7p561-4

Yoneyama Y, et al. Serum adenosine deaminase activity in women with hyperemesis gravidarum
Clinica Chimica Acta (Oct 2002)v324n1-2p141-5

Yoneyama Y, et al. The T-helper 1/T-helper 2 balance in peripheral blood of women with hyperemesis gravidarum.
Am J Obstet Gynecol (Dec 2002)v187n6p1631-5

Gallbladder Problems

Cruikshank D, et al. Maternal Physiology in Pregnancy
Obstetrics: Normal & Problem Pregnancies; Gabbe, 2nd Edition
p126

Helicobacter pylori

Bagis T, et al. Endoscopy in hyperemesis gravidarum and Helicobacter pylori infection
Int J Gynaecol Obstet (Nov 2002)v79n2p105-9

Berker B, et al. Serologic assay of Helicobacter pylori infection. Is it useful in hyperemesis gravidarum?
J Reprod Med (Oct 2003)v48n10p809-12

Cevrioglu AS, et al. Efficient and non-invasive method for investigating Helicobacter pylori in gravida with hyperemesis gravidarum: Helicobacter pylori stool antigen test. J Obstet Gynaecol Res (Apr 2004)v30n2p136-41

El Younis CM, et al. Rapid marked response of severe hyperemesis gravidarum to oral erythromycin Am J Perinatol (1998)v9p533-4

Erdem A, et al. Detection of Helicobacter pylori seropositivity in hyperemesis gravidarum and correlation with symptoms. Am J Perinatol (Feb 2002)v19n2p87-92

Frigo P, et al. Hyperemesis Gravidarum Associated With Helicobacter pylori Seropositivity Obstet Gynecol (Apr 1998)v91n4p615-17

Hayakawa S, et al. Frequent Presence of Helicobacter Pylori Genome In the Saliva of Patients With Hyperemesis Gravidarum Am J Perinatol (2000)v17n5p243-7

Jacobson GF, et al. Helicobacter pylori seropositivity and hyperemesis gravidarum J Reprod Med (Aug 2003)v48n8p578-82

Jacoby EB, et al. Helicobacter pylori infection and persistent hyperemesis gravidarum Am J Perinatol (1999)v16n2p85-8

Karaca C, et al. Is lower socio-economic status a risk factor for helicobacter pylori infection in pregnant woman with hyperemesis gravidarum?
Turk J Gastroenterol (Jun 2004)v15n2p86-9

Kazerooni T, et al. Helicobacter pylori seropositivity in patients with hyperemesis gravidarum
Int J Gynaecol Obstet (Dec 2002)v79n3p217-20

Kocak I, et al. Helicobacter pylori seropositivity in patients with hyperemesis gravidarum
Int J Gynecol Obstet (Sept 1999)v66n3p251-4

Larraz J, et al. Lack of relationship between infection by Helicobacter pylori and vomiting that usually occurs during pregnancy, although possible relationship with severe forms of emesis.
Rev Esp Enferm Dig (Jul 2002)v94n7p417-22

Reymunde A, et al. Helicobacter pylori and Severe Morning Sickness
Am J Gastroenterol (Jul 2001)v96n7p2279-80

Salimi-Khayati A, et al. Helicobacter pylori seropositivity and the incidence of hyperemesis gravidarum
Med Sci Monit (Jan 2003)v9n1CR12-5

Home Treatment

Cowan MJ Hyperemesis gravidarum: implications for home care and infusion therapies
J Intraven Nurs (Jan-Feb 1996)v39n1p46-58

Heaman M Antepartum home care for high-risk pregnant women
AACN Clin Issues (Aug 1998)v9n3p362-76

Naef RW, et al. Treatment for hyperemesis gravidarum in the home: an alternative to hospitalization
J Perinatol (Jul-Aug 1995)v15n4p289-92

O'Brien P High-risk pregnancy and neonatal care
Crit Care Nurs Clin North Am (Sep 1998)v10n3p347-55

Hospitalization
Necessity of
Adams MM, et al. Antenatal Hospitalization Among Enlisted Servicewomen, 1987-1990
Obstet & Gynecol (July 1994)v84n1p35-9

Anderson AS, et al. Managing pregnancy sickness and hyperemesis gravidarum
Prof Care Mother Child (Jan-Feb 1994)v4n1p13-15

Fell DB, et al. Risk factors for hyperemesis gravidarum requiring hospital admission during pregnancy
Obstet Gynecol (Feb 2006)v107n2(part1)p277-84

Levy BT, et al. Nausea and vomiting in pregnancy
University of Iowa Family Practice Handbook
Chapter 8: Obstetrics

Nelson-Piercy C, et al. Randomised, double-blind, placebo-controlled trial of corticosteroids for the treatment of hyperemesis gravidarum
BJOG (Jan 2001)v108n1p9-15

Nelson-Piercy C. Treatment of nausea and vomiting in pregnancy. When should it be treated and what can be safely taken?
Drug Saf (1998)v19n2p155-64

Peleg D, et al. Prescribing antiemetic therapy during pregnancy
Contemp OB/GYN (Jun 1997)p164-71

Simpson SW, et al. Psychological factors and hyperemesis gravidarum
J Women's Helath Gend Based Med (Jun 2001)v10n5p471-7

Denial of (for monetary reasons)
Buttino L, et al. Home Subcutaneous Metoclopramide Therapy for Hyperemesis Gravidarum
J Perinatol (Sep 2000)v20n6p359-62

Hydration
Johnson DR, et al. Dehydration and orthostatic vital signs in women with hyperemesis gravidarum
Acad Emerg Med (Aug 1995)v2n8p692-7

Hypnotherapy
Baram DA Hypnosis in Reproductive Health Care: A Review and Case Reports
Birth (March 1995)v22n1p37-42

Frankel F Comment on Torem's "Hypnotherapeutic Techniques in the Treatment of Hyperemesis Gravidarum" (And a response from Torem)
Am J Clin Hypn (Oct 1994)v37n2p160

Simon EP Hypnosis in the Treatment of Hyperemesis Gravidarum (Correspondence)
Am Fam Phys (Jul 1999)v60n1p56-7

Simon EP, et al. Medical Hypnosis for Hyperemesis Gravidarum
Birth (Dec 1999)v26n4p248-54

Torem MS Hypnotherapeutic techniques in the treatment of hyperemesis gravidarum
Am J Clin Hypn (Jul 1994)v37n1p1-11

Impact of Nausea/Vomiting

Arsenault MY, et al. The management of nausea and vomiting of pregnancy.
J Obstet Gynaecol Can (Oct 2002)v24n10p817-31

Attard CL, et al. The burden of illness of severe nausea and vomiting of pregnancy in the United States
Am J Obstet Gynecol (May 2002)v186n5pS220-7

Erick M Morning sickness impact study
Midwifery Today Int Midwife (Fall 2001)n59p30-2

Koren G, et al. Motherisk-PUQE (pregnancy-unique quantification of emesis and nausea) scoring system for nausea and vomiting of pregnancy
Am J Obstet Gynecol (May 2002)v186n5pS226-31

Magee LA, et al. Development of a health-related quality of life instrument for nausea and vomiting of pregnancy
Am J Obstet Gynecol (May 2002)v186n5pS232-8

Mazzota P, et al. Psychosocial morbidity among women with nausea and vomiting of pregnancy: prevalence and association with antiemetic therapy
J Psychosom Obstet Gynecol (Sep 2000)v21n3p129-36

Smith C, et al. The impact of nausea and vomiting on women: a burden of early pregnancy
Aust N Z J Obstet Gynaecol (2000)v40n4p397-401

Liver Problems (Jaundice)
Ch'ng CL, et al. Prospective study of liver dysfunction in pregnancy in Southwest Wales
Gut (Dec 2002)v51n6p876-80

Conchillo JM, et al. Liver enzyme elevation induced by hyperemesis gravidarum: etiology, diagnosis and treatment
Neth J Med (Oct 2002)v60n9p340-2

Orazi G, et al. Jaundice induced by hyperemesis gravidarum
Int J Gynecol Obstet (May 1998)v61n2p181-3

HG Mimics
Aggarwal R, et al. Esophageal achalasia presenting during pregnancy
Indian J Gastroenterol (Apr 1997)v16n2p72-3

Chong W, et al. Unsuspected thyrotoxicosis and hyperemesis gravidarum in Asian women
Postgrad Med J (Apr 1997)v73n858p234-6

Coukos G, et al. Complete hydatidiform mole: A disease with a changing profile
J Reprod Med (Aug 1999)v44n8p698-704

Gaither K, et al. Pregnancy complicated by autoimmune polyglandular syndrome type II
J Matern Fetal Med (May0Jun 1998)v7n3p154-6

Kokrdova Z Pregnancy and primary hyperparathyreoidism
Ceska Gynekol (May 2004)v69n3p186-9

Levy C, et al. Solid pseudopapillary pancreatic tumor in pregnancy. A case report.
J Reprod Med (Jan 2004)v49n1p61-4

Ozbey N, et al. Clinical course of a pituitary macroadenoma in the first trimester of pregnancy: probable lymphocytic hypophysitis
Int J Clin Pract (Sep 1999)v53n6p478-81

Miscarriage/Stillbirth (Reduced Risk)

Bashiri A, et al. Hyperemesis gravidarum: epidemiologic features, complications and outcome
Euro J Obstet Gynecol Reprod Biol (Dec 1995)v63n2p135-8

Peleg D, et al. Prescribing antiemetic therapy during pregnancy
Contemp OB/GYN (Jun 1997)p164-71

Wolf J Liver Disease In Pregnancy
Med Clin North Am (Sept 1996)v80n5p1167-87

Miscellaneous

Medina MJ Treatment of hyperemesis gravidarum by husband's blood transfusion. 1948
Ginecol Obstet Mex (Aug 2003)v71p436-9

Parenteral Feeding (TPN/Hyperalimentation)

Brimacombe J Midazolam and Parenteral Nutrition in the Management of Life-threatening Hyperemesis Gravidarum in a Diabetic Patient
Anaesth Intens Care (Apr 1995)v23n2p228-30

Brown RO, et al. One-year experience with a pharmacist-coordinated nutritional support clinic
Am J Health-Syst Pharm (Nov 1999)v56p2324-2330

Folk J, et al. Hyperemesis Gravidarum: Pregnancy Outcomes and Complications Among Women Nutritionally Supported with and Without Parenteral Therapy
Obstet Gynecol (April 2001)v97supplement4s42

Folk JJ, et al. Hyperemesis gravidarum: outcomes and complications with and without total parenteral nutrition
J Reprod Med (Jul 2004)v49n7p497-502

Hamaoui E, et al. Nutritional assessment and support during pregnancy
Gastroenterol Clin North Am (Mar 2003)v32n1p59-121,v

Hasbun J, et al. Total parenteral nutrition in severe hyperemesis gravidarum
Rev Chil Obstet Ginecol (1994)v59n5p378-82

Ireton-Jones C, et al. Clinical pathways in home nutrition support
J Am Diet Assoc (Sep 1997)v97n9p1003-7

Jeejeebhoy KN, et al. Parenteral Nutrition
Harrison's Principles of Internal Medicine 11ᵗʰ Edition p406-10

Katz VL, et al. Mycobacterium chelonae sepsis associated with long-term use of an intravenous catheter for treatment of hyperemesis gravidarum. A case report
J Reprod Med (Jul 2000)v45n7p581-4

Levine MG, et al. Total parenteral nutrition for the treatment of severe hyperemesis gravidarum: maternal nutritional effects and fetal outcome
Obstet Gynecol (Jul 1988)v72n1p102-7

Maccarrone G, et al. Total parenteral nutrition in pregnancy
Minerva Ginecol (May 1998)v50n5p185-9

Russo-Stieglitz KE, et al. Pregnancy outcome in patients requiring parenteral nutrition
J Matern Fetal Med (Jul-Aug 1999)v8n4p164-7

Shparago NI, et al. Systemic Malassezia furfur infection in an adult receiving total parenteral nutrition
J Am Osteopath Assoc (Jun 1995)v95n6p375-7

Subramaniam R, et al. Total Parenteral Nutrition (TPN) and Steroid Usage in the Management of Hyperemesis Gravidarum
Aust. NZ J Obstet Gynaecol (Aug 1998)v38n3p339-41

Turrentine MA, et al. Right atrial thrombus as a complication of total parenteral nutrition in pregnancy
Obstet Gynecol (Oct 1994)v84n4(Pt 2)p675-7

Physician Humanism
Munch S A Qualitative Analysis of Physician Humanism: Women's Experiences With Hyperemesis Gravidarum
J Perinatol (Dec 2000)v20n8 (part 1)p540-7

Soltani H, et al. Changing attitudes and perceptions to hyperemesis gravidarum
Midwives (Dec 2003)v6n12p520-4

Pregnancy Outcome
Czeizel AE, et al. Protective effect of hyperemesis gravidarum for nonsyndromic oral clefts
Obstet Gynecol (Apr 2003)v101n4p737-44

Dodds L, et al. Outcomes of pregnancies complicated by hyperemesis gravidarum
Obstet Gynecol (Feb 2006)vn2(part 1)p285-92

Erick M. Hyperolfaction and hyperemesis gravidarum: What is the relationship?
Nutrition Reviews (Oct 1995)v53n10p289-95

Goodwin TM. Hyperemesis Gravidarum
Clin Obstet Gynecol (Sept 1998)v41n3p597-605

Hallak M Hyperemesis gravidarum. Effects on fetal outcome
J Repred Med (Nov 1996)v41n11p871-4

Russo-Stieglitz KE, et al. Pregnancy outcome in patients requiring parenteral nutrition
J Matern Fetal Med (Jul-Aug 1999)v8n4p164-7

Seto A, et al. Pregnancy outcome following first trimester exposure to antihistamines: meta-analysis
Am J Perinatol (Mar 1997)v14n3p119-24

Tsang IS, et al. Maternal and fetal outcomes in hyperemesis gravidarum
Int J Gynaecol Obstet; (Dec 1996)v55n3p231-5

Private Room (Justification For)
Sanders S, et al. Metabolic Support Team Hyperemesis Gravidarum Protocol: Treatment of Hyperemesis Gravidarum With Nasogastric Feeding
copy of protocol obtained by writing S. Sanders, MS, RD at Cedars-Sinai Medical Center, 8700 Beverly Blvd, Los Angeles, CA 90048-1869, Attn: Department of Medicine, GI 7511

Hyperolfaction (Additional Justification)
Erick M Hyperolfaction and Hyperemesis Gravidarum: What Is the Relationship?
Nutrition Reviews (Oct 1995)v53n10p289-95

Heinrichs L Linking olfaction with nausea and vomiting of pregnancy, recurrent abortion, hyperemesis gravidarum, and migraine headache.
Am J Obstet Gynecol (May 2002)v185n5(Suppl Understanding)pS215-9

Physical v. Psychogenic

Bashiri A, et al. Hyperemesis gravidarum: epidemiologic features, complications and outcome
Euro J Obstet Gynecol and Repro Biol (1995)v63n2p135-8

Bjelica A, et al. Persistent hyperemesis gravidarum as a psychosomatic dysfunction: case report
Med Pregl (Mar-Apr 2003)v56n3-4p183-6

Bogen, JT Neurosis: A Ms-Diagnosis
Perspect Biol Med (Winter 1994)v37n2p263-74

Buckwalter JG, et al. Psychological factors in the etiology and treatment of severe nausea and vomiting in pregnancy
Am J Obstet Gynecol (May 2002)v186n5pS210-4

Child TJ Management of hyperemesis in pregnant women
Lancet (Jan 23 1999)v353n9149p325

Coverdale MB, et al. Clinical Implications of Respect for Autonomy in the Psychiatric Treatment of Pregnant Patients With Depression
Psychiatric Services (Feb 1997)v48n2209-12

Erick M Nausea & Vomiting In Pregnancy
ACOG Clin Review (May/Jun 1997)v2n3p1-2, 14-6

Field J Hyperemesis gravidarum: a short case study
Nurs Times (Aug 2001)v97n32p55

Franko, et al. Detection and management of eating disorders during pregnancy
Obstet Gynecol (Jun 2000)v95n6, part 1,p942-6

Iancu J, et al. Psychiatric Aspects of Hyperemesis gravidarum
Psychoter Psychosom (1994)v61n3-4p143-9

Josephs L Women and trauma: A contemporary psychodynamic approach to traumatization for patients in the OB/GYN psychological consultation clinic
Bulletin of the Menninger Clinic (Winter 1996)v60n1p22-38

Kawarabayashi T, et al. Analysis of relationship between personality and emesis gravidarum in pregnant women
Nippon Sanka Fujinka Gakkai Zasshi (Jun 1995)v80n2p547-52

Lub-Moss MM, et al. Clinical experience with patients suffering from hyperemesis gravidarum (severe nausea and vomiting during pregnancy): thoughts about subtyping of patients, treatment and counseling models
Patient Educ Couns (May 1997)v31n1p65-75

Matteson S, et al. The role of behavioral conditioning in the development of nausea
Am J Obstet Gynecol (May 2002)v186n5pS239-43

Munch S Chicken or the egg? The biological-psychological controversy surrounding hyperemesis gravidarum
Soc Sci Med (Oct 2002)v55n7p1267-78

Munch S Women's experiences with a pregnancy complication: causal explanations of hyperemesis gravidarum
Soc Work Health Care (2002)v36n1p59-76

Neri A, et al. Nausea and vomiting in pregnancy: a review of the problem with particular regard to psychological and social aspects
Br J of Obstet Gynaecol (Aug 1995)v102n8p671

Rabinerson D, et al. Hyperemesis gravidarum during Ramadan
J Psychosom Obstet Gynecol (2000)v21n4p189-91

Rech F, et al. The role of chorionic gonadotropin in transient hyperthyroidism in hyperemesis gravidarum
Minerva Ginecol (Jun 1998)v50n6p261-4

Riely CA Hepatic Disease in Pregnancy
Am J Med (Jan 17, 1994)v96suppl1Ap1A-18S

Simpson SW, et al. Psychological factors and hyperemesis gravidarum
J Womens Health Gend Based Med (Jun 2001)v10n5p471-7

Swallow BL, et al. Psychological health in early pregnancy: relationship with nausea and vomiting.
J Obstet Gynaecol (Jan 2004)v24n1p28-32

Tzeng YL Unraveling the myths about nausea and vomiting during pregnancy
Hu Li Za Zhi (Jun 2004)v51n3p89-93

Vaiva G, et al. Value of a consultation center and crisis intervention in addressing psychiatric disorders in the perinatal period
Encephale (Jan-Feb 2002)v28n1p71-6

Rare Complications
Boerhaave's Syndrome
Harrison's Principles of Internal Medicine
Part One: Cardinal Manifestations of Disease:p174-5

Central Pontine Myelinolysis
Robinson JN, et al. Coagulopathy secondary to vitamin K deficiency in hyperemesis gravidarum
Obstet Gynecol (Oct 1998)v92n4 part 2p673-5

Tonelli J, et al. Central pontine myelinolysis induced by hyperemesis gravidarum
Medicina (1999)v59n2p176-8

Esophageal Rupture
Eroglu A, et al. Spontaneous esophageal rupture following severe vomiting in pregnancy.
Dis Esophagus (2002)v15n3p242-3

Liang SG, et al. Pneumomediastinum following esophageal rupture associated with hyperemesis gravidarum.
J Obstet Gynaecol Res (Jun 2002)v28n3p172-5

Gallstones
Gouldman JW, et al. Laparoscopic cholecystectomy in pregnancy
Am Surg (Jan 1998)v64n1p93-7

Kidney Failure
Hill JB, et al. Acute renal failure in association with severe hyperemesis gravidarum
Obstet Gynecol (Nov 2002)v100n5(part 2)p1119-21

Pneumomediastinum
Gorbach JS, et al. Spontaneous pneumomediastinum secondary to hyperemesis gravidarum
J Emerg Med (Sep-Oct 1997)v15n5p639-43

Yamamoto T, et al. Pneumomediastinum secondary to hyperemesis gravidarum during early pregnancy
Acta Obstet Gynecol Scand (Dec 2001)v80n12p1143-5

Porphyria
Shenhav S, et al. Acute intermittent porphyria precipitated by hyperemesis and metoclopramide treatment in pregnancy
Acta Obstet Gynecol Scand (1997)v76p484-5

Rhabdomyolysis
Fukada Y, et al. Rhabdomyolysis secondary to hyperemesis gravidarum
Acta Obstet Gynecol Scand (1999)v78p71-3

Splenic Avulsion
Kanayama N, et al. Vasospasms of cerebral arteries in hyperemesis gravidarum
Gynecol Obstet Invest (Aug 1998)v46n2pg139-41

Nguyen N, et al. Splenic avulsion in a pregnant patient with vomiting
Can J Surg (Oct 1995)v80n2p464-5

Wernicke's Encephalopathy
Accetta SG, et al. Memory loss and ataxia after hyperemesis gravidarum: a case of Wernicke-Korsakoff syndrome.
Eur J Obstet Gynecol Reprod Biol (Apr 2002)v102n1p100-1

Chataway J, et al. Thiamine in Wernicke's syndrome-how much and how long
Postgrad Med J (Apr 1995)v71n83p249-53

Chiossi, G, et al. Hyperemesis gravidarum complicated by Wernicke's encephalopathy: background, case, report, and review of the literature
Obstet Gynccol Surv (April 2006)v61n4p255-68

Dickson MJ Management of hyperemesis in pregnant women
Lancet (Jan 23, 1999)v353n9149p325

Gardian G, et al. Wernicke's encephalopathy induced by hyperemesis gravidarum
Acta Neurol Scand (Mar 1999)v99n3p196-8

Hillbom M, et al. Pregnant, vomiting, and coma
Lancet (May 1999)v353n9164p1584

Iwamoto Y, et al. Beneficial effect of steroid pulse therapy on Wernicke-Korsakoff syndrome due to hyperemesis gravidarum
Rinsho Shinkeigaku (Jun 1994)v80n2p599-601

Manji H Neurological cases for MRCP:1
Br J Hosp Med (May 21-Jun 3 1997)v57n10p500-1

Ohkoshi Norio, et al. Wernicke's Encephalopathy Induced by Hyperemesis gravidarum, Associated with Bilateral Caudate Lesions on Computed Tomography and Magnetic Resonance Imaging
Eur Neurol (1994)v34n3p177-80

Olindo S, et al. Gayet-Wernicke encephalopathy and centropontine myelionolysis induced by hyperemesis gravidarum
Rev Neurol (Jul 1997)n6-7p427-9

Omer SM, et al. Acute Wernicke's encephalopathy associated with hyperemesis gravidarum: magnetic resonance imaging findings
J Neuroimaging (Oct 1995)v5n4p251-3

Otsuka F, et al. Gestational thyrotoxicosis manifesting as wernicke encephalopathy: a case report
Endocr J (Jun 1997)v44n3p447-52

Rabenda-Lacka K, et al. Wernicke's encephalopathy due to hyperemesis gravidarum
Ginekol Pol (Aug 2003)v74n8p633-7

Rastenyte D, et al. Wernicke's encephalopathy induced by hyperemesis gravidarum
Medicina (Kaunas) (2003)v39n1p56-61

Rees JH, et al. Two pregnant women with vomiting and fits
Am J Obstet Gynecol (Dec 1997)v177n6p1539-40

Rotman P Wernicke's encephalopathy in hyperemesis gravidarum: association with abnormal liver function
Isr J Med Sci (1994)v30p225-8

Sakakibara R, et al. Micturitional disturbance in Wernicke's encephalopathy
Neurourol Urodyn (1997)v16n2p111-5

Spruill SC, et al. Hyperemesis gravidarum complicated by Wernicke's encephalopathy
Obstet Gynecol (May 2002)v99n5(part 2)p875-7

Tesfaye S, et al. Pregnant, vomiting, and going blind
Lancet (Nov 1998)v352n9140p1594

Togay-Isikay C, et al. Wernicke's encephalopathy due to hyperemesis gravidarum: an under-recognised condition
Aust N Z J Obstet Gynaecol (Nov 2001)v41n4p453-6

Sex of Child
Askling J, et al. Sickness in pregnancy and sex of child (Correspondence)
Lancet (Dec 11, 1999)v354n9195p2053

Basso O, et al. Sex ratio and twinning in women with hyperemesis or pre-eclampsia.
Epidemiology (Nov 2001)v12n6p747-9

Schiff MA, et al. The sex ratio of pregnancies complicated by hospitalization for hyperemesis gravidarum
BJOG (Jan 2004)v111n1p27-30

Sorensen H, et al. Hyperemesis gravidarum and sex of child (correspondence)
Lancet (Jan 29, 2000)v355n9201p407

Testes Cancer
Henderson BE, et al. An explanation for the increasing incidence of testis cancer: decreasing age at first full-term pregnancy (Correspondence)
J National Cancer Inst (Jun 4, 1997)v89n11p818-9

Thyroid Function
ACOG practice bulletin. Thyroid disease in pregnancy. Number 37, August 2002. American College of Obstetrics and Gynecology.
Int J Gynaecol Obstet (Nov 2002)v79n2p171-80

Asakura H, et al. Correlations between interscapular deep temperature and plasma free fatty acid levels in pregnant women with hyperemesis gravidarum
Arch Gynecol Obstet (Apr 2003)v268n1p35-40

Burgun SJ, et al. Pernicious Vomiting in Two Pregnant Women
Hospital Practice (Oct 1997)v32n10p197-8, 200, 202

Caffrey TJ Transient Hyperthyroidism of Hyperemesis Gravidarum: A Sheep in Wolf's Clothing
J Am Board Fam Pract (Jan-Feb 2000)v13n1p35-8

Chan NN Thyroid function in hyperemesis gravidarum (Correspondence)
Lancet (Jun 1999)v353n9174p2243

Chihara H, et al. Basal metabolic rate in hyperemesis gravidarum: comparison to normal pregnancy and response to treatment.
Am J Obstet Gynecol (Feb 2003)v188n2p434-8

Colin JF, et al. Hyperthyroidism: a possible factor of cholestasis associated with hyperemesis gravidarum of prolonged evolution
Gastroenterol Clin Biol (1994)v18n4p378-80

Deruelle P, et al. Hyperemesis in the first trimester of pregnancy: role of biological hyperthyroidism and fetal sex
Gynecol Obstet Fertil (Mar 2002); v30n3p204-9

Fantz CR, et al. Thyroid Function during Pregnancy
Clin Chem (Dec 1999)v45n12p2250-8

Garro A Hyperemesis gravidarum and hyperthyroidism
Acta Med Port (Sep-Oct 2003)v16n5p337-8

Girling JC Thyroid disease in pregnancy
Hosp Med (Dec 2000)v61n12p834-40

Goodwin, et al. Hyperthyroidism Due to Inappropriate Production of human chorionic gonadotropin
Clin Obstet Gynecol (Mar 1997)v40n1p32-44

Hiroi H, et al. Hyperemesis gravidarum associated with thyrotoxicosis and a past history of an eating disorder.
Arch Gynecol Obstet (Nov 2001)v265n4p228-30

Kopp P Human Genome and Diseases: Review; The TSH receptor and its role in thyroid disease
Cell Mol Life Sci (Aug 2001)v58n9p1301-22

Krentz AJ, et al. Hyperthyroidism associated with hyperemesis gravidarum
Br J Clin Pract (Mar-Apr)v48n2p75-6

Kuscu NK, et al Hyperemesis gravidarum: current concepts and management
Postgrad Med J (Feb 2002)v78n916p76-9

Lazarus JH, et al. Thyroxine excess and pregnancy
Acta Med Austriaca (1994)v21n2p53-6

Leunen M, et al. Is there a relationship between hyperemesis gravidarum and hyperthyroidism?
Acta Clin Belg (Mar-Apr 2001)v56n2p78-85

Leylek OA, et al. Hyperthyroidism in hyperemesis gravidarum
Int J Gynaecol Obstet (Oct 1996)v55n1p3307

Mestman JH Diagnosis and management of maternal and fetal thyroid disorders
Curr Opin Obstet Gynecol (Apr 1999)v11n2p167-75

Mestman, JH Hyperthyroidism in pregnancy
Endocrinal Metab Clin North Am (Mar 1998)v27n1p127-49

Nader S, et al. Recurrent hyperthyroidism in consecutive pregnancies characterized by hyperemesis
Thyroid (Oct 1996)v46n1p465-6

Rebordao MA, et al. Transient hyperthyroidism and hyperemesis gravidarum
Acta Med Port (Oct 1997)v10n10p729-30

Rech F, et al. The role of chorionic gonadotropin in transient hyperthyroidism in hyperemesis gravidarum
Minerva Ginecol (Jun 1998)v50n6p261-4

Rodien P, et al. Abnormal stimulation of the thyrotrophin receptor during gestation
Hum Reprod Update (Mar-Apr 2004)v10n2p95-105

Tan JY, et al. Transient hyperthyroidism of hyperemesis gravidarum.
BJOG (Jun 2002)v109n6p683-8

Tareen AK, et al. Thyroid hormone in hyperemesis gravidarum
J Obstet Gynaecol (Oct 1995)v21n5p497-501

Watanabe S, et al. Alterations of thermoregulation in women with hyperemesis gravidarum
Arch Gynecol Obstet (Feb 2003)v267n4p221-6

Yoshimura M, et al. Thyrotropic action of human chorionic gonadotropin
Thyroid (Oct 1995)v5n5p425-34

Vitamins

Czeizel AE Prevention of hyperemesis gravidarum is better than treatment (Correspondence)
Am J Obstet Gyneco; (May 1996)v174n5p1667

van Stuijvenberg M, et al. The nutritional status and treatment of patients with hyperemesis gravidarum
Am J Obstet Gynecol(May 1995)v172n5p1585-91

X-Ray

American College of Obstetricians and Gynecologists, Committee on Obstetric Practice. Guidelines for diagnostic imaging during pregnancy
ACOG Committee Opinion (Sep 1995)n158p32-35

ENDNOTES

One:

[1] Nageotte MP, et al. Droperidol and diphenhydramine in the management of hyperemesis gravidarum
Am J Obstet Gynecol (June 1996)v174n6p1801-6

[2] Eliakim R, et al. Hyperemesis Gravidarum: A current Review
Am J Perinatol (2000)v17n4p207-18

[3] Fantz CR, et al. Thyroid function during pregnancy
Clin Chem (Dec 1999)v45n12p2250-8

[4] Goodwin TM. Hyperemesis Gravidarum
Clin Obstet Gynecol (Sept 1998)v41n3p597-605

[5] Erick M Hyperolfaction and hyperemesis gravidarum: What is the relationship?
Nutrition Reviews (Oct 1995)v53n10p289 95

[6] ibid.

[7] Nageotte MP, et al.

[8] ibid.

[9] Erick M Morning sickness impact study
Midwifery Today Int Midwife (Fall 2001)n59p30-2

[10] Mazzota P, et al. Factors associated with elective termination of pregnancy among Canadian and American women with nausea and vomiting of pregnancy
J Psychosom Obstet Gynecol (Mar 2001)v22n1p7-12

[11] Erick M More on NVP
Midwifery Today (Summer 1997)n42pMT-7

[12] Gardner DK Hyperemesis gravidarum

Pharmacist (Aug 1997)p47-66

[13] Hallak, et al. Hyperemesis gravidarum: Effects on fetal outcomes
J Reprod Med (Nov 1996)v41n11p871-4

[14] Eliakim R, et al.

[15] van de Ven CJ Nasogastric enteral feeding in hyperemesis gravidarum
Lancet (Feb 1997)v349n9050p445(2)

[16] Gawande A A Queasy Feeling
The New Yorker (July 5, 1999)p34-41

Two:

[17] Jewell D, et al. Interventions for nausea and vomiting in early pregnancy
Cochrane Database Syst Rev (2002)n1:CD000145

[18] Strong TH Alternative therapies of morning sickness
Clin Obstet Gynecol (Dec 2001)v44n4p653-60

[19] Sherman PW, et al. Nausea and vomiting of pregnancy in an evolutionary perspective
Am J Obstet Gynecol (May 2002)v186n5pS190-7

[20] Czeizel AE Prevention of hyperemesis gravidarum is better than treatment
Am J Obstet Gynecol (May 1996)v174n5p1667

[21] Rochelson B, et al. Low prepregnancy ideal weight/height ratio in women with hyperemesis gravidarum
J Reprod Med (Jun 2003)v48n6p422-4

[22] Gardner DK Hyperemesis gravidarum
Pharmacist (Aug 1997)p47-66

[23] ibid.

[24] Mazzota P, et al. Therapeutic abortions due to severe morning sickness

Can Fam Phys (Jun 1997)v43p1055-7

[25] ibid.

[26] Henderson BE, et al. An explanation for the increasing incidence of testis cancer: decreasing age at first full-term pregnancy
J National Cancer Inst (Jun 4, 1997)v89n11p818-9

[27] Vilming B, et al. Hyperemesis gravidarum in a contemporary population in Oslo
Acta Obstet Gynecol Scand (Aug 2000)v79n8p640-3

[28] Tan JY, et al. Transient hyperthyroidism of hyperemesis gravidarum.
BJOG (Jun 2002)v109n6p683-8

[29] Munch S Chicken or the egg? The biological-psychological controversy surrounding hyperemesis gravidarum
Soc Sci Med (Oct 2002)v55n7p1267-78

[30] Hallak M, et al. Hyperemesis gravidarum: effects on fetal outcome
J Repred Med (Nov 1996)v41n11p871-4

[31] Tsang IS, et al. Maternal and fetal outcomes in hyperemesis gravidarum
Int J Gynaecol Obstet (Dec 1996)v55n3p231-5

[32] Czeizel AE, et al. Protective effect of hyperemesis gravidarum for nonsyndromic oral clefts
Obstet Gynecol (Apr 2003)v101n4p737-44

[33] Snell LH, et al. Metabolic crisis: hyperemesis gravidarum
J Perinat Neonat Nurs (Sept 1998)v12n2p26-37

[34] Erick M Maternity—morning sickness
The Boston Parents' Paper (June 1995)

[35] Peleg D, et al. Prescribing antiemetic therapy during pregnancy
Contemp OB/GYN (Jun 1997)p164-71

[36] van de Ven CJ Nasogastric enteral feeding in hyperemesis gravidarum
Lancet (Feb 1997)v349n9050p445(2)

[37] Snell, LH, et al.

[38] Erick M Hyperolfaction and hyperemesis gravidarum: What is the relationship?
Nutrition Reviews (Oct 1995)v53n10p289-95

[39] ibid.

[40] Gardner DK

[41] Nageotte MP, et al. Droperidol and diphenhydramine in the management of hyperemesis gravidarum
Am J Obstet Gynecol (June 1996)v174n6p1801-6

[42] Askling J, et al. Sickness in pregnancy and sex of child
Lancet (Dec 11, 1999)v354n9195p2053

[43] Gardner DK

[44] Krentz AJ, et al. Hyperthyroidism associated with hyperemesis gravidarum
Br J Clin Pract (Mar-Apr)v48n2p75-6

[45] Goodwin, et al. Hyperthyroidism due to inappropriate production of hCG
Clin Obstet Gynecol (Mar 1997)v40n1p32-44

[46] ibid.

[47] op. cit.

[48] Snell LH, et al.

[49] Sekizawa A, et al. Cell-free fetal DNA is increased in plasma of women with hyperemesis gravidarum
Clin Chem; (Dec 2001)v47n12p2164-5

[50] Yoneyama Y, et al. Serum adenosine deaminase activity in women with hyperemesis gravidarum
Clinica Chimica Acta (Oct 2002)v324n1-2p141-5

[51] Snell LH, et al.

[52] ibid.

[53] Teksen F, et al. Copper, zinc and magnesium status in hyperemesis gravidarum
J Obstet Gynaecol (2001)v21n1p46-8

[54] op. cit.

[55] Black FO Maternal susceptibility to nausea and vomiting of pregnancy: Is the vestibular system involved?
Am J Obstet Gynecol (May 2002)v186n5pS204-9

[56] Nageotte MP, et al.

[57] Trogstad LI, et al. Recurrence risk in hyperemesis gravidarum
BJOG (2005)v112n12p1641-5

[58] Munch S

[59] Snell LH, et al.

[60] Gardner DK

[61] ibid.

Three:

[62] Goodwin, TM Hyperemesis Gravidarum
Clin Obstet Gynecol (Sept 1998)v41n3p597-605

[63] Attard CL, et al. The burden of illness of severe nausea and vomiting of pregnancy in the United States
Am J Obstet Gynecol (May 2002)v186n5pS220-7

[64] Crotti M, et al. Evaluation and treatment of hyperemesis gravidarum
Minerva Ginecol (Dec 2001)v53n6p413-9

[65] Buttino L, et al. Home subcutaneous metoclopramide therapy for hyperemesis gravidarum
J Perinatol (Sep 2000)v20n6p359-62

[66]Munch S A qualitative analysis of physician humanism: women's experiences with hyperemesis gravidarum
J Perinatol (Dec 2000)v20n8 (part 1)p540-7

Four:

[67] Nageotte MP, et al. Droperidol and diphenhydramine in the management of hyperemesis gravidarum
Am J Obstet Gynecol (June 1996)v174n6p1801-6

[68] Goodwin TM Hyperemesis gravidarum
Clin Obstet Gynecol (Sept 1998)v41n3p597-605

[69] Czeizel AE Prevention of hyperemesis gravidarum is better than treatment
Am J Obstet Gynecol (May 1996)v174n5p1667

[70] Signorello LB, et al. Saturated fat intake and the risk of severe hyperemesis gravidarum
Epidemiology (Nov 1998)v9n6p636-40

[71] El Younis CM, et al. Rapid marked response of severe hyperemesis gravidarum to oral erythromycin
Am J Perinatol (1998)v9p533-4

[72] Kocak I, et al. Helicobacter pylori seropositivity in patients with hyperemesis gravidarum
Int J Gynecol Obstet (Sept 1999)v66n3p251-4

[73] Bagis T, et al. Endoscopy in hyperemesis gravidarum and helicobacter pylori infection
Int J Gynaecol Obstet (Nov 2002)v79n2p105-9

[74] El Younis CM, et al.

[75] Snell LH, et al. Metabolic crisis: Hyperemesis gravidarum
J Perinat Neonat Nurs (Sept 1998)v12n2p26-37

Five:

[76] Erick M Maternity: Morning sickness
The Boston Parents' Paper (June 1995)

[77] Knight B, et al. Effect of acupuncture on nausea of pregnancy: A randomized, controlled trial
Obstet Gynecol (Feb 2001)v97n2p184-188

[78] Carlsson C, et al. Manual acupuncture reduces hyperemesis gravidarum: A placebo-controlled, randomized, single-bind, crossover study
J Pain Symptom Manage (Oct 2000)v20n4p273-9

[79] Golaszewski TM, et al. Treatment of hyperemesis gravidarum by electrical stimulation of the vestibular system
Am J Obstet Gynecol (Aug 1994)v171n2p577

[80] Slotnick RN Safe, successful nausea suppression in early pregnancy with P-6 acustimulation
J Reprod Med (Sep 2001)v46n9p811-4

Six:
[81] Koren G, et al. The teratogenicity of drugs for nausea and vomiting of pregnancy: perceived versus true risk
Am J Obstet Gynecol (May 2002)v186n5pS248-52

[82] ibid.

[83] Godfrey KM, et al. Fetal nutrition and adult disease
Am J Clin Nutr (May 2000)v71n5p1344s-52s

[84] Seto A, et al. Pregnancy outcome following first trimester exposure to antihistamines: meta-analysis
Am J Perinatol (Mar 1997)v14n3p119-24

[85] Strong TH Alternative therapies of morning sickness
Clin Obstet Gynecol (Dec 2001)v44n4p653-60

[86] Gardner DK Hyperemesis gravidarum
Pharmacist (Aug 1997)p47-66

[87] Niebyl JR, et al. Overview of nausea and vomiting of pregnancy with an emphasis on vitamins and ginger
Am J Obstet Gynecol (May 2002)v186n5pS253-5

[88] Sahakian V, et al. Vitamin B6 is effective therapy for nausea and vomiting of pregnancy: a randomized, double-blind placebo-controlled study
Obstet Gynecol (Jul 1991)v78n1p33-6

[89] Sullivan CA, et al. A pilot study of intravenous ondansetron for hyperemesis gravidarum
Am J Obstet Gynecol (1996)v174n5p1565-8

[90] Gardner DK

[91] op. cit.

[92] Goodwin TM. Hyperemesis Gravidarum
Clin Obstet Gynecol (Sept 1998)v41n3p597-605

[93] Safari HR, et al. Experience with oral methylprednisolone in the treatment of refractory hyperemesis gravidarum
Am J Obstet Gynecol (May 1998)v178n5p1054-8

[94] Ozdemir I, et al. A case of primary Addison's disease with hyperemesis gravidarum and successful pregnancy
Eur J Obstet Gynecol Reprod Biol (Mar 2004)v113n1p100-2

[95] Goodwin TM.

[96] Moran P, et al. Management of hyperemesis gravidarum: the importance of weight loss as a criterion for steroid therapy
QJM (Mar 2002)v95n3p153-8

[97] Nelson-Piercy C, et al. Complications of the use of corticosteroids for the treatment of hyperemesis gravidarum (Authors' Reply)
Br J Obstet Gynaecol (Jun 1995)v102n6p508-9

[98] ibid.

[99] op. cit.

[100] Subramaniam R, et al. Total parenteral nutrition (TPN) and steroid usage in the management of hyperemesis gravidarum

Aust. NZ J Obstet Gynaecol (Aug 1998)v38n3p339-41
[101] Park-Wyllie L, et al. Birth Defects After Maternal Exposure to Corticosteroids: Prospective Cohort Study and Meta-Analysis of Epidemiological Studies
Teratology (2000)v62p385-392
[102] op. cit.
[103] Nelson-Piercy C, et al. Randomised, double-blind, placebo-controlled trial of corticosteroids for the treatment of hyperemesis gravidarum
BJOG (Jan 2001)v108n1p9-15
[104] ibid.
[105] Moran P, et al.
[106] Goodwin TM

Seven:
[107] (n.a.) (2002) Ireland's OWN History: List of dead and other hunger strikers: The hunger strike of 1981
Retrieved on June 21, 2003 from
http://www.irelandsown.net/HungerStrikeList.html
[108] Peleg D, et al. Prescribing antiemetic therapy during pregnancy
Contemp OB/GYN (Jun 1997)p164-71
[109] Levy BT, et al. Nausea and vomiting in pregnancy
University of Iowa Family Practice Handbook; Chapter 8: Obstetrics

Eight:
[110] Greenspoon JS, et al. Hyperemesis gravidarum protocol: treatment of hyperemesis gravidarum with nasogastric feeding

correspondence from Cedars-Sinai in Los Angeles, California

[111] Sanders SL, et al. New protocol to manage hyperemesis gravidarum
J AM Diet Ass; (Dec 1994)v94n12p1367-8

[112] Hsu JJ, et al. Nasogastric enteral feeding in the management of hyperemesis gravidarum
Obstetrics and Gynecology (Sept 1996)v88n3p343-6

[113] ibid.

[114] Sanders SL, et al.

[115] Cosmas JM Van de Ven. Nasogastric enteral feeding in hyperemesis gravidarum (Commentary)
Lancet (Feb 1997)v349n9050p445(2)

[116] Hsu JJ

[117] Pearce CB, et al. Enteral nutrition by nasojejunal tube in hyperemesis gravidarum
Clin Nutr (Oct 2001)v20n5p461-4

[118] op. cit.

[119] American College of Obstetricians and Gynecologists, Committee on Obstetric Practice. Guidelines for diagnostic imaging during pregnancy
ACOG Committee Opinion (Sep 1995)n158p32-35

[120] Harrison's Principles of Internal Medicine 11th Edition: Alternation of the feeding route
p400-1, 403-4

[121] Hsu JJ

[122] (n.a.) (1994) American Gastroenterological Association: Medical position statement: Guidelines for the use of enteral nutrition
Retrieved on June 21, 2003 from http://www3.us.elsevierhealth.com/gastro/policy/v108n4p1280.html#REF1

Nine:

[123] Harrison's Principles of Internal Medicine 11ᵗʰ Edition page 403-4

[124] Garcia-Luna PP, et al. PEG and PEG-J for nutrition support in pregnancy (Correspondence)
JPEN J Parenter Enteral Nutr (Nov-Dec)v23n6p367-8

[125] Irving PM, et al. Percutaneous endoscopic gastrostomy with a jejunal port for severe hyperemesis gravidarum
Eur J Gastroenterol Hepatol (Sep 2004)v16n9p937-9

[126] Harrison's

[127] Godil A, et al. Percutaneous endoscopic gastrostomy for nutrition support in pregnancy associated with hyperemesis gravidarum and anorexia nervosa
J Parenter Enteral Nutr (Jul-Aug 1998)v22n4p238-41

[128] Hsu JJ, et al. Nasogastric Enteral Feeding in the Management of Hyperemesis Gravidarum
Obstetrics and Gynecology (Sept 1996)v88n3p343-6

Ten:

[129] Sanders SL, et al. New protocol to manage hyperemesis gravidarum
J AM Diet Ass; (Dec 1994)v94n12p1367-8

[130] Jeejeebhoy KN, et al. Parenteral Nutrition
Harrison's Principles of Internal Medicine 11ᵗʰ Edition p406-10

[131] Russo-Stieglitz KE, et al. Pregnancy outcome in patients requiring parenteral nutrition
J Matern Fetal Med; (Jul-Aug 1999)v8n4p164-7

[132] op. cit.

[133] Hsu JJ, et al. Nasogastric enteral feeding in the management of hyperemesis gravidarum

Obstetrics and Gynecology; (Sept 1996)v88n3p343-6

[134] American College of Obstetricians and Gynecologists, Committee on Obstetric Practice. Guidelines for diagnostic imaging during pregnancy
ACOG Committee Opinion (Sep 1995)n158p32-35

[135] Maccarrone G, et al. Total parenteral nutrition in pregnancy
Minerva Ginecol (May 1998)v50n5p185-9

[136] Ireton-Jones C, et al. Clinical pathways in home nutrition support
J Am Diet Assoc (Sep 1997)v97n9p1003-7

[137] Godil A, et al. Percutaneous endoscopic gastrostomy for nutrition support in pregnancy associated with hyperemesis gravidarum and anorexia nervosa
J Parenter Enteral Nutr (Jul-Aug 1998)v22n4p238-41

[138] Safari H, et al. Experience with oral methylprednisolone in the treatment of refractory hyperemesis gravidarum
Am J Obstet Gynecol (May 1998)v178n5p1054-8

[139] Greenspoon JS, et al. Physician's script for placing the nasogastric feeding tube
correspondence from Cedars-Sinai in Los Angeles, California

Twelve:

[140] Mazzota P, et al. Factors associated with elective termination of pregnancy among Canadian and American women with nausea and vomiting of pregnancy
J Psychosom Obstet Gynecol; (Mar 2001)v22n1p7-12

[141] Miller F Nausea and vomiting in pregnancy: The problem of perception-Is it really a disease?
Am J Obstet Gynecol; (May 2002)v186n5pS182-3

[142] Panesar N, et al. Are thyroid hormones or hCG responsible for hyperemesis gravidarum? A paired study in pregnant Chinese women
Acta Obstet Gynecol Scand; (2001)v80n6p519-24

[143] Field J Hyperemesis gravidarum: a short case study
Nurs Times; (Aug 2001)v97n32p55

[144] Mazzota P, et al. Therapeutic abortions due to severe morning sickness: unacceptable combination
Can Fam Phys (Jun 1997)v43p1055-7

[145] (n.a.) Lilly Centre for Women's Health: Depression: Sidebar
Retrieved on June 22, 2003 from http://www.lillywomenshealth.com/depression/postmenohealth.html

[146] Buckwalter JG, et al. Psychological factors in the etiology and treatment of severe nausea and vomiting in pregnancy
Am J Obstet Gynecol (May 2002)v186n5pS210-4

[147] Bogen JT Neurosis: A Ms Diagnosis
Perspect Biol Med (Winter 1994)v37n2p263-74

[148] Mazzota P, et al. Therapeutic abortions due to severe morning sickness: unacceptable combination

[149] Snell LH Metabolic crisis: hyperemesis gravidarum
J Perinat Neonat Nurs (Sept 1998)v12n2p26-37

[150] Simon EP, et al. Medical hypnosis for hyperemesis gravidarum
Birth; (Dec 1999)v26n4p248-54

[151] Bogen JT

[152] Mathews-Green F The bitter price of choice.
Washington Times; December 22, 1989. May also be found online at:
Feminists For Life. Retrieved on June 16, 2003 from http://www.feministsforlife.org/FFL_topics/after/pricchoc.htm

[153] Torres A, et al. Why do women have abortions?
Fam Plan Perspect; (Jul/Aug 1988)v20n4p170

[154] Child TJ Management of hyperemesis in pregnant women
Lancet; (Jan 23 1999)v353n9149p325

[155] Munch S Chicken or the egg? The biological-psychological
controversy surrounding hyperemesis gravidarum
Soc Sci Med (Oct 2002)v55n7p1267-78

[156] God.

Holy Bible; Old Testament: Book of Job

[157] Bogen JT

[158] Hallak, et al. Hyperemesis gravidarum: Effects on fetal
outcomes
J Reprod Med (Nov 1996)v41n11p871-4

[159] Seto, et al. Pregnancy outcome following first trimester
exposure to antihistamines: Meta-analysis
Am J Perinatol (Mar 1997)v14n3p119-24

[160] Eliakim, et al. Hyperemesis gravidarum: a current review
Am J Perinatol (2000)v17n4p207-18

Fourteen:

[161] Erick M Hyperolfaction and hyperemesis gravidarum: What
is the relationship?
Nutrition Reviews (Oct 1995)v53n10p289-95

[162] Erick M Battling morning (noon and night) sickness
J Am Diet Ass (Feb 1994)v94n2p147-8

[163] Greenspoon JS, et al. Hyperemesis gravidarum protocol:
treatment of hyperemesis gravidarum with nasogastric
feeding
correspondence from Cedars-Sinai in Los Angeles, California

[164] Sanders SL, et al. New protocol to manage hyperemesis
gravidarum
J AM Diet Ass; (Dec 1994)v94n12p1367-8

Sixteen:

[165] Eroglu A, et al. Spontaneous esophageal rupture following severe vomiting in pregnancy
Dis Esophagus (2002)v15n3p242-3

[166] Yamamoto T, et al. Pneumomediastinum secondary to hyperemesis gravidarum during early pregnancy
Acta Obstet Gynecol Scand (Dec 2001)v80n12p1143-5

[167] Spruill SC, et al. Hyperemesis gravidarum complicated by Wernicke's encephalopathy
Obstet Gynecol (May 2002)v99n5(part 2)p875-7

[168] ibid.

[169] op. cit.

[170] Hill JB, et al. Acute renal failure in association with severe hyperemesis gravidarum
Obstet Gynecol (Nov 2002)v100n5(part 2)p1119-21

Seventeen:

[171] Mazzota P, et al. Factors associated with elective termination of pregnancy among Canadian and American women with nausea and vomiting of pregnancy
J Psychosom Obstet Gynecol (Mar 2001)v22n1p7-12

[172] Siu SS, et al. Treatment of intractable hyperemesis gravidarum by ondansetron
Eur J Obstet Gynecol Reprod Biol (Oct 2002)v105n1p73-4

[173] Mazzota P, et al. Therapeutic abortions due to severe morning sickness: unacceptable combination
Can Fam Phys (Jun 1997)v43p1055-7

[174] Munch S Chicken or the egg? The biological-psychological controversy surrounding hyperemesis gravidarum

Soc Sci Med (Oct 2002)v55n7p1267-78

[175] Erick M Hyperolfaction and Hyperemesis Gravidarum: What is the relationship?

Nutrition Reviews (Oct 1995)v53n10p289-95

[176] Wong CY, et al. Complications of the use of corticosteroids for the treatment of hyperemesis gravidarum

Br J Obstet Gynaecol (Jun 1995)v102n6p508; letter

[177] Sanders SL, et al. New protocol to manage hyperemesis gravidarum

J AM Diet Ass (Dec 1994)v94n12p1367-8

[178] Goodwin, TM Hyperemesis Gravidarum

Clin Obstet Gynecol (Sept 1998)v41n3p597-605

[179] Moran P, et al. Management of hyperemesis gravidarum: the importance of weight loss as a criterion for steroid therapy

QJM (Mar 2002)v95n3p153-8

Eighteen:

[180] Torres A, et al. Why do women have abortions?

Fam Plan Perspect (Jul/Aug 1988)v20n4p170

[181] Arizona Republic; Woman begged for help before her abortion killed her

(Jan 30, 2001)

[182] Elford K, et al. Novel treatment of a patient with secondary infertility

Fertility and Sterility (Apr 2003)v79n4p1028-1030

[183] Thorp, et al. Long-term physical and psychological health consequences of induced abortion: review of the evidence.

Obstet Gynecol Survey (2003)v58n1p67-79

[184] Rooney B, et al. Induced abortion and risk of later premature births

J Am Phys Surgeons (Summer 2003)v8n2p46-9

[185] Ansfeld L, et al. The replacement child. Variations on a theme in history and psychoanalysis.
Psychoanal Study Child (2000)v55p301-18

[186] Willke JC, et al. Abortion: Questions and Answers
Cincinnati, OH: Hayes Publishing Company, 1988

[187] Gissler M, et al. Pregnancy-associated deaths in Finland 1987-1994: Definition problems and benefits of record linkage
Acta Obset Gynecol Scand (1997)v76p 651-657

[188] (n.a.) Coalition on abortion/breast cancer: Homepage
Retrieved November 4, 2006 from
http://www.abortionbreastcancer.com

[189] Malec K The abortion-breast cancer link: How politics trumped science and informed consent
J Am Phys Surgeons (Summer 2003)v8n2p41-45

[190] Daling JR, et al. Risk of breast cancer among young women: relationship to induced abortion
Am J Epidemiol (Aug 15 1996)v144n4p373-80

[191] Willke JC The deadly after effect of abortion: breast cancer
(Brochure) Hayes Publishing Company, Cincinnati, 2000

[192] Russo J, et al. Susceptibility of the mammary glad to carcinogenesis.II Pregnancy interruption as a risk factor in tumor incidence
Am J Pathol (Aug 1980)v100n2p497-512

[193] Brind J, et al. What every woman in the world has a right to know!
(Brochure) Endeavour Forum, Inc. (Toorak, Victoria, Australia) and the Abortion-Breast Cancer Quarterly Update (Poughkeepsie, NY)

[194] Reardon D Women at risk: abortion and the high risk patient
Pediatrics (1981)v68n5p670

[195] Thorp, et al.

[196] Gissler M, et al.

[197] McFadden A The link between abortion and child abuse
Family Resources Center News (January 1998) 20

[198] Reardon D Psychological reactions reported after abortion
The Post-Abortion Review (Fall 1994)v2n3p4-8

[199] Tischler C Adolescent suicide attempts following elective abortion
Pediatrics (1981)v68n5p670

[200] Reardon D Women at risk: abortion and the high risk patient
Retrieved August 22, 2004 from
http://www.afterabortion.org/women_a.html

[201] Gissler M, et al.

[202] Ney PG, et al. The effects of pregnancy loss on women's health
Soc Sci Med (1994)v48n9p1193

Nineteen:

[203] Nall D (n.d.)Welcome to the Shadowlands. HuGs: Hyperemesis gravidarum survivors
Retrieved June 16, 2003 from
http://www.angelfire.com/nt/hugs/shadowlands.html

Appendix B

[204] Many of these great resources and ideas were found in The American Feminist, Fall 2001, v8n3.

Made in the USA